The Structural Basis of Neurobiology

The Structural Basis of Neurobiology

Edward G. Jones

James L. O'Leary Division of Experimental Neurology and Neurological Surgery
Washington University School of Medicine

with a chapter on The Cell by Leon Weiss

Elsevier
New York • Amsterdam • Oxford

Cover picture: Oligodendrocytes commencing myelination of axons in the corpus callosum of a six-day-old rat. Scanning electron micrograph by Karen L. Valentino.

Chapters 1 and 8 have been taken in total from *Histology: Cell and Tissue Biology,* fifth edition. Leon Weiss, editor. New York: Elsevier Science Publishing Co., Inc., 1983.

Published by:

Elsevier Science Publishing Co., Inc.
52 Vanderbilt Avenue, New York, New York 10017

Sole distributors outside the USA and Canada:

Scientific and Medical Division of Macmillan Press, Ltd.
London and Basingstoke, UK

Library of Congress Cataloging in Publication Data

Jones, Edward G., 1939–
     The structural basis of neurobiology.

     Consists of chapters 1 and 8 from Histology: cell and tissue biology, with an additional new chapter added.

     Includes bibliographies and index.
     1. Nerve tissue. 2. Nerves. 3. Neurons. I. Histology. II. Weiss,
     Leon. III. Title. [DNLM: 1. Histology, Cell and tissue biology. 2. Nervous system—
     Cytology. 3. Cells—Cytology. WL 101 J76s]
QM575.J66   1983   611'.0188   83-11553
ISBN 0-444-00795-4

Manufactured in the United States of America

For Steve, Jean, Stewart, Chiiko, Karen, David, and Mary Kay

Contents

Foreword

The textbook *Histology: Cell and Tissue Biology*, fifth edition, is a collaborative effort of thirty-three scientists to present to the student of medicine a comprehensive but manageable account of the structure and function of the tissues of the body. Because some readers will find certain chapters or groups of chapters useful but may not require the whole text, we are providing a number of monographs drawn from *Histology: Cell and Tissue Biology* and dealing with selected areas.

This book, THE STRUCTURAL BASIS OF NEUROBIOLOGY, is the first of these monographs. It consists of Chapter 8, The Nervous Tissue, from *Histology: Cell and Tissue Biology*, to which a new account of the special sense organs, Chapter 8A, has been added. Chapter 1, The Cell, has also been provided as an introduction to cells in general. In order to expedite publication and to keep the monograph price as low as possible, Chapters 1 and 8 are reproduced exactly from the original negatives so that the original text—including reference to other chapters—and the original pagination are retained. A new index has also been included.

Leon Weiss

Preface

This book attempts to fill a perceived need in the Neural Sciences. Though this singularly active field has recently seen the publication of several new textbooks, these have tended to be lengthy treatises, often derived from integrated courses for medical students, and attempting to cover in a comprehensive manner the anatomy, physiology, chemistry, and even the clinical aspects of the discipline. Other shorter books that have tried to emphasize only the principles of neurobiology have tended to concentrate on a more limited range of topics and have commonly adopted a viewpoint based upon the fundamental electrophysiological properties of nerve cells and other excitable membranes. There appear to have been few attempts to write from the viewpoint of nerve cell structure in order to elucidate these principles. Such accounts as have been written in standard textbooks of neuroanatomy have generally been overwhelmed by details of the gross morphology and fiber connections of the brain and spinal cord. Accounts of neurocytology in textbooks of histology have been, for understandable reasons, rather brief and are commonly lost to readers other than medical students by forming part of a systematic account of all the body tissues and organs. Even so, accounts of neurohistology are rarely integrated with the accounts of modern cell biology that accompany them in textbooks of histology and the functional attributes that nerve cells have in common with other cells are rarely pointed out.

In the present work, I have sought to provide a comprehensive account of neurocytology that is unencumbered by descriptive morphology and by accounts of nervous pathways. Instead, the morphological basis for the functions of individual cells is emphasized and only the broad principles of their organization into groups and systems with common or diverse functions are drawn out. As such, the book still provides a thorough account of neurohistology suitable for medical students but it should serve as a base for graduate and undergraduate students entering the field of neurobiology who wish to know about nerve cells but to whom, on the one hand, the wiring of the brain and, on the other, the finest biophysical details of nerve function are for the time being less relevant. The book also incorporates a chapter on the biology of cells in general, kindly provided by Leon Weiss. I feel that this may be unique in books on the Neural Sciences and serves the important purpose of providing the details of the structure and function of those organelles that the cells of the nervous system have in common with the cells of other tissues. It is an account that can serve as a source of reference for those whose primary interest is in the nervous system, or on its own as an introduction to fundamental cell biology.

The core of the book, Chapters 1 and 8, is formed by chapters taken without change in pagination from the fifth edition of *Histology: Cell and Tissue Biology*, edited by Leon Weiss. The reader who finds some unevenness in the book as a consequence, will be more than adequately compensated by a significant reduction in the price of the book. Chapter 8 is derived from a chapter written some years ago in collaboration with Doctor W. Maxwell Cowan and I am, as always, grateful for his many contributions. Chapter 8A is a new account of the special sense organs. Without the prompting and careful editorial assistance of Leon Weiss the original chapter probably would not have been converted into the present monograph. It is a pleasure also to acknowledge the generosity of several individuals who provided illustrations. Their names are mentioned at appropriate places in the text. It is also my privilege to thank Ms. Margo Gross for her devotion to the secretarial side of preparing the book and Doctor James Fleshman, Jr., Mr. William Kraft, and Mr. Ronald Steiner for their contributions to the preparation of the illustrations.

Edward G. Jones

St. Louis, Missouri

The Structural Basis
of Neurobiology

The Cell

Leon Weiss

General Properties

The cell is the unit of living structure. The tissues that form the body consist entirely of cells and of extracellular material elaborated by cells. The cell, moreover, can carry out an independent existence whereas none of its constituents can do so. Indeed, an entire phylum, the Protozoa, is unicellular, and isolated metazoan cells may be maintained in tissue culture.

Most mammalian cells are microscopic, although in some instances they reach macroscopic visibility. The limits of cell size are exemplified by bacteria or bacteria-like organisms, which may be less than 1 μm in their largest dimension, and by avian egg cells, measured in centimeters (Table 1–1).

A cell is a complex, aqueous gel made of protein, carbohydrate, fat, nucleic acids, and inorganic material. Protein alone or in combination with fat, as lipoprotein, or with carbohydrate, as glycoprotein, mucoprotein, or proteoglycan, constitutes the substantive structural element both of the cell and of extracellular substances. Enzymes, large molecules that catalyze metabolic reactions, are proteins. Products and secretions of cells may be proteins. Carbohydrate is the major source of energy in mammalian cells. Among the principal carbohydrates are glucose, a monomeric utilizable form, and glycogen, a polymeric storage form. Carbohydrates built into complexes with protein may play a role in linking cells together, are major components of extracellular tissues, are significant structural elements within cells, and serve as distinctive receptors on the cell surface. Fat, too, may be a source of energy to the cell. Moreover, fatty acids, which constitute the principal storage form of fat, provide the cell with efficient depots of energy. Lipids have major structural properties. Phospholipids and sphingolipids are important in the structure of biological membranes, making them preferentially permeable to fats; they also control the orientation and mobility of proteins in the membranes.

Inorganic materials occur in cells in a variety of combinations. They may be associated with enzymes and with other proteins or fats, or they may be free of organic chemicals. They influence the adhesiveness and other physical properties of cells and extracellular materials in many different ways. Thus calcium contributes to the rigidity of bone; to the adhesiveness of the constituents of the subcellular particles, the ribosomes; to the capacity of cells to aggregate; and to the capacity of muscle to relax.

One of the achievements of microscopic anatomy is the ability to induce selective chemical reactions that reveal the location of different chemical moieties in tissue prepared for examination under the microscope. Chapter 2 is devoted to histochemistry, the term given to this division of histology, and histochemical findings are presented throughout this book.

There are two major classes of cells: prokaryotes and eukaryotes. *Prokaryotes*, exemplified by bacteria, contain nucleoprotein that may be segregated in the protoplasm as a *nuclear body* or *nucleoid* but is not enveloped in membrane. In *eukaryotes*, represented by fungi and higher forms, a true membrane-bounded nucleus is present. In fact, the eukaryotic cell is distinguished by well-developed membrane systems that not only envelope the nucleus but compartmentalize many cellular functions such as protein and steroid synthesis (the membranes of endoplasmic reticulum), respiration (the membranes of mitochondria), and secretion (the membranes of the Golgi complex).

The nucleus is typically a prominent ovoid structure lying near the center of the cell (Figs. 1–1 and 1–2). In it are chromosomes that contain *deoxyribonucleic acid (DNA)*, which encodes the genetic information. With the microscope, DNA appears as densely stained particles termed, in aggregate, *chromatin*. A nucleus may contain one or more *nucleoli*, typically spherical structures representing specialized modifications of chromosomes. There are several forms of a second type of nucleic acid, *ribonucleic acid (RNA)*. RNAs read the genetic code built into DNA and then play the central role in synthesizing the proteins encoded in the DNA. RNAs, themselves encoded in the DNA, are generated in the nucleus and are distributed in both nucleus and cytoplasm. Their complex structures and functions are discussed below.

The nucleus is surrounded by cytoplasm, the realm of protoplasm that expresses most differentiated cellular functions. The cytoplasm contains many highly organized, distinctive organ-

TABLE 1–1 Equivalent measurements

10 angstroms (Å) =	1 millimicrometer (mμm)
	or 1 nanometer (nm)
10,000 angstroms =	1 micrometer (μm)
1,000 microns =	1 millimeter (mm)
10 millimeters =	1 centimeter (cm)
100 centimeters =	1 meter (m)

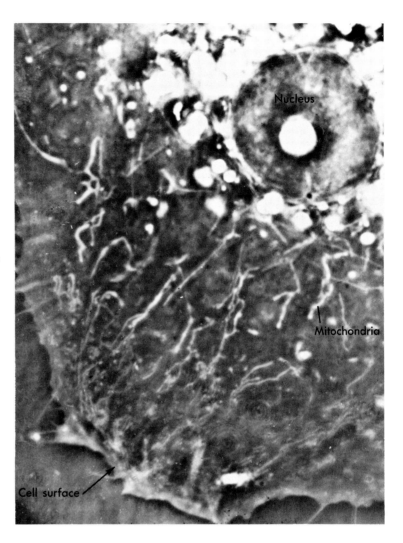

1–1 Hela cells, living in tissue culture; phase-contrast photomicrograph. Hela cells were derived by Dr. George Gey from a carcinoma of the uterine cervix explanted in tissue culture. They are maintained as a cell strain in tissue culture and used in a variety of experimental procedures. The cell border is ruffled and in places retracted, resulting in spinelike processes. The nucleus is spherical, surrounded by refractile clear bodies. Mitochondria are evident as irregular linear structures. × 1200. (From the work of Dr. G. Gey.)

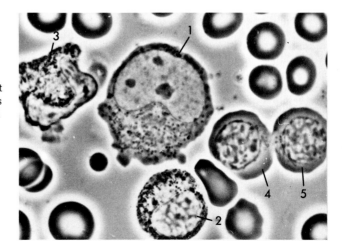

1–2 Human bone marrow cells, phase contrast microscopy. Developing white blood cells are present. They are myelocytes (1 and 2) and a metamyelocyte (3). Developing erythroblasts are also present (4 and 5) as are mature erythrocytes (unnumbered). See Chap. 12. × 1300. (From the work of G. A. Ackerman.)

4

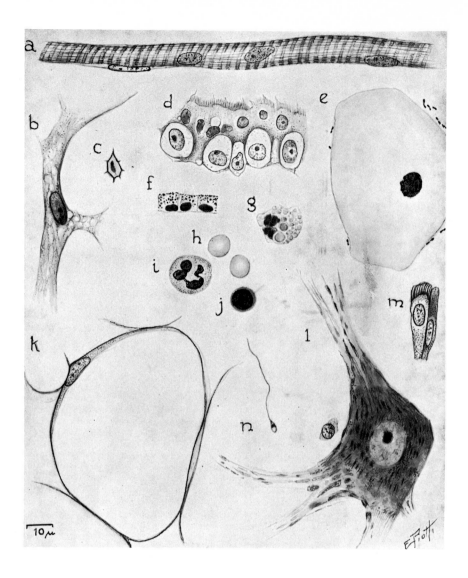

1–3 Variety of cells from the human body. **a,** portion of a striated muscle fiber. **b,** fibroblast from the umbilical cord. **c,** osteocyte within a bone lacuna. **d,** portion of the placental chorion, showing syncytial trophoblast and underlying cytotrophoblast cells. **e,** squamous epithelial cell and bacteria from a vaginal smear. **f,** three pigmented epithelial cells from the first layer of the retina. **g,** macrophage in bone marrow, which has ingested masses of blood pigments. **h,** two red blood cells. **i,** polymorphonuclear neutrophil; and **j,** small lymphocyte, all from a blood smear. **k,** fat cell from loose connective tissue. **l,** large motor neuron and adjacent small glial cell (process not revealed) from a hypoglossal nucleus in the medulla. **m,** adjacent ciliated and secretory epithelial cells from the oviduct. **n,** mature spermatozoon from semen. Cells a and d are multinucleate; g is binucleate; e has a pycnotic nucleus; c, f, j, and n have dense nuclei; the nucleus of l is extremely vesicular; i has a lobulated nucleus; the nuclei of a, g, and k are displaced by the cell contents. Some of the cells are rounded or polygonal, but a is extremely elongate, b and c have short processes, and the neuron in l has long processes (cut off here). The syncytium in d has a brush border; one cell in m has cilia; n has a flagellum. Cells a and l display cytoplasmic fibrils; f, pigment granules; g, phagocytized masses; l, specific granules; k, a space left by dissolved fat; j and the neuron in l, conspicuous amounts of cytoplasmic basophilia. [The diameter of the red blood cells (approximately 7.5 μm) provides a useful measure of the other cells.] All × 700. (Prepared by H. W. Deane and E. Piotti.)

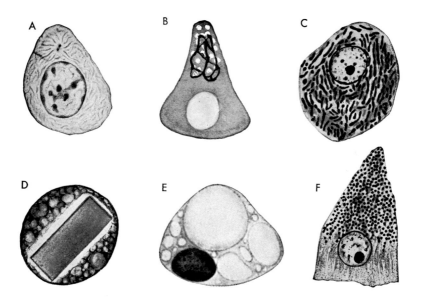

elles. These organelles include mitochondria, lysosomes, the Golgi apparatus, endoplasmic reticulum, centrioles, microtubules, microfilaments, ribosomes, secretory granules, and other structures that will be considered below. In addition, the cytoplasm contains such simple structures as glycosomes and lipid vacuoles. The cytoplasm is limited by a membrane called the *cell membrane, plasma membrane,* or *plasmalemma* (Figs. 1–2 to 1–5).

In metazoan or multicellular organisms, cells show marked specialization (Figs. 1–3 to 1–5). We speak of these cells as differentiated. In mammals cells vary in shape and size, exemplified by anucleate discoid pigmented blood cells 7 μm in diameter and branched nerve cells whose processes may reach a meter or more in length. Cell types may display pronounced internal variation. Striated muscle cells are packed with cross-banded filaments that slide on one another causing cellular contraction. Adipose cells are distended with fat, and secretory cells are filled with secretory granules. Osteoclasts may contain 25 or more nuclei, interstitial cells of the testis are packed with smooth endoplasmic reticulum, parietal cells of the stomach have rich infoldings of plasma membrane, renal tubular cells and brown fat contain extraordinarily large numbers of mitochondria, and immature erythrocytes are unusually rich in ribosomes. Keratinocytes in the skin may lose virtually all of their organelles and become scalelike structures packed with tough keratin filaments. So much has been

1–4 Various cytoplasmic organelles and cell inclusions. Because of their specific physical and chemical properties, these objects are not generally demonstrated by routine methods and are rarely revealed together. **A.** Cytocentrum in a cell of grasshopper testis, showing paired centrioles. **B.** Golgi material in a pancreatic cell of guinea pig, as demonstrated with osmic acid fixation. [Redrawn from Cowdry, E. V. (ed.) 1932. Special Cytology, 2d ed. New York: Paul B. Hoeber.] **C.** Mitochondria in a hepatocyte of a dog, stained with hematoxylin. (Weatherford.) **D.** Crystal within the nucleus of a hepatocyte of a dog. (Weatherford.) **E.** Spaces in a young fat cell left by dissolved fat. **F.** Secretory granules in a human pancreatic cell. Below and lateral to the nucleus lies ergastoplasm.

learned of the functions of the various cell constituents, in fact, that the function of a cell may be inferred from knowledge of its subcellular constituents. Indeed, such variations in cell structure and function constitute the backbone of this book.

The diversely differentiated cells that make up the complex metazoan body have clearly established a division of labor: the functions of the body are divided among them. Keratinocytes of the skin combine to form a tough protective barrier facing the outside environment. Erythrocytes of the blood, having developed chromoprotein pigment, carry the respiratory gases O_2 and CO_2. Muscle cells contract, nerve cells conduct, and bone cells provide a stable skeleton. The cells of the eye permit vision; those of the ear,

6

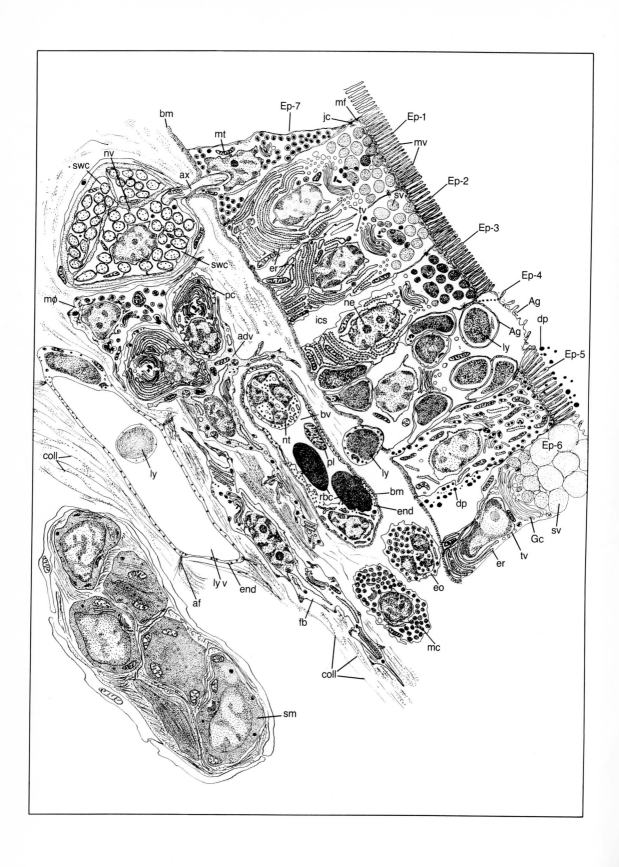

1–5 This drawing depicts a variety of cell types organized into an "imaginary" tissue that includes features of the gastrointestinal tract.

A major feature is the presence of epithelial cells lying side by side forming a surface that faces on a lumen. On their basal surface the epithelial cells rest upon a basement membrane **(bm)**. (Epithelium is discussed in Chap. 3.) These epithelial cells (Ep–1 to Ep–7) are bound together by junctional membranous complexes (Chap. 3) near their luminal or apical surface, while at their lateral surfaces below the junctional complexes **(jc)** the cells diverge somewhat, creating intercellular space **(ics)**. Epithelial cells Ep–1 to Ep–3 are secretory cells. They produce membrane-bounded secretory vesicles **(sv)** and release them at the luminal surface. These cells contain those cell organelles associated with secretion, viz: nucleoli **(ne)** euchromatin, endoplasmic reticulum **(er)**, transport vesicles **(tv)**, Golgi complex **(Gc)**, and condensing, storage, and secretory vesicles. See discussions of these organelles in this chapter and discussion of secretion in Chaps. 3, 20, and 21. The apical surface of each of these cells bear microvilli **(mv)**. Microfilaments **(mf)** form a terminal web beneath the microvilli and extend into them, conferring a contractile capacity upon them. Ep–5, also a secretory cell, produces mucous. Its secretory vesicles accumulate in the apical portion of the cell, but they are a good deal larger than those of Ep–1 to Ep–3 and they tend to coalesce. The Golgi complex is particularly well developed. Note that the outer nuclear membrane in the secretory cells is part of the endoplasmic reticulum and that the nuclear cisterna is dilated. The basal and lateral aspects of the cells may contain mitochondria **(m)**, which are often "pocketed" by infoldings of the basal and lateral plasma membrane. Ep–1 is an absorptive cell that takes up substances in the lumen, often modifying them, transports them across the cell, and releases them to the subjacent tissues where they may be metabolized or picked up by blood or lymphatic vessels and carried to metabolic centers such as the liver. Droplets **(dp)** at the luminal surface are taken through the microvillous border and enter the cell (endocytosis) in pinocytic vesicles (p. 52). These are conveyed to the lateral margin of the cell where they are released (exocytosis). They then travel extracellularly through the basement membrane to the subjacent connective tissue. Ep–4 is a highly specialized cell, the M cell, which is part of the immune system (Chap. 19). Lymphocytes **(ly)**, small immunologically competent cells that are responsible for such immunological processes as antibody formation, regularly enter and leave the M cell, lying in "pockets" of plasma membrane on its basal and lateral surfaces. The M cell takes up foreign material (antigen) from the lumen and conveys it, via pinocytotic vesicles, to the lymphocyte-containing pockets. M cells thereby present antigen to the lymphocytes initiating an immune response (Chap. 11). Ep–7 is a truncated epithelial cell resting upon the basement membrane but not reaching to the lumen. It contains granules that, on release, can influence the activity of nearby cells. A type of endocrine or paracrine cell, it may be part of the APUD system (see text). Note that it is penetrated by an axon **(ax)** that emerges from a small nerve **(nv)**. The nerve consists of a large cell, Schwann cell **(swc)**, whose cytoplasm carries many nerve fibers.

A stratum of connective tissue (Chap. 4) underlies the epithelium. It supports the epithelium and contains nerves, blood vessels **(bv)**, lymphatic vessels **(lyv)**, and free cells as macrophages **(mφ)**, plasma cells **(pc)**, fibroblasts **(fb)**, eosinophils **(eo)**, and mast cells **(mc)**. Connective tissue is characterized by abundant extracellular substance. This extracellular material often includes strong, supporting collagen fibers **(coll)**. The various cell types present in the connective tissues confer certain capacities on the tissue: plasma cells, antibody production; macrophages, phagocytosis; fibroblasts, collagen formation; eosinophils, phagocytosis, antiparasitic and antiinflammatory actions; mast cells, inflammation. Consult Chap. 4 (Connective Tissues) and Chap. 11 (Blood) for discussion. The blood vessel is a capillary whose wall is made of an endothelial cell **(end)** lying upon a basement membrane and an "outside" cell or adventitial cell **(adv)** (see Chap. 10). The capillary contains blood cells: a neutrophil **(nt)**, red cells **(rbc)**, and a platelet **(pl)**. The wall of the lymphatic capillary consists of endothelium alone **(end)**. The vessel contains a lymphocyte **(ly)** and its lumen is kept patent by the anchoring filaments **(af)** attached to the outside of the endothelium (Chap. 15).

Peripheral to the connective tissue layer is a fascicle of smooth muscle **(sm)**, which imparts contractile functions to the tissue.

hearing; those of kidney, excretion, and so on, as this book attempts to show. Implicit in such differentiation is the formation of tissues of diverse cells to effect these functions. Nerves conduct impulses, but they form a complex tissue. Included in this tissue are fibroblasts that produce collagen to support the nerve cells, glial cells to insulate them, endothelial cells to form blood vessels to carry blood to them, and other nerves to connect with them. Thus, specialized cells exist with other specialized cells forming specialized tissues that carry out specialized functions. The dominant or distinctive cells in such tissues are recognized as *parenchyma* (e.g., the nerve cells in nervous tissue) whereas the supporting cells can be designated as *stroma*. The *vasculature*, another essential "service" part of a tissue, may be included with the stroma.

It is further implicit in the existence of the diverse tissues working together to constitute a structurally and functionally coherent body that there are integrating systems. The classic integrating systems are the nervous system (Chap. 8) and the endocrine system (Chap. 21), which coordinate such complex events as reproduction, respiration, locomotion, etc. Histology is undergoing a revolution—no other term will do—because as additional actions of the classic systems are being newly discovered, hitherto unknown integrating systems are simultaneously being recognized. For example, a fair number of substances long known as regulators in other systems are now being uncovered as neural mediators as well. Prolactin, newly discovered as a central nervous system neurotransmitter has been known for years as a hormone produced in the pituitary gland and targeting the mammary glands where it induces the production and release of milk. There are, moreover, systems of *paracrine secretion* wherein peptides released by cells lying within a tissue govern the activity of other cells in that tissue. In contrast to the *endocrine system* in which hormones released from an endocrine organ typically travel some distance via the blood stream to reach a target organ, paracrine secretion is released and diffuses locally to affect local cells. Thus, paracrine cells in the epithelium of the gut release peptides that regulate motility, absorption, and secretion of nearby cells in the gut wall (Chap. 19). Some of these paracrine cells are fired by connecting nerves. A common characteristic of a subpopulation of such secretory cells in the gastrointes-

tinal, respiratory, and several other systems is that they form their peptides or other low-molecular weight agents by taking up amine precursors and decarboxylating them. These types of cells have therefore been collectively termed the *APUD system* (Amine Precursor Uptake and Decarboxylation), further discussed in Chaps. 19 and 29. Still another network of cells with regulatory function is that of T lymphocytes, as discussed in Chaps. 11, 12, and 14. T lymphocytes have a controlling role over lymphocytes, macrophages, and related cells in inflammation and immune reactions. They may have a rather broad role in regulating cellular differentiation in other contexts.

Despite pronounced variations in cell structure, most cells do have much in common. Before exploring the general features of cells, we shall first consider some techniques widely used by morphologists.

Microscopy

In the most common types of microscopy of biological material, light or electrons are sent through a slice of tissue. The light or electrons are modified by the tissue as they pass through it. This modification contains information inherent in the specimen, and the function of the lens systems in any microscope is to amplify and convert that information to a form, an *image*, discernible by eye.

The human eye is sensitive to the contrast of light and dark and to differences in color. A light train may be represented as electromagnetic sine waves, color being a function of wavelength and intensity a function of amplitude. To render visible the disturbance in the light train induced by a biological preparation, the light must be modified in color or intensity. Some wave frequencies must be absorbed more than others so that the preparation will be seen to contain materials of different colors, or there must be a change in the amplitude of a wave so that the preparation will be seen to consist of dark and light parts. Thus, if the rim of a nucleus is darker than the surrounding structure, the nucleus is delineated and can be recognized (Figs. 1–3 and 1–4). If such structures as mitochondria or glycosomes can be distinctively colored, they can be recognized. Perhaps the primary role of the microscope is to permit the identification of different structures within tissues. Beyond such simple identification, however, there is considerable physical, chemical, and ultrastructural information inherent in tissues that can be revealed by specialized methods of microscopic analysis. These methods depend on various types of microscope, which we shall now consider.

Bright-field Microscopy

The bright-field microscope is a complex optical instrument consisting of three lens systems, a stage on which to place the preparation, and controls to permit focus.

The light is focused on the preparation by the condenser lens system. It passes through the specimen, where it is modified, and this modified beam enters the objective lens system. An image is formed in the focal plane of the objective. In that image lies whatever resolution the instrument is capable of providing. The bright-field microscope is theoretically capable of resolving points approximately 0.2 μm apart. The ocular or eyepiece then magnifies the image formed by the objective, presenting it to the eye as a visible magnified image.

The primary purpose in staining histological preparations is to induce differential absorption of light so that various structures may be seen in distinguishing colors. Staining has expanded from this elementary function until it has become possible to stain many chemical compounds selectively and specifically (Chap. 2).

Phase-contrast Microscopy

Although unstained tissue does not absorb light, it does affect light by retarding some wave trains more than others. Thus light may enter a specimen in phase, that is, with peaks and troughs of the component sine waves in register. However, the components of the specimen, having different optical densities, retard the sine waves differentially, putting them out of phase with one another. These phase differences are not perceivable by the eye. The function of the phase microscope is to convert phase differences into amplitude differences by matching the retarded waves with out-of-phase waves so as to cancel or diminish the amplitude of the retarded waves. The phase microscope thus permits one to observe considerable detail in unstained material and hence is suited to the study of living cells (Figs. 1–1 and 1–2).

Dark-field Microscopy

The dark-field microscope is also able to provide contrast in unstained material. Its effectiveness depends on excluding the central light train that comes into the objective from the condenser in the conventional bright-field microscope. Instead, the specimen is illuminated by light coming in from the side. Should there be objects of greater optical density than their surroundings in the field, such as bacteria moving in a fluid medium, they will deflect light into the microscopic objective and appear as light objects against a dark background. Little or no internal structure of the lighted particles is revealed. This technique has largely been superseded by phase-contrast microscopy.

Interference Microscopy

The interference microscope provides not only contrast in unstained preparations but additional information on the physical properties and the submicroscopic organization of tissue. Like the phase microscope, the interference microscope relies on phase differences induced in transmitted light by differences in optical densities in the parts of the biological preparation. However, the interference microscope is a quantitative instrument in which the light trains subject to phase retardation are compared with a reference beam. Because the optical density and phase retardation are in proportion to specimen mass, the mass of different components of the cell may be calculated.

Fluorescence Microscopy

The fluorescence microscope depends on exciting the emission of visible light in a specimen irradiated with ultraviolet light. Certain biological substances, such as vitamin A, are *autofluorescent*; that is, they can absorb light of one frequency and emit light of another. In practice, light within one frequency range, usually in the ultraviolet spectrum, is focused on the specimen, care being taken to protect the observer's eyes from this damaging radiation. This light is absorbed by certain structures in the specimen, which then emit light within the visible range, the wavelength of the emitted light depending on the chemical nature of the emitting substance. Although the autofluorescence of materials like

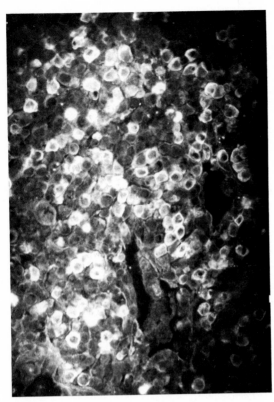

1–6 Fluorescence microscopy. A lymph node of a rabbit in the fourth day of a secondary antibody response to the antigen bovine serum albumin. The antibody, which has been tagged with a fluorescent tracer and is white in this photomicrograph, is present in the cytoplasm of plasma cells and lymphocytes. The nuclei are seldom stained and are present as negative (dark) images. See Chaps. 2 and 15. × 500. (From the work of A. H. Coons.)

vitamin A permits the use of this microscope with unstained material, the value of the technique is enormously enhanced by staining the tissue with fluorescent reagents (see Fig. 1–6 and Chaps. 2, 15, and 16).

Ultraviolet Microscopy

The ultraviolet microscope, like the fluorescence microscope, is built around the use of ultraviolet light instead of visible light. Its optical system is usually made of quartz, which efficiently transmits ultraviolet light. The image-bearing ultraviolet light coming from the ocular of the ultraviolet microscope is recorded on a photographic film, because ultraviolet light is both invisible and damaging to the eye. The value of the ultraviolet microscope lies in the fact that certain highly significant cellular structures, notably those containing nucleic acids, absorb ultraviolet light of specific wavelengths and can therefore be demonstrated. Because the wavelength of ultraviolet is shorter than that of visible light, this microscope offers somewhat higher resolution than the bright-field microscope.

Polarizing Microscopy

The polarizing microscope permits one to determine whether biological materials have different refractive indices along different optical axes. Such materials are *birefringent* or *anisotropic*. They are able to convert a beam of linear polarized light to elliptical polarized light, one axis of which can be transmitted by an analyzer and visualized. In the polarizing microscope, light is polarized below the stage of the microscope by a Nicol quartz prism or other suitable polarizer. The polarizer is made of material capable of transmitting only polarized light in one plane or axis. By rotating the analyzer, the polarization of the light transmitted by the specimen may be determined and any change from the character of polarization of the source detected. Substances incapable of affecting polarized light are termed *isotropic*. For biological material to change linear to elliptical polarized light, submicroscopic particles that are asymmetric must be present, and these particles must be oriented in an ordered nonrandom manner. Thus, the ability of biological material to change linear to elliptical polarized light indicates that its submicroscopic structure consists of oriented asymmetric molecules.

Filaments, fibers, and linear proteins are typically birefringent. Lipoprotein complexes, such as those composing membranes, may display complex polarizing properties. Typically, the orientation of the lipid molecules, and hence their rotation of polarized light, is at right angles to that of the protein component. Polarization optics have been fruitfully applied to the study of muscle, connective tissue fibers, cell membranes, and the achromatic mitotic apparatus (Fig. 1–7).

Transmission Electron Microscopy

The transmission electron microscope (TEM), in contrast to light microscopes, uses a beam of electrons in place of a beam of light. Additional

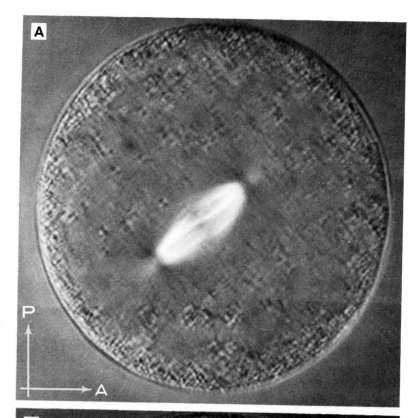

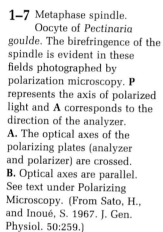

1–7 Metaphase spindle.
Oocyte of *Pectinaria goulde*. The birefringence of the spindle is evident in these fields photographed by polarization microscopy. **P** represents the axis of polarized light and **A** corresponds to the direction of the analyzer.
A. The optical axes of the polarizing plates (analyzer and polarizer) are crossed.
B. Optical axes are parallel. See text under Polarizing Microscopy. (From Sato, H., and Inoué, S. 1967. J. Gen. Physiol. 50:259.)

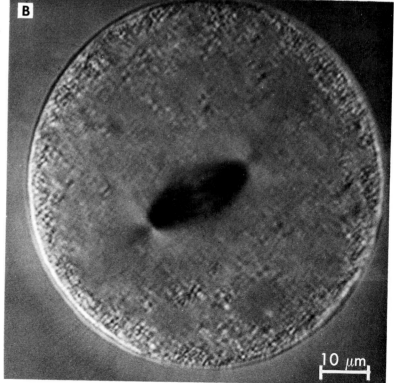

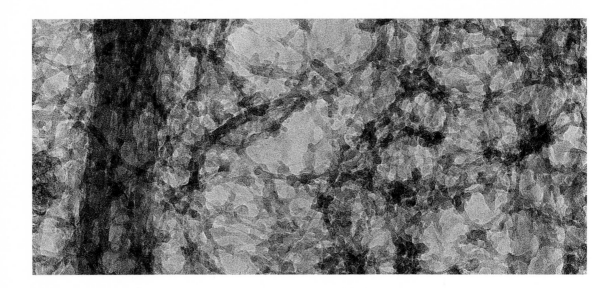

1–8 High-voltage electron micrograph. The electron beam, impelled at higher voltage, penetrates thicker sections and provides greater resolution than that in conventional transmission electron microscopes. This field includes the ground cytoplasm (hyaloplasm or cell sap). The ground substance of the cytoplasm contains a lattice of microtrabeculae. These form an irregular lattice which is continuous with the actin fibers (on the left) and support polysomes at their junction points. The microtrabeculae are about 30 to 50 Å in diameter and highly variable in length. The intertrabecular spaces provide for the rapid diffusion of water soluble metabolites. × 145,000. (Courtesy of John Wolosewick and Keith Porter.)

differences follow from the special properties of electrons. Electron beams are streams of negatively charged particles incapable of passing through glass. Hence, the lenses of an electron microscope are electromagnetic coils that surround the beam at different levels, somewhat like a set of collars. The strength of these electromagnetic lenses may be changed by varying the current passing through their coils. By varying the strength of the projector lens (the counterpart of the ocular of the light microscope), the magnification of the image formed by the objective lens is changed.

Electrons are charged particles, and because collision with charged molecules of air will absorb and deflect electrons and distort the beam, the optical system of an electron microscope must be evacuated of air. A vacuum of 10^{-4} mm Hg is commonly required. The electron stream is produced by heating a tungsten filament. The electrons are directed and impelled by moderately high voltage, usually ranging from 40,000 to 100,000 V. The higher voltages produce electron streams with shorter wavelengths, which are more penetrating and produce an image with less contrast but with higher resolution than lower voltages. Because electron beams are invisible to the eye, the images they form must be revealed by causing them to strike a fluorescent screen, and they are then recorded on a photographic plate.

Stability of the specimen is always a major consideration, and efforts must be made to protect the specimen against sublimation, distortion, and other damage by the electron beam or the vacuum. The specimen must be extremely thin for the electrons, so easily absorbed, to pass through it and create an image. Electron-microscopic sections are approximately 0.025 µm (250 Å) thick. Obtaining sections of tissues this thin has required the development of special slicing machines, *ultramicrotomes*, and a special technology of fixing and embedding tissues. Because thin sections have little intrinsic contrast, they must be stained with electron-absorbing heavy metals to provide the contrast necessary to reveal details of cell structure.

The value of the electron microscope lies in its great resolving power. Resolution of a microscope, measured as the distance between the closest two points it can distinguish as separate, depends on the wavelength of the radiation. An electron train has wave characteristics in addition to the characteristics of charge and mass. Its wavelength is small enough so that resolution of about 2 Å is possible and about 30 Å is routine. Consequently, a useful magnification of more than 500,000 is possible. The bright-field microscope, in contrast, has a resolution of approximately 0.2 μm and a useful magnification of 2,000. It has not yet proved practicable to examine living tissue by electron microscopy because of the vacuum and the damaging effects of electrons. Techniques that make it possible to obtain histochemical information at electron-microscopic resolutions have made electron microscopy increasingly productive. Moreover, quantitative analytic methods are available.

Variations on the TEM have been made. High-voltage electron microscopes capable of exceptionally high resolution exist. With accelerating voltages of a million electron-volts, they provide greater resolution and greater penetrating power of the electron beam and, therefore, the capacity to use thicker sections than is possible by conventional TEMs (Fig. 1–8).

Scanning Electron Microscopy

Scanning electron microscopy (SEM) provides a beautiful three-dimensional high-resolution image of cells and tissues (Figs. 1–9, 13–7, and 16–19). Moreover, cytochemical features can be localized on the image.

In SEM the surface of the tissue is studied. Whole mounts of tissue cultures or pieces of tissue are placed on the stage of the SEM. A slender electron beam or probe plays upon the surface, going back and forth in a regular way scanning the preparation. As the electron probe strikes the surface of the specimen, it generates several different kinds of signals. These signals include electrons (the so-called secondary electrons) and x rays. The secondary electrons may be focused on a cathode-ray tube or photographic film to form the three-dimensional image. X rays are generated when the electron probe strikes atoms having a mass greater than that of sodium. Each element is the source of x rays of distinctive wavelengths. The magnitude of the x rays generated is a function of the concentration of the element. Analysis of the x ray pattern of a tissue thus provides information on the concentration and distribution of elements.

Tissues prepared for SEM are fixed and dried. Drying at *critical point* has become the preferred method. The tissue is introduced into a suitable fluid and that fluid brought to its critical point, which is the combination of pressure and temperature at which the fluid and gaseous phases exist together without an interface or meniscus. Thus, there is no surface tension. The presence of surface tension during drying is disruptive to a tissue and causes visible distortions. After

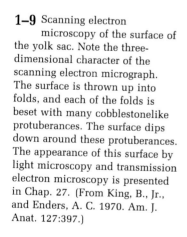

1–9 Scanning electron microscopy of the surface of the yolk sac. Note the three-dimensional character of the scanning electron micrograph. The surface is thrown up into folds, and each of the folds is beset with many cobblestonelike protuberances. The surface dips down around these protuberances. The appearance of this surface by light microscopy and transmission electron microscopy is presented in Chap. 27. (From King, B., Jr., and Enders, A. C. 1970. Am. J. Anat. 127:397.)

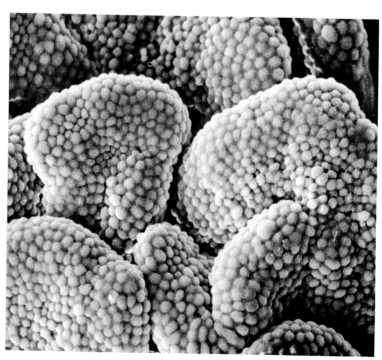

drying, the surface of the tissue is commonly coated in a vacuum with an electrically conductive coat of gold, gold–palladium, or carbon.

The SEM's resolution is inversely proportional to the diameter of the electron probe. Accordingly, SEMs possess very narrow, very coherent electron beams. Resolution of the SEM in the images generated by secondary electrons is 25 to 75 Å.

Biological Microscopic Preparations

Living Cells

Living cells may be maintained in tissue culture for long periods and examined by microscopy while undisturbed in culture. Tissue culture permits control of the environment and isolation of single cells or of *clones*, which are colonies derived from the proliferation of a single cell.

Maintaining cells in tissue culture requires considerable attention, involving nutritive media, control of atmospheric gases, and sterility. For short-term investigation, living cells such as leukocytes in a drop of blood may be placed on a clean slide, covered with a coverslip, sealed with petroleum jelly to prevent evaporation, placed on a warming stage, and studied under the microscope. This type of preparation is called *supravital* in distinction to more stable, longer-lasting preparations, such as whole animals or long-term tissue cultures, which are called *vital preparations*. Thus living cells may be observed with the conventional bright-field microscope or with the phase, interference, polarizing, or fluorescence microscopes. Living material may be studied unstained or it may be stained and remain alive, but such vital or supravital staining offers limited structural detail and damages the cells. Although it is valuable in special situations, as in the staining of the reticulocytes of the blood (Chap. 11), it is seldom used.

The nucleus, cytoplasm, mitochondria, Golgi apparatus, and centrioles may all be observed in the living state, as may such activities as motility of whole cells and the movement of structures within the cell.

The plasma membrane may be in active movement, associated with such processes as pinocytosis and phagocytosis (discussed under cytoplasmic vesicles, below). The study of living material offers certain satisfactions. Any scientific study induces artifacts, or departures from the natural state. A question that a scientist must always consider is whether or not the artifacts are consistent, repeatable, and significant—and therefore useful. Intuitively, one thinks that what is seen in the living cell is less apt to be an uncontrolled or misleading artifact and nearer to the typical, undisturbed life of the cell than what can be inferred from killed, sectioned, and stained tissue.

In order to obtain greater resolution and more chemical and other information about cells, it is necessary to kill them by fixation, section them into thin slices, and stain them. We shall now consider these procedures.

Fixation

Fixation is a procedure wherein a given cellular structure or activity is preserved or stabilized, often at the expense of other structures, for subsequent viewing with the microscope. Fixation is most commonly achieved by immersing the tissue in a solution of chemicals, but it may be accomplished by physical means, such as heat denaturation, freezing, or air drying. Although there are fixatives of general use, fixation may be quite selective. Thus, to study the structure of fat droplets, the tissues must be fixed in formaldehyde or other chemicals that stabilize the fat, and alcohol or other organic solvents that extract fats must be avoided. Fixatives that fix or coagulate protein are widely used because they preserve the general structure of nucleus and cytoplasm. Greater resolution and less distortion of cellular structures are obtained with a fixative that produces a fine coagulum than with one that produces a coarse one. Thus glutaraldehyde and osmium tetroxide, which cause a very fine precipitation of protein, permit high resolution without appreciable distortion of structure. They are the most widely used fixatives for electron microscopy. Phosphotungstic acid is a coarse protein precipitator that causes protoplasm to be thrown into heavy strands. For general work, therefore, it is used infrequently, but its drastic action may expose more reactive groups. More sulfhydryl groups are free to react after the coarse fixation with phosphotungstic acid than with fixatives that induce a finer coagulation of protein. For the special purpose of detecting sulfhydryl groups in tissue section, this otherwise unsatisfactory chemical may be the fixative of choice.

Fixation induces chemical change in tissue.

Thus fixatives containing heavy metals, such as Zenker's fluid, which contains mercuric chloride, may react with the carboxyl groups of tissue proteins and influence their subsequent staining. Aldehyde-containing fixatives, such as formaldehyde and gluteraldehyde, may react with amino groups in tissue and block them. Reagents such as bromine in the fixative may saturate double bonds and influence the stability and staining of lipids. Staining methods are available that detect enzyme activity. The fixative used for this purpose must be very gentle; most chemical fixatives tend to damage enzymes so much that they become inoperative and therefore undetectable.

Although fixation is commonly required in preparation for microscopic study, it must sometimes be avoided or its effects minimized because of unwanted chemical change. Some living tissues, such as a drop of blood or tissue cultures, lend themselves directly to microscopy and need not be fixed. The deleterious effects of fixation may be minimized by such maneuvers as freezing the tissue or using very dilute fixatives for very short times (see below and Chap. 2).

Embedding and Sectioning

After the tissue is fixed, it usually must be sectioned into sufficiently thin slices so that its details can be revealed by microscopy. Only in exceptional cases, as in spreading out a drop of blood on a slide, can the required thinness be obtained without slicing. The slices must be thin enough to transmit light (or electrons in electron microscopy). Moreover, since the depth of focus of microscopic objectives is shallow, clarity of detail is favored by thin sections. For light microscopy, section thickness varies from less than 1 μm to about 100 μm. Most preparations are about 5 μm thick. Slices this thin are made with an instrument known as a *microtome*, which consists of a chuck that holds the tissue, a knife, and an advance mechanism. However, tissue after fixation is often pulpy or brittle and impossible to cut into thin slices. It must be infiltrated with a stiff material that can be cut. Most of these infiltrating or embedding agents are fatty waxes, immiscible with the aqueous cytoplasm. Most fixing solutions, moreover, are aqueous. Therefore, to be embedded in the most commonly used embedding agents, which are paraffin or celloidin for light microscopy and the acrylic or epoxy

resins for electron microscopy, the fixed tissues must be dehydrated. To this end the tissues are passed through a series of increasingly concentrated aqueous solutions of ethyl alcohol, acetone, or other dehydrating agents that are miscible with both water and fat. Thus the tissue may be passed through solutions of 50, 70, 80, and 95% ethanol, and then into absolute ethanol. Next, either directly or through an intermediate organic solvent like toluene, the tissue is placed in the embedding agent in a liquid phase. The embedding agent replaces the solvent and thoroughly infiltrates the tissue.

Paraffin is made fluid by temperatures above the melting point, usually about 60°C, and the dehydrated tissue is allowed to steep in molten paraffin. The preparation is then cooled. Having infiltrated the interstices of the tissue, the paraffin becomes solid, forming a block that can be cut.

In plastic embedding for electron or light microscopy, the plastic is introduced in the fluid monomeric state. With sufficient steeping, it infiltrates the tissue. Then, by means of heat or ultraviolet light, the plastic is polymerized and becomes, like paraffin, a solid in which the tissue lies thoroughly infiltrated and embedded.

However, a price must be paid to obtain such stable infiltrated blocks of tissue. The alcohols used to dehydrate tissues before infiltration extract fat, coagulate protein, and cause other chemical changes in a tissue. In order to infiltrate with paraffin, moreover, the tissue must be subjected to temperatures high enough to inactivate many enzymes. As plastic polymerizes, heat is given off and may damage the tissue. Paraffin and other embedding agents shrink and thereby distort the tissues. For these reasons, alternatives to these convenient types of embedding can be used. Water-soluble embedding agents are available that circumvent the need for dehydration so that fatty materials may be preserved.

Some enzymatic activities, however, are so fugitive that they do not withstand infiltration with an embedding agent. In such circumstances the tissue may be frozen, and the frozen block of tissue has the physical properties to permit sectioning. Freezing saves the time required for embedding. Tissues can be frozen and sections made, stained, and read in minutes, as is common practice in a surgical operating room.

Freeze-drying is a significant refinement over fixation by freezing or chemical means because it allows minimal distortion and displacement of tissues, minimal chemical extraction, and maximal preservation of enzyme activity for light microscopy. A small block of tissue is quick-frozen or quenched by immersion in isopentane in liquid nitrogen at a temperature of $-150°$ to $-160°C$. It is then placed in a vacuum and dried by sublimation of H_2O, thereby avoiding liquid H_2O, which causes displacement and extraction of cellular components. The dried tissue, while still in vacuo, may be infiltrated with molten paraffin.

In tissues that have been quenched, the sublimated water may be replaced by a chemical fixative in vapor form; this type of fixation is called *free substitution*. It offers the results of freeze-drying coupled with chemical fixation. An electron-microscopic technique, freeze-fracture-etch, has proved so valuable that it is described in detail below.

Mounting and Staining

After the tissue is sectioned for light microscopy, it is usually mounted on a glass slide and stained, although it is possible with phase-contrast or interference microscopy to study unstained tissue.

Freeze–Fracture–Etch

The technique of freeze-fracture-etch has become an invaluable method in cell biology for studying membranes (Figs. 1–10 to 1–14; Fig. 1–27). The technique avoids embedding and sectioning of tissue and may even avoid fixation. It demonstrates heterogeneity in biological membranes and illuminates the nature of cell junctions. Its applications have not been restricted to the study of membranes, however. Useful information has also been obtained on particles, filaments, ground substance within the cell, and extracellular substances. Freeze-fracture-etch depends on the rather simple fact that when a tissue is frozen and fractured, the fracture line tends to travel within membranes so as to separate them into inner and outer leaflets, thereby revealing structures previously hidden. This technique is carried out in steps (Table 1–2):

1. The tissue is removed from the body and fixed, although fixation may be eliminated.

2. After suitable rinses the tissue is transferred to glycerol. The glycerol infiltrates the tissue and protects against artifacts due to ice-crystal formation in the subsequent freezing.

3. The tissue is cut into small pieces and placed on metal (temperature conductive) discs.

4. The tissue is then plunged into a bath of isopentane, held in a temperature-conductive vessel partially immersed in liquid nitrogen. Temperature is low ($-160°C$) so that the tissue is almost immediately quenched or frozen below the eutectic point of water. This is most important because it permits freezing without ice-crystal formation in glycerated tissue. As ice crystals form, they rotate and literally cut apart the tissue, causing visible artifacts.

5. The frozen tissue is quickly transferred to the chamber of a freeze–fracture–etch machine, where a number of operations can be carried out. The chamber can be cooled to a low temperature. It contains a razor on an adjustable swinging arm that can intersect the tissue. It can be pumped out to achieve high vacuum (approximately 10^{-8} mm of mercury). Moreover, it is equipped with platinum electrodes so that platinum can be evaporated to form a film over the specimen. Within the freeze–fracture–etch machine the tissue is maintained frozen and under vacuum through the production of a platinum replica (step 8).

6. The tissue, positioned on its disc, is now fractured by the razor blade on the swinging arm. The cutting edge of the blade strikes the tissue and starts a fracture rift. The free piece of tissue above the fracture flies off and is lost. The lower part of the tissue affixed to the disc now has an exposed fracture face. The face is relatively smooth, with glasslike frozen water surrounding the tissue and filling in the spaces between membranes, particles, and other cellular and extracellular structures.

7. The freshly fractured face of tissue is kept under vacuum for a short time, usually a matter of minutes. This represents the etching phase of the process, during which some of the frozen water at the fracture face sublimates into the vacuum. As a result, membranes, granules, and other cellular structures on the fractured surface now stand out in relief, the level of the frozen water table being below them.

8. Current is passed through the platinum electrodes and a layer of platinum is evaporated over the frozen-fracture-etched surface of the tissue. This platinum layer forms a tough membranous replica of the surface. The platinum is evaporated from a point source and reaches the tissue from a given direction. The platinum covers the tissue very much as snow falling from a certain direction covers a landscape. It piles up

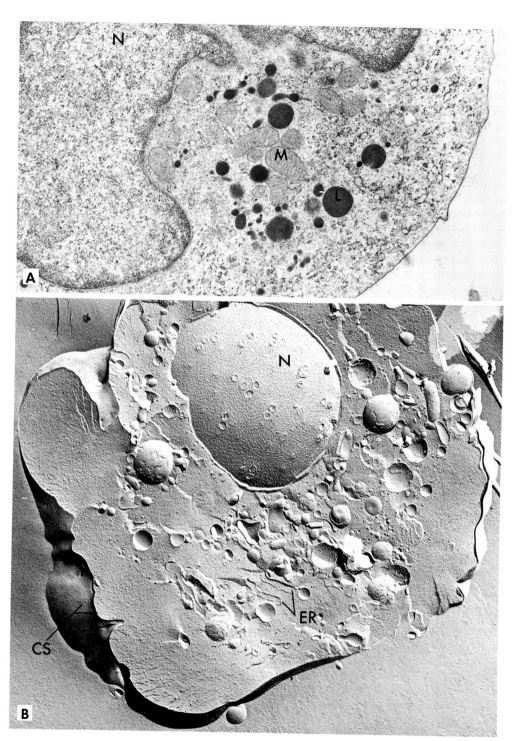

1–10 Guinea pig macrophage. **A,** A cell which has been fixed and sectioned and photographed in the electron microscope after staining with heavy metals. Nucleus **(N),** mitochondria **(M),** lysosomes **(L),** and the plasma membrane are visible by this standard technique. × 13,500. **B,** A freeze-fractured-etched macrophage, showing the nucleus **(N),** bearing nuclear pores, numerous globular profiles, two cisternae of the ER **(ER),** and an invagination **(arrow)** at the cell surface **(CS),** × 19,000. [From Daems, W. Th., and Brodero, R. *In* R. van Furth (ed.), Mononuclear Phagocytes. Philadelphia: F. A. Davis, p. 29.]

Table 1–2 Freeze–Fracture–Etch (Prepared by Dr. Maya Simionescu)

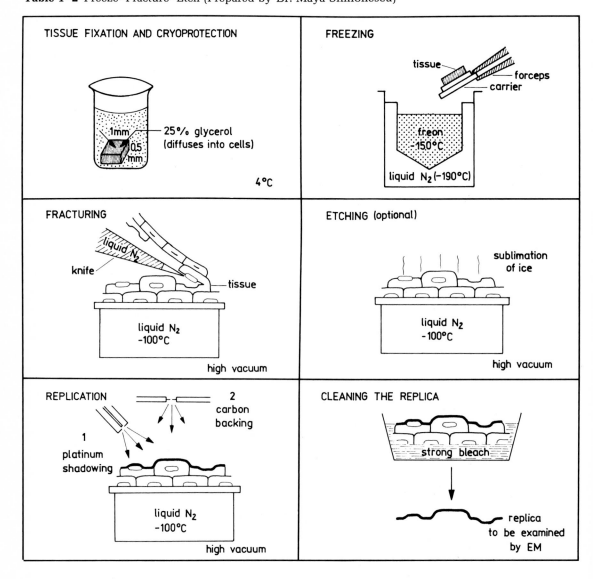

on the near side of structures that rise from the surface and leaves a clear space or shadow on the far side. A carbon film is evaporated on the back of the platinum replica to strengthen it.

9. The vacuum is broken, the chamber is opened, and the disc bearing the tissue covered with a platinum replica is removed from the machine.

10. The replica is freed from the tissue by digesting the tissue away and is caught on a grid that fits into a TEM. Under the electron microscope, the grain of the platinum permits resolution to better than 30 Å.

Isolation of Whole Cells and Parts of Cells

Techniques are available for isolating cells from complex tissues and for disrupting cells to isolate their constituent parts.

A single cell type can be purified in a viable state from a complex tissue containing many cell types. For example, hepatocytes, the distinctive parenchymal cell type of liver, can be isolated from blood vessels, lymphatics, nerves, fibroblasts, macrophages, extracellular substances, and other cells and extracellular materials of the liver. The first step is to prepare a cell suspension of the tissue. In a few tissues, such as blood, this is not necessary, because the cells already are in suspension in the liquid plasma. In a solid tissue, however, such as the liver and kidney, the tissue is usually cut into pieces and subjected to enzyme digestion while it is shaken. *Trypsin,* a proteolytic enzyme produced by the pancreas, will digest virtually any protein substrate and is widely used in cell-separation procedures. With judicious application, extracellular substances will be destroyed or depolymerized and intercellular junctional complexes will be loosened without too much cell destruction. (A valuable related use of trypsin is for harvesting cells in tissue culture that are adherent to the flask walls. Brief treatment loosens the cells; overlong treatment digests and destroys them.) *Collagenase* is especially useful in freeing cells enmeshed in collagen. *Neuriminidase* can remove a sticky extrinsic carbohydrate, *sialic acid,* from the cell surface. (This example highlights a refined use of enzymes in cell biology in which certain receptors or other molecules can be specifically removed from the cell surface, such as *fucose* by *fucase.*)

After enzymatic treatment and mechanical agitation, a solid tissue is reduced to a suspension of diverse cell types and debris. A given cell type may be separated by one or more techniques. Cells will migrate differently in a countercurrent or in an electrophoretic system, and a given cell type may thereby be removed. In certain instances cells may be selectively eliminated, for example, by destroying erythrocytes with hypotonic solutions or destroying other cells with anticell antibodies. Cells may have different affinities for surfaces. If a suspension of macrophages and lymphocytes is poured through a column of glass wool, the macrophages will adhere to the glass fibers (from which they can later be removed) and the lymphocytes will go through. This technique may be refined by coating a surface with reactants that can hold certain cell types by interacting with specific cell surface receptors.

The major method for separating cells, however, is centrifugation, whereby the cells are subjected to pulls greater than gravity. (The number of gravities, or g, is a function of the speed of rotation and the distance from the center of rotation to the material in the centrifuge tube.) The rate at which a structure reaches the bottom of the centrifuge tube depends on its density and volume. Cells or other particles may thus be separated differentially by varying the time of centrifugation, with the denser and more voluminous structures coming down first. When centrifugation is complete, moreover, the larger denser structures are on the bottom of the tube and the smaller lighter ones lie on top of them. This is the technique of *differential centrifugation.* For example, the density of red cells is approximately 1.077 and that of white cells, 1.033. As a result, on differential centrifugation, the red cells and white cells are separated so that the red cells are below and the white cells above. (The sedimentation of red cell is enhanced by their tendency to aggregate into *rouleaux,* thereby increasing their effective unit volume.) However, separation may be cleaner by interposing a density barrier. That is, a suspension of blood cells may be layered carefully over a solution of bovine albumin or sucrose whose density is between that of red and white cells. The red cells go through the density barrier and the white cells do not, and hence a better separation is achieved. This is the principle of *density-gradient* separation. The technique may be refined by using a number of layers of varying density, or going gradually from low to high density without steps, resulting in continuous, or linear, density-gradient centrifugation. If the range of densities in such multiple or continuous density barriers encompasses the densities of the cells being centrifuged into them, the cells will come to rest in the layer whose density equals its own. This technique is *isopycnic centrifugation.*

In the separation and analysis of constituent parts of a cell, the main elements of the procedure are as follow. Fresh tissue is shred into small pieces or run through a grinder. Cells are then disrupted in a blender, or with a mortar and pestle, or ground by fine sand or in a mill by a closely fitting piston riding in a test tube. The tissue is thereby reduced to a pulpy heterogenous liquid containing disrupted cells and their constitutent parts, extracellular material, and debris. This homogenate is centrifuged and its different components are isolated. The nucleus is a relatively large, heavy structure and is concentrated in fields of low gravity. Mitochondria, ribosomes, lysosomes, and other cellular elements may also be separated differentially. An isolated component may be studied by electron microscopy to confirm its nature and to determine the damage done during its concentration and the cleanness of separation.

Microchemistry and Histochemistry

Microchemical methods developed as refinements of chemical methods. With them it has become possible to take a section of a tissue, study it with the microscope, and then take the section next to it and analyze it for inorganic salts, oxidative enzymes, or other components. It is possible, moreover, to dissect sections and carry out chemical analyses on small groups of similar cells or even on single cells.

Histochemistry, the visualization of chemical reactions in microscopic preparations, is so valuable that it is accorded a full chapter (Chap. 2).

The Structure of the Cell

Biological Membranes

Membranes are essential to cells. They are metabolically active sheets that enclose the cell as the plasma membrane. They also occur within the metazoan cell as nuclear membranes, endoplasmic reticulum, Golgi membranes, and as the membranes enclosing lysosomes, pinocytotic and phagocytic vacuoles, and many other structures. Membranes thus bound the cell and compartmentalize its elements. The organization and many of the functions of the cell, such as secretion of protein, synthesis of fat, detoxification of drugs, phagocytosis, respiration, and active transport depend on membranes.

The plasma membrane is the outer limit of the living cell and its face to the environment. It controls the ease with which substances enter the cell, providing it with selective permeability. The plasma membrane contains many and diverse molecules in its surface, which confer the capacity to interact with other cells and the extracellular environment. The fluidity of the membrane is determined by its ratio of cholesterol to phospholipid. Its permeability is also dependent on its lipid content. The membrane contains enzymatic pumps that control the levels of Na^+, K^+, Ca^{++}, and other ions both in the cell and its environment. It contains the enzyme adenosine triphosphatase (ATPase), which breaks down adenosine triphosphate (ATP) to the diphosphate (ADP), thereby providing energy for active transport (pumping), endocytosis, and other energy-costing membrane functions. (See discussion under Mitochondria.)

Some of the molecules that extend from the surface of the plasma membrane are *receptors* capable of selectively linking with substances outside the cell, including receptors on other cells. Many essential cell functions are receptor-mediated, such as conduction, phagocytosis, antibody production, antigen recognition, hormone-induced activities, and other cellular interactions in embryogenesis, cell homing, and cell sorting. Some receptors are shared by many cell types, such as insulin receptors needed in carbohydrate metabolism (Chap. 22). Other receptors are quite restricted to cell type, such as the *erythropoietin receptors* on erythroblasts, needed to capture the hormone *erythropoietin*, which drives the proliferation and differentiation of red cell precursors (Chap. 12). A cell type may show a succession of receptors as it differentiates, each stage of differentiation characterized by a distinctive set of cell surface receptors or markers, well exemplified by lymphocytes (Chaps. 11 and 14).

The phenomenon of *contact inhibition* is related to properties of the cell surface. Normal cells, as can be shown in tissue culture, cease to grow or move away when they establish contact with other cells; they show contact inhibition. Malignant cells, on the other hand, are not inhibited but move over other cells.

Most cells of the body contain an array of molecules on their surfaces, distinctive to cell type, encoded by major histocompatibility complex (MHC), the "supergene" on chromosome 6 in human beings that governs many cellular interactions, including immune-related actions (Chap. 12). Although not all of these MHC-determined molecules have been characterized or their formation determined, many of them seem to possess receptor functions. Cells, particularly those that are metabolically active, must literally bristle with surface molecules, an expression of the extraordinary importance of these molecules in regulating cell function. This discussion will be carried further after the chemistry and modeling of the plasma membrane are considered.

Plasma membranes, like other membranes, are complex and diverse. Their composition and functions have been studied by a number of techniques. They can be isolated by cell disruption followed by differential centrifugation and studied by x-ray diffraction, freeze-fracture-etch, and microchemistry. The erythrocyte plasma membrane has been extensively studied because large amounts can be easily prepared. As is the case with most membranes, it is preponderantly protein (50–60% of dry weight). This composition reflects high metabolic activity and structural stability. A notable exception is the lipid-

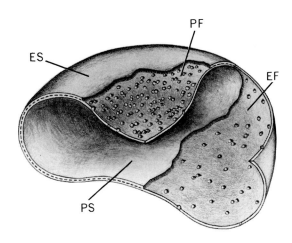

1-11 Diagrammatic representation of the four membrane "faces" that can be studied with the freeze-fracture-etch technique as shown on an erythrocyte. Note the terms used to designate the four surfaces: **ES**, the true outside surface of the plasma membrane; **PS**, the true inside surface of the plasma membrane; **PF**, the split surface of the plasma membrane which faces away from the cytoplasm; **EF**, the split surface of the plasma membrane which faces toward the cytoplasm. Particles, representing protein molecules, are shown only on faces PF and EF. (From Weinstein, R. S. 1974. The Red Blood Cell. New York: Academic Press, Inc., p. 247.)

rich membrane of myelinated nerves, whose high concentration of myelin appears to serve as an insulator. Most proteins associated with cell membranes are regarded as intrinsic to the membrane because they can be removed only by drastic procedures of extraction, digestion, or denaturation. The rest of the proteins are easily removed and thus considered extrinsic. Intrinsic or extrinsic proteins include structural proteins, enzymes, and receptor substances. Many of these proteins, notably the intrinsic ones, appear to be amphipathic, that is, asymmetric or polarized with hydrophilic groups at one pole and hydrophobic groups at the other. The implications of amphipathety are discussed below.

Lipids constitute 20 to 30% of the dry weight of erythrocyte membranes. Because lipid determines the permeability of plasma membrane, fat-soluble compounds readily enter cells, dissolving in the membrane, whereas fat-insoluble compounds enter by more complex mechanisms. The dominant lipid in the cell membrane is phospholipid, which is amphipathic: the glycerol end is water-soluble, carrying phosphate and other ionized groups, whereas the fatty acid end is not, being lipid-soluble and hydrophobic. Other lipids include cholesterol and a minor component linked to protein or carbohydrate as lipoprotein or liposaccharide. Carbohydrate accounts for less then 10% of the weight of plasma membranes in most cells studied. It may be free as oligosaccharide or linked to protein or fat.

By TEM of sectioned tissue, the plasma membrane is approximately 75 Å in thickness with a range of about 60 to 90 Å. As with most intracellular membranes, it is seen as a trilaminar structure, termed the *unit membrane,* with outer

darker lines approximately 20 Å wide and an inner lighter line, approximately 35 Å wide (Fig. 1-12). With high resolution, suggestions of bridges across the lucent central zone or of granular structures within the membrane may be present, but usually little or no specialization is evident. By negative staining some membranes, such as mitochondrial membranes, display distinctive structures (see below); but plasma membranes do not. A valuable technique in revealing structural heterogeneity in membranes is *freeze-fracture-etch* described above. By this method membranes are typically split into outer and inner leaflets, the split tending to occur in the central lucent zone (Figs. 1-11 and 1-14). As a result of this split there are four surfaces. The original surface facing to the exterior is the *E face* and the original surface facing to the interior, or protoplasm, of the cell is the *P face.* The fracture face on the exterior leaflet is the *EF* (Exterior Fracture) *face* while the fracture face on the interior leaflet is the *PF* (Protoplasmic Fracture) *face.* Particles may be seen on the split surfaces (Fig. 1-13). The number, size, and pattern of these particles differ from place to place in a given membrane and from membrane to membrane. By the use of labeled antibodies or other cytochemical procedures, it is evident that at least some of these particles are enzymes such as ATPase and adenylate cyclase.

A number of models for the organization of the plasma membrane have been put forth. That of Singer and Nicholson has received wide support (Fig. 1-14). Like other models, it postulates a lipid bilayer consisting primarily of phospholipid molecules oriented with their hydrophilic ends directed both to the outside and to the in-

1–12 Erythrocyte, peripheral cytoplasm. Note the
trilaminar character of the plasmalemma, there
being two dark laminae separated by a light one. This
membrane is a unit membrane. × 280,000. (From the
work of J. D. Robertson.)

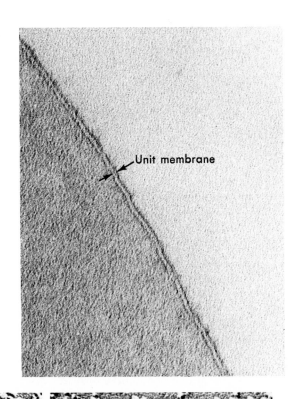

1–13 Replicas of freeze-fractured human red cell
membranes. **A.** Freeze-fracture face PF
originating from within the interior of the membrane
shows more or less randomly distributed membrane-
associated particles **(MAP),** which may represent sites
of integral membrane proteins. × 120,000. **B.** Face-EF
has fewer MAP than face-PF. × 140,000. **C.** Freeze-
etching has exposed the true exterior surface of the
red cell membrane **(*),** which appears barren and
smooth. The fracture has entered the membrane
(arrows) and exposed a PF-face for replication.
× 100,000. **D.** Small fibrils **(arrows)** apparently
extend from the cytoplasm of intact cells into the
interior of the cell membrane. × 90,000. (From
Weinstein, R. S. 1974. The Red Blood Cell. New York:
Academic Press, Inc.) ▽

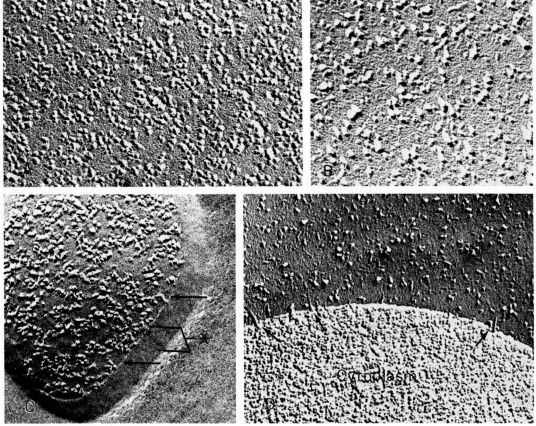

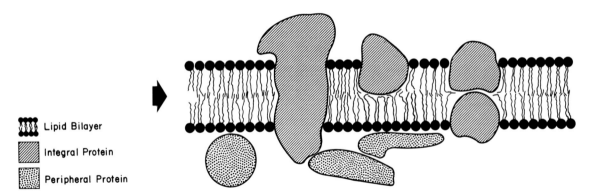

Lipid Bilayer

Integral Protein

Peripheral Protein

side surfaces. Being hydrophilic, the surfaces of the membrane interact with watery environments. Within the membrane, on the other hand, lie the long-chain nonpolar hydrocarbon portions of the fatty acid constituents of the phospholipid bilayer. The internum of the membrane is, therefore, fatty and hydrophobic. The phospholipid constituents of the outside and inside surfaces of the membrane, moreover, are somewhat different. Cholesterol molecules are dispersed throughout the membrane. Lying in the phospholipid bilayer like "icebergs in a lipid sea" are the proteins. They are most likely amphipathetic with their hydrophobic ends lying within the membrane among the hydrophobic fatty acids and hydrophilic pole protruding from the outside or inside hydrophilic surface of the membrane. Certain intrinsic proteins are longer than the width of the membrane and therefore cross it, protruding from both inside and outside surfaces. These proteins are presumably hydrophilic at the ends and hydrophobic in the center. There are places in membranes, such as in the synaptosome of nerve and junctional complexes, unusually rich in proteins, which may be linked to one another. Proteins may be fixed in the membrane or may be rather loosely attached and move about in the plane of the membrane. Such movement can be demonstrated by an experiment in which certain receptors in the plasma membrane of mouse cells are stained with a fluorescent marker of one color and those of human cells stained with a fluorescent marker of another color. The plasma membranes, and thereby the cells, are then fused by the action of sendai virus. At first the labeled receptor substances remain apart, but within 40 min they appear completely intermixed. The mixing is temperature-dependent, occurring at physiological temperature but inhibited at 4°C. This temper-

1–14 Fluid mosaic model of cell membrane. The bulk of the phospholipids (**solid circles** represent polar head groups and **wavy lines** their fatty acid chains) are organized in a discontinuous lipid bilayer. Intrinsic or integral proteins are embedded in the bilayer but can protrude from the membrane. Extrinsic or peripheral proteins may bind to phospholipid polar head groups or to the membrane via protein-protein interactions. The **arrow** shows the position of the natural cleavage plane within the center of a lipid bilayer in freeze-fracture-etch techniques. (From Weinstein, R. S. 1974. The Red Blood Cell. New York: Academic Press, Inc., p. 239.)

ature-dependence suggests simple diffusion as the basis of mixing.

In addition to proteins intrinsic to the membrane, there are peripheral proteins, the extrinsic proteins, that are linked to the membrane. The contractile protein *actin* lies directly beneath the plasma membrane in microvilli and other places and appears linked to intrinsic proteins. As a result, the plasma membrane of the microvilli is moved when actin contracts. *Spectrin* is a linear structural protein that forms a bridgework beneath the plasma membrane of erythrocytes and inserts into the underside of the membrane. This membrane-associated protein both strengthens the plasma membrane, protecting it against the shearing forces of the circulation, and anchors many of those intrinsic membrane proteins that extend into the subjacent cytoplasm. Spectrin is in the class of structural filaments known as *intermediate filaments* (page 60). A further example of membrane-associated proteins are the *cytochromes*, which are rather loosely attached to the surface of the plasma membrane. Carbohydrates are often attached to the outside of the plasma membrane. Among them are sialic acid and other glyco- or mucoproteins. The carbohydrate-rich extrinsic coat may be so heavy as to be

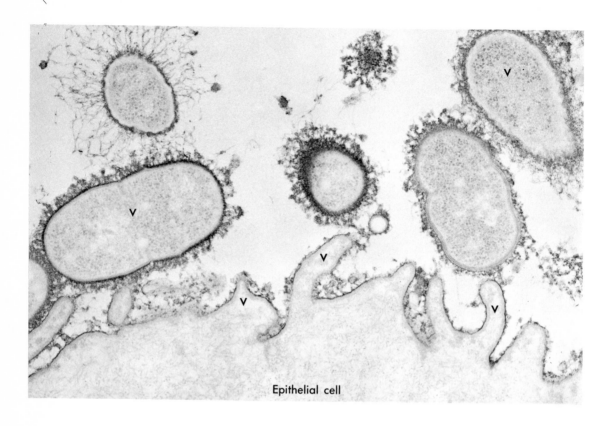

Epithelial cell

1–15 Cell surface, human buccal epithelium; electron micrograph. The free surface of an epithelial cell having large and small villi **(v)** is shown. A surface coat has been stained selectively with the dye ruthenium red. The coat, where it lies upon the plasmalemma, is relatively dense. On its free surface, on the other hand, the surface coat has a flocculent or filamentous character. × 40,000. (From Luft, John. 1971. Anat. Rec. 171:347.)

visible as a fuzzy layer called the *glycocalyx* and can be selectively stained by ruthenium red or lanthanum (Fig. 1–15). If sufficiently thick, it can be visible by light microscopy when stained by the periodic acid Schiff procedure. The sarcolemma of muscle and basal laminae in general may be regarded as sites of large-scale accumulation of proteoglycans extrinsic to the plasma membrane.

The Nucleus

The nucleus is the fundamental part of a cell that encodes the information from which the structure and function of the organism derive. The information is encoded in the genetic material

DNA, complexed to simple basic proteins, histones, to form deoxyribonucleoprotein (DNP). With some exceptions, notably mitochondria, DNA lies exclusively in the nucleus. DNA is capable of replicating itself, thereby providing precise copies of the genetic code that are passed on to daughter cells by cellular division.

The nucleus also plays a central role in synthesizing proteins and polypeptides from the genetic information it carries. All the nucleated cells of the body contain the same genes, yet cells differ in their structure, function, and products. The nucleus differentially controls the use of this information from cell to cell by repressing or derepressing the action of various genes. The nucleus initiates the translation of its encoded information into the synthesis of proteins by mean of RNAs, a group of nucleic acids that differ from DNA primarily in base composition. Some RNAs are complexed to proteins to form ribonucleoprotein (RNP). The RNAs are produced in or under the control of the nucleus and are released to the cytoplasm where they engage in protein synthesis. The "machine" that assembles proteins from amino acids is a complex of RNAs and protein, the *ribosome*, whose constituents are produced in a nuclear component, the *nucleolus*. Other RNAs are *messenger RNA* (mRNA), which links ribosomes into working units called *polyribosomes*, and *transfer RNA* (tRNA), which carries amino acids to the polyribosomes to initiate protein synthesis.

A nucleus is present in virtually all differentiated metazoan cells, being absent only from mammalian erythrocytes and a few other end-stage cell types. Certain cell types have many nuclei or are polyploid (see below); the number of genes and other elements in the protein-synthesizing apparatus of a cell is thus multiplied and the cell is able to produce a greater volume of product. Hepatocytes, particularly with age, may develop two or more nuclei, and renal tubular cells may be binucleate. Osteoclasts or foreign-body giant cells may contain 25 or more nuclei. A mechanism for increasing nuclear function without increasing nuclear number is polyploidy, an increase in the number of chromosomal pairs within a single nucleus. Most somatic cells are diploid (2n), having one pair of each chromosome characterizing its species, but cells may develop two pairs (4n) or more. Hepatocytes tend to increase in ploidy with age; in old rats they are often 8n and 16n. Megakaryocytes, giant cells of the bone marrow containing a giant polymorphous nucleus may become 32n or 64n. A more restricted mechanism for increasing nuclear components is an increase in the number of nucleoli in certain oocytes, with a concomitant increase in production of ribosomal RNA.

The nucleus may occur in a dividing (mitotic or meiotic) state, during which it reproduces itself, or in a nondividing or interphase state. The interphase nucleus is most frequently encountered, because nuclear division takes approximately 1 h whereas, even in actively dividing cells, 6 h or more elapse between divisions. Many cells of the body seldom divide (e.g., hepatocytes) or never divide (e.g. nerve cells). (See section below on Life Cycle of Cells.)

In most cell types the interphase nucleus is an ovoid structure several micrometers in diameter (Figs. 1–10 and 1–16 to 1–18). In the leukocytes of blood and connective tissues, the nucleus is lobulated and hence termed polymorphous (see Chaps. 11 and 12). The nucleus is deformable and may therefore be pressed into a reniform or horseshoe shape. In contracted smooth muscle, it may be twisted like a corkscrew (Fig. 1–18).

The interphase nucleus is bounded by a nuclear envelope and typically contains several distinctive structures. These structures include chromatin, nuclear sap or karyolymph, and one or more nucleoli. The protoplasm of the nucleus is termed *nucleoplasm* or *karyoplasm*.

Chromatin. Chromatin, by light microscopy, consists of irregular clumps or masses that, although not highly constant, tend to be characteristic in texture, quantity, and size for any given cell type. These clumps, sometimes called *karyosomes*, have an affinity for basic dye because chromatin contains DNA. DNA confers distinctive staining reactions on chromatin. Thus, chromatin is specifically stained in the Feulgen reaction. It selectively binds methyl green. In Romanovsky preparations, which are stained with methylene blue and azures, chromatin is stained violet (Chap. 11). These distinctive DNA staining reactions are abolished by pretreating the specimen with the enzyme *deoxyribonuclease*.

Chromatin is the embodiment in the interphase nucleus of the DNP of chromosomes. The chromosomes in the interphase nucleus are very slender, long, threadlike structures lying in a rather tangled mass. It is impossible to delineate individual chromosomes from this tangle. Indeed, it was at one time thought that this mass was a continuous single thread instead of individual interlaced chromosomes, and the name *spireme* was applied to it.

Chromosomes may be either coiled or uncoiled along their length. Whenever the tight coiling of the chromosome forms clumps greater than 0.2 μm in dimension, they are visible with the light microscope. Chromosomes in this form constitute the *heterochromatin*. The karyosomes are heterochromatin. In many cells, moreover, heterochromatin is also applied against the inner surface of the nuclear envelope, forming an outer rim of the nucleus interrupted only by nuclear pores (Figs. 1–10, and 1–17 to 1–19). There is also nuclear membrane–associated chromatin. Because the chromatin in uncoiled chromosomes, the *euchromatin*, is below the limit of resolution of the light microscope, euchromatin is "invisible" and cannot be differentiated from the nuclear sap. The proportions of euchromatin and heterochromatin and the distribution of heterochromatin can be quite characteristic for a given cell type. In fact, in the interphase nucleus, chromosomes may be tightly coiled in certain segments and uncoiled in other segments. Cells

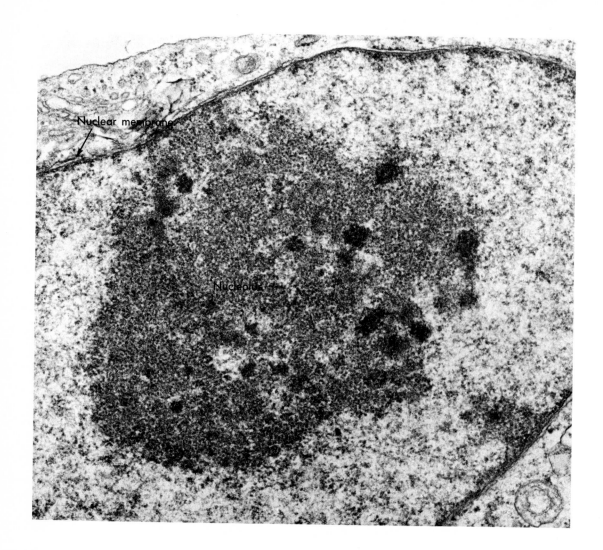

Nuclear membrane

Nucleolus

1–16 Rhesus kidney cell (strain MA 104) in culture.
The nucleolus, stained with uranyl acetate and lead, is well developed. It touches the inside surface of the nuclear membrane. Heterochromatin, densely stained, is present as a rim against the inside surface of the inner nuclear membrane. Most of the chromatin is dispersed and presents as euchromatin. The outer nuclear membrane (nuclear membrane) stands out clearly. It is part of the endoplasmic reticulum and, at places, bears ribosomes on its surface. See Fig. 1–25. × 40,000. (From the work of A. Monneran.)

with large blocks of heterochromatin tend to be relatively inactive in an early stage of protein synthesis, the production of mRNA. The uncoiled chromosomes are in the functional state that enables transcription of DNA through the formation of mRNA. The uncoiled chromosomes serve as a *template* for transcription of information to mRNA. This messenger leaves the nucleus and enters the cytoplasm. There, in concert with tRNA and the ribosomal RNA (rRNA) of the ribosomes, it synthesizes proteins whose structure was encoded in the DNA. Thus cells whose nuclei are relatively rich in euchromatin tend to be quite active in the transcription phase of protein synthesis. In cells of females a characteristic mass of heterochromatin lying against the nuclear membrane represents one of the female sex chromosomes, an X chromosome, which remains tightly coiled through interphase. It is called *sex chromatin* or, after its discoverer, the *Barr body* (Fig. 1–20). It enables the genetic sex of an individual to be determined, a procedure of value in certain endocrinopathies or congenital disturbances in which the genetic sex may not be ap-

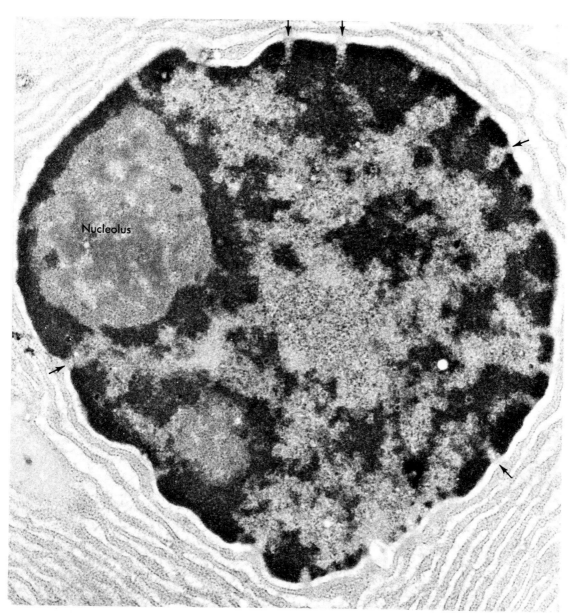

Nucleolus

1–17 Pancreatic acinar cell. The nucleus of this cell,
       which secretes digestive enzymes, has been
selectively treated to enhance the staining of DNA and
to reduce the staining of the nucleoli and other RNA-
containing structures. Chromatin is densely stained.
Much of it is marginated on the inner surface of the
nuclear membrane. Nuclear pores are prominent
(arrow), their location marked by the lightly stained
aisles between heterochromatin masses. The section
was treated with picric acid, uranyl acetate, and lead.
× 30,000. (From the work of A. Monneron.)

1–18 Contracted muscle cell. The nucleus has been
       twisted into a corkscrew spiral. On relaxation,
the nucleus will untwist and be cigar-shaped.

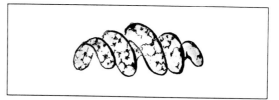

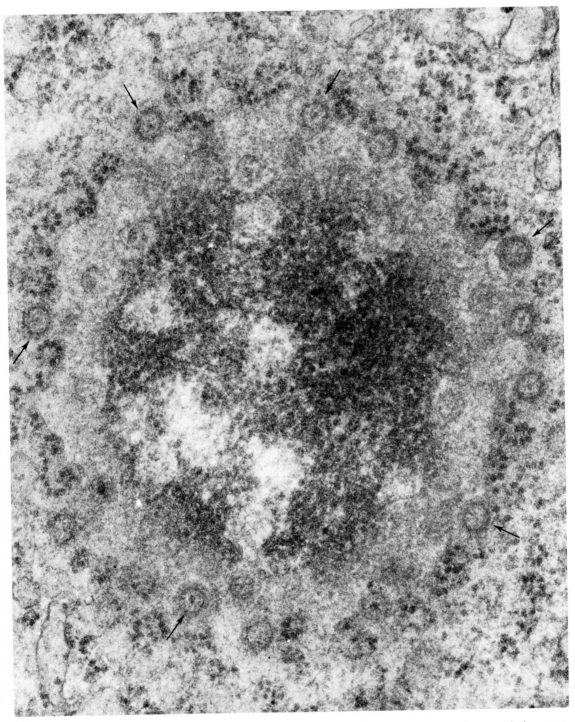

1–19 Rat hepatocyte. This is a tangential section of the nucleus, revealing nuclear pores all around **(arrow)**, some with a dark central granule. Note that polyribosomes are in close association with the pores. This preparation is stained with uranyl acetate and lead. × 140,000. (From the work of A. Monneron.)

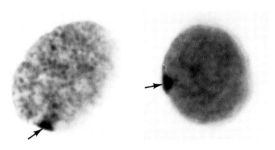

1–20 Sex chromatin of a human female. The chromatin lies against the nuclear membrane **(arrows)**. This formation of sex chromatin appears to be due to the persistent coiling in interphase in one of the X chromosomes. Human buccal mucosa. × 4000. (From the work of B. R. Migeon.)

parent. The Y (male) chromosome may be demonstrated in interphase nuclei by a special fluorescence staining method.

The elements of the interphase nucleus—namely, chromatin, nucleoli (see below), karyolymph, and nuclear membranes—are readily identified by electron microscopy. However, the correlation of electron-microscopic observations of interphase nuclei with what is inferred of the structure of chromosomes and other nuclear components from genetic and other data remains rudimentary. It is known, for example, that an uncoiled chromosome may be of the order of 10,000 times the largest dimension of the nucleus. But it is difficult to gain any appreciation from sections of nuclei of the nature of the immense folding and coiling that the chromosomes must undergo. Such inferences as electron microscopy affords come from preparations in which chromosomes are floated out of disrupted nuclei, dried down on supporting membranes, and examined whole. In these preparations high degrees of coiling and folding are evident. Pure DNA may be prepared and examined as whole, unsectioned filaments by electron microscopy. These filaments are approximately 20 Å in diameter. DNA can be identified in sectioned interphase nuclei on the basis of selective staining. It is present in filaments of varying diameter, that of the slimmest being about 100 Å. The greater thickness of DNA in sections may be due to such factors as coiling, folding, or intertwining of DNA filaments or complexing of DNA with histones or other substances.

Nucleolus. A nucleolus is a discrete intranuclear structure consisting largely of protein and RNA, which synthesizes the major components of ribosomes. The nucleolus is well developed in cells active in protein synthesis. Such cells may contain several nucleoli. In cells synthesizing little protein, such as spermatocytes, neutrophils, and muscle cells, a nucleolus may not be evident. Nucleoli appear at certain specific sites, the *nucleolar organizing sites* in certain chromosomes (Fig. 1–21). These sites represent secondary constrictions in the chromosomes. At these sites on the chromosomes, the gene sequences *(cistrons)* are located that encode the genetic information for the synthesis of rRNA. Nucleoli remain attached to the chromosomes at nucleolar organizing sites.

Nucleoli by light microscopy are usually spherical, up to 1 μm in diameter, but may be oval or even bow-tie shaped. They are usually compact and sharply outlined, but they may be porous with fuzzy borders. Nucleoli may lie at random or against the inside of the nuclear membrane, an efficient location for discharging substances into the cytoplasm (Figs. 1–3 and 1–4).

Nucleoli are rich in RNA. Thus they absorb ultraviolet light at a wavelength of 2,600 Å, and can thereby be identified by ultraviolet microscopy. Nucleoli may be stained with pyronin in the methyl green-pyronin mixture and blue in Romanovsky blood stains. Staining of nucleoli is abolished by treating the section with *ribonu-*

1–21 Chromosomes containing nucleolar organizing sites from the clawed toad *Xenopus laevis.* They are taken from the metaphase karyotype (see text). Each of the chromosomes in the wild type contains very slender zones, the nucleolar organizing sites. In the heterozygote, on the other hand, only one pair of chromosomes contains this site. The resultant heterozygote, as discussed in the text, is nucleolar-deficient mutants. (From the work of D. D. Brown.)

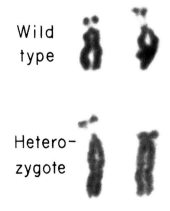

Wild type

Hetero-zygote

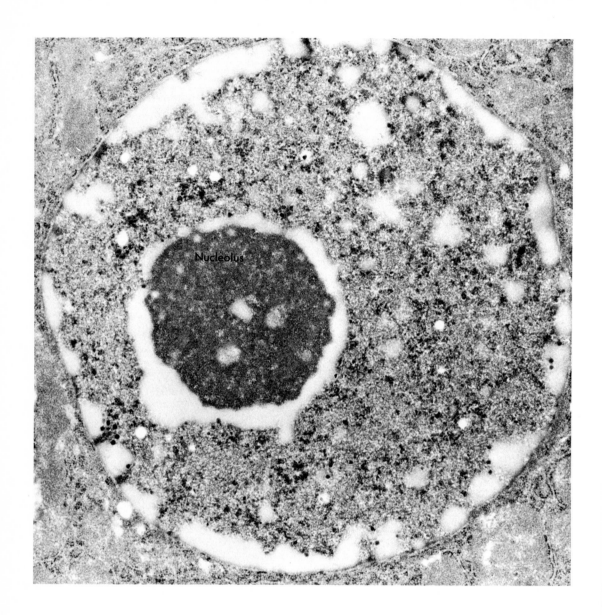

1–22 Hepatocyte. In this preparation RNP is preferentially stained and chromatin is bleached. The nucleolus stands out sharply. Stained granules, presumably containing RNA, lie outside the nucleolus in association with the chromatin. There are large (400 to 500 Å) perichromatin granules and small (200 Å) interchromatin granules. × 27,000. (From the work of A. Monneron; see also Bernhard, W. 1969. J. Ultrastruct. Res. 27:250.)

clease. RNA contains the nucleotide base *uridine.* (*Thymidine* is the DNA base counterpart to uridine.) Therefore, if radioactive uridine is given to an animal, autoradiography of its cells shows positive nucleoli (Fig. 1–23).

By electron microscopy, nucleoli contain two forms of RNA (Figs. 1–16, 1–17, 1–22, and 1–23). One is granular, approximately 150 Å in diameter, and represents maturing forms of RNP particles. This is typically the dominant nucleolar structure. The second form of RNA is fibrillar, 50 to 80 Å in thickness, and is probably a precursor to the granules.

Nucleoli are not the only sites of RNP in the nucleus. Particles of different sizes and filaments of RNP lie against and between chromatin. It is likely that some of this widely dispersed nuclear RNA is mRNA (see below) produced on extended segments of DNA (euchromatin).

DNA is a component of the nucleolus, desig-

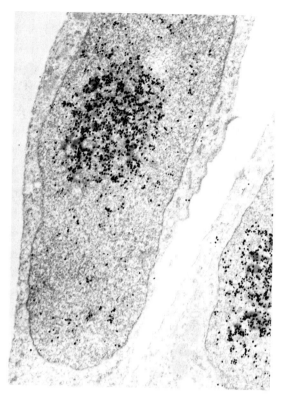

1–23 Monkey kidney cells (strain BSC). These cells, in tissue culture, were exposed to [³H] uridine (a precursor of RNA) for 30 min and then fixed and processed for EM autoradiography. The distribution of silver grains is only over the nucleus and mainly over the nucleolus. ×25,000. (From A. Monneron, J. Burglen, and W. Bernhard. 1970. J. Ultrastruct. Res. 32:370.)

produce the subunits of ribosomes and release them to the cytoplasm. The release to the cytoplasm may be facilitated by the nucleolus moving against the nuclear membrane and discharging through nuclear pores. In the cytoplasm, the nucleolar-produced ribosomal components may mature further, perhaps by adding protein, and combine to form ribosomes.

Support for the role of nucleoli in ribosomal synthesis comes from the work of Brown and his associates on amphibian mutants lacking nucleoli. The embryo of the clawed toad *Xenopus laevis* synthesizes few ribosomes before the tail bud stage, the ribosomes from the oocyte serving until that time. A lethal anucleolate mutant of *Xenopus* may be bred from a spontaneously occurring heterozygote mutant with but one nucleolus per cell, instead of the normal two. Development of the anucleolate embryos is retarded after hatching. The embryos are microcephalic and edematous and die before feeding. The mutation that prevents the formation of a normal nucleolus also prevents synthesis of 28S and 18S rRNA, as well as high molecular-weight precursor molecules of ribosomes.

The correlation between ribosome production and nucleoli is evident in multinucleolate amphibian oocytes where the DNA specifying the sequences for 28S and 18S rRNAs is selectively replicated. As many as 1,000 autonomously functional nucleoli may occur per oocyte (Fig. 1–24).

nated *nucleolar chromatin* of the nucleolar organizing site of the chromosome. It occurs in twisted or single filaments 200 to 300 Å in diameter.

Poorly defined granular material, probably protein, occurs throughout nucleoli. Rarefied vacuolar zones, not membrane-bounded, may be present.

The nucleolus is a center for the synthesis of ribosomes. The size and number of nucleoli depend on the level of rRNA synthesis. In actively secretory cells (pancreatic acinar cells) nucleoli are large and multiple, whereas in cells showing a low level of protein synthesis (muscle cells, certain small lymphocytes) nucleoli may be small or absent.

Ribosomes have several subunits (see section on Ribosomes). On the basis of isolation and sedimentation analysis it appears that nucleoli

1–24 Nucleus isolated from an oocyte of *Xenopus laevis*. The nucleus was dissected from the oocyte, flooded with cresyl violet stain, and photographed. The deeply stained spots are those of the hundreds of nucleoli which are in the plane of focus. (From Brown, D. D., and Dawid, I. B. 1968. Science 160:272.)

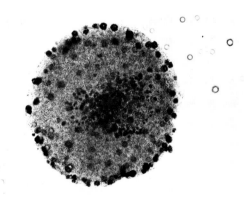

Nuclear Envelope. The nuclear envelope consists of two concentric unit membranes (Fig. 1–5). Each is approximately 70 Å in thickness, the inner one somewhat thinner. The space of the cisterna between inner and outer nuclear membranes varies in size and content. It is commonly about 150 Å wide and lucent. The outer nuclear membrane is continuous with the endoplasmic reticulum (ER), both rough and smooth. The cytoplasmic character of nuclear membrane is underscored in reformation in the telophase. The nuclear membranes are clearly formed by segments of ER, which line up around the reconstituted nuclear mass. In cells synthesizing protein, the nuclear envelope may, like the rough ER, contain the protein product. Thus, in antibody-producing cells the nuclear envelope may be distended with antibody and, indeed, is among the first places antibody accumulates. In the interphase nucleus the inner nuclear membrane is reinforced on its inner surface by a closely applied finely granular *lamina*. A subset of heterochromatin lies against the inner surface of the lamina, and, in places, penetrates it and reaches to the inner nuclear membrane (Figs. 1–25 and 1–26). This heterochromatin forms a rim around the nucleus, interrupted by nuclear pores (Figs. 1–10 and 1–16 to 1–19). During the first meiotic prophase, chromosomes may be attached to the inner surface of the inner membrane and nucleoli may lie there. Although the nuclear envelope cannot be resolved by light microscopy, its location is often revealed as a definite line representing the sum of the nuclear membranes, nuclear cisterna, and lamina.

Nuclear pore complexes represent interruptions in the nuclear membranes. At a pore complex the inner and outer nuclear membranes appear to fuse and their margins thicken to form an annulus as great as 1,000 Å in outside diameter and 600 Å inside. On surface view it is circular or octagonal in outline. By low-power electron microscopy the pore complex may appear as an aperture in the nuclear membranes with a thickened annulus, closed by a thin diaphragm that often contains a central granule. At high resolution the complex appears to be a granular and filamentous structure with eight regularly spaced granules, each about 100 Å in diameter, lying in the rim of the pore. There are, in fact, two sets of eight granules, one set lying at the outer rim associated with the outer nuclear membrane, the other at the inner rim, associated with the inner nuclear membrane (Fig. 1–25). The central gran-

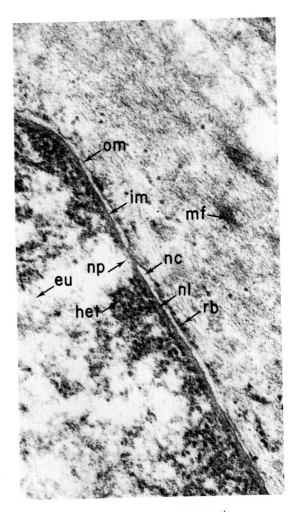

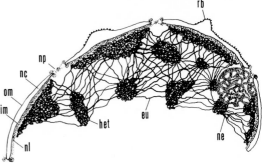

1–25 Above, an electron micrograph of a reticular cell, equine spleen, the nucleus on the left, the cytoplasm on the right. **om** outer nuclear membrane; **im** inner nuclear membrane; **nc** nuclear cisterna; **nl** nuclear lamina; **np** nuclear pore complex; **eu** euchromatin; **het** heterochromatin; **rb** ribosome; **mf** plaque of microfilaments. Courtesy of Fern Tablin. × 42,000. Below, schema of nuclear structures showing, in addition, **ne** nucleolus.

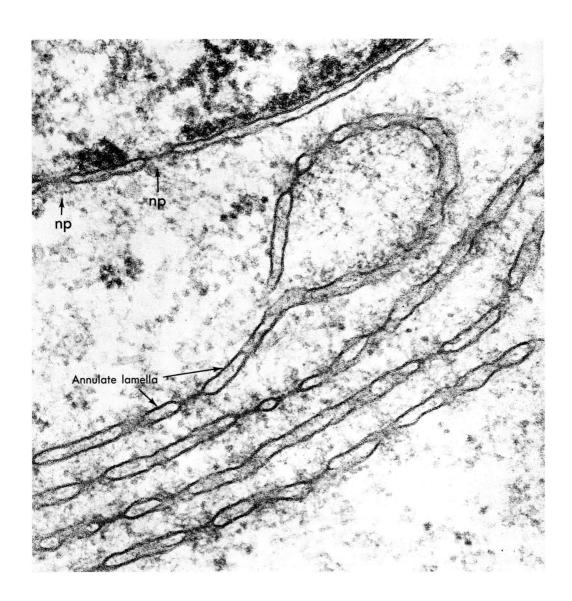

ule is connected by filaments to the wall of the pore complex and to the annular granules. The granules and filaments may be surrounded by a particulate material. The central granule may be traversed by a slender aperture, connecting nucleoplasm with cytoplasm (Fig. 1–19).

There are very few cell types, such as the spermatozoa of bulls, that have few or even no nuclear pore complexes. In other cell types, 3 to 35% of the nuclear surface may be covered by complexes. They may be distributed over the whole nuclear surface or clustered. They may lie irregularly or regularly, falling into square or hexagonal arrays.

Nuclear pore complexes would seem to rep-

1–26 Nuclear pores and annulate lamellae. The nucleus in the left upper corner is bounded by a double membrane, each component consisting of a unit membrane (see text). Within the nucleus, densely stained chromatin is arranged against the nuclear membrane, in which two nuclear pores **(np)** are present. Within the cytoplasm, occupying much of the field, are stacks of annulate lamellae. These appear identical in structure with the nuclear membrane and, like the nuclear membrane, have frequently spaced pore complexes. × 65,000. (From Maul, G. 1970. J. Cell Biol. 46:604.)

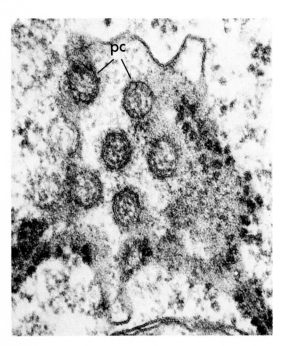

1–27 Annulate lamellae. In this face-on section, surface views of the pore complexes **(pc)** are presented. The pores appear limited by a unit membrane and have a complex, regular internal structure. × 65,000. (From Maul, G. 1970. J. Cell. Biol. 46:604.)

resent passageways, albeit restricted ones, between nucleus and cytoplasm.

Annulate Lamellae. In many cell types stacks of membranes that exactly resemble portions of nuclear membranes, pore complexes and all, may be found in the cytoplasm (Figs. 1–26 and 1–27). In germ cells they may also be present in nucleoplasm. These membranes are termed *annulate lamellae* and are especially common in germ cells and in some tumor cells. They may be continuous with ER. Their significance is not known.

The Cytoplasm

The cytoplasm surrounds the nucleus and is bounded peripherally by the plasma membrane. The cytoplasm expresses most of the functions of the cell. It is dependent on the nucleus for direction, renewal, and regeneration. Thus, isolated units of cytoplasm, exemplified by blood plate-

lets and mature erythrocytes, are capable of protein synthesis and of such specific functions as respiration and the retraction of blood clots. The cytoplasmic structures, however, such as membranes, granules, and microfilaments, which are the basis of such cytoplasmic functions, were originally synthesized and accumulated in the cytoplasm from ribosomes and other materials derived from a viable nucleus that was present at an early phase in the life cycle of these anucleate structures. The volume of cytoplasm in proportion to the nucleus, the nuclear–cytoplasmic ratio, varies considerably from cell type to cell type. In some cells, such as spermatozoa and small lymphocytes, the cytoplasm is scant. In most cells the cytoplasm is relatively abundant and exceeds the nuclear volume by a factor of 3 to 5 or more. The cytoplasm possesses distinctive organelles with specialized functions that lie in the ground substance or hyaloplasm.

Cytoplasm in the center of the cell next to the nucleus, may be gelated. It contains the centrioles and centrosphere but is usually clear of other organelles. It may be bounded by microtubules and surrounded by the Golgi apparatus. Often it pushes the nucleus aside, indenting it. This zone is called the *cell center* or *cytocentrum*. Peripheral to this zone is a solvated part of the cell containing vacuoles and granules, mitochondria, and elements of the ER. Cytoplasmic streaming occurs here, carrying the cytoplasmic organelles in rapid movement. This zone is called *endoplasm*. The peripheral cytoplasm in many cell types, particularly in free or motile cells, is gelated and often rich in microfilaments but free of other organelles. This zone is the *ectoplasm*. It is capable of rapid sol-gel transformation. Gelated ectoplasm may become liquid, particularly in motile cells or cells extending pseudopodial processes, and the already liquid endoplasm bearing organelles then flows in.

The structural protein of the hyaloplasm has a reticulated character visible in high-voltage electron micrographs (Fig. 1–8), which underscores the importance in providing the framework of the cell. Fat occurs in macromolecular micelles that may be visible. Fat sometimes coalesces to form larger fatty vacuoles, *not* bound by membrane, that are visible by electron and light microscopy (Chap. 5). Granules of glycogen may lie in the hyaloplasm, in clusters termed *alpha particles* (Fig. 1–28). However, the predominant structures carried in the hyaloplasm

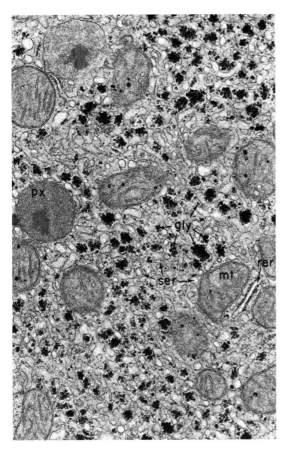

1–28 Glycogen. This electron microscopic field contains particles of glycogen **(gly)**. The individual particles are termed beta particles. Ten to fifteen beta particles form an alpha particle. When glycogen is present in lysosomes, presumably to be broken down to glucose and utilized, the glycogen–lysosome structure may be termed *glycosome*. The field also contains peroxisomes **(px)**, mitochondria, and endoplasmic reticulum. Most of the endoplasmic reticulum is smooth **(ser)** and contains the glycogen, a finding suggesting that smooth er has a role in glycogen synthesis. × 23,000. (From the work of Robert R. Cardell, Jr.)

are complex organelles fashioned of membranes, filaments, tubules, and granules, which we shall consider now.

Mitochondria. Mitochondria are membranous cytoplasmic organelles capable of trapping chemical energy released by oxidation of compounds derived from food. They then fix that en-

ergy in a form, *adenosine triphosphate (ATP)*, that is readily utilizable by the cell. They are present as punctate or linear structures just within the resolving power of the light microscope (Figs. 1–4 and 1–29). By electron microscopy, mitochondria are tubular or spherical structures bounded by one membrane called the *outer membrane* and containing a second internal folded membrane termed the *inner membrane* (Figs. 1–30 and 1–31).

A cell obtains energy from substrates derived from food. Thus amino acids derived from protein, fatty acids from fat, and glucose from carbohydrate may be sources of energy. The major source, however, is glucose. Glucose is broken down in the cell by glycolytic enzymes to form pyruvic acid, which is then oxidized to acetyl coenzyme A. This compound then proceeds to a cycle of further oxidations, the Krebs tricarboxylic acid cycle, whose end products are carbon dioxide and water. Approximately 690,000 calories of energy per mole lie in the chemical bonds of glucose. Its breakdown to pyruvate yields approximately 40,000 calories per mole, but its complete oxidation to carbon dioxide and water through the Krebs cycle yields another 650,000 calories per mole. The energy-capturing mechanism of cells is at best only about 50% efficient, however, because half of the energy is lost as heat. Therefore, the total caloric content of glucose is never available.

Only about 350,00 calories per mole are useful to the cell. The glycolytic breakdown of glucose is anaerobic—that is, it does not use oxygen. In contrast, the mechanism of the Krebs cycle does require oxygen and is therefore respiratory in nature. The oxidation through the Krebs cycle is of the greatest importance, as indicated by its caloric yields; indeed, it is necessary to life. Blocking this system, as can be done with fluoracetate, causes death. *The Krebs cycle enzymes are present in mitochondria.*

The energy resulting from the oxidation of pyruvate to carbon dioxide and water would, by itself, yield only heat. For this energy to be of value to the metabolism of the cell, it must first be chemically fixed or stored in certain molecules and then be readily released from these molecules as needed. The cell accomplishes this by means of a distinctive enzyme system coupled into the Krebs cycle: the electron-transfer system of cytochromes. This system accepts the energy liberated in each of the steps of the Krebs

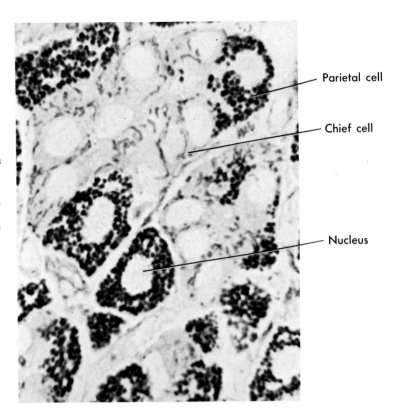

Parietal cell

Chief cell

Nucleus

1–29 Light micrograph of a portion of the stomach lining. The preparation has been stained for NAD⁺-dependent isocitric dehydrogenase activity (consult Chap. 2). This constitutes a selective stain for mitochondria. Nuclei are present in negative image. Two cell types are present. One, the parietal cell, is rich in granular mitochondria and carries out active transport. The second, the chief cell, has relatively few filamentous mitochondria and is concerned with the synthesis of protein. These cell types are discussed in Chap. 19. × 1,500. (From the work of D. G. Walker.)

cycle and incorporates it into so-called high-energy phosphate compounds, notably ATP. This is done by the conversion of *adenosine diphosphate (ADP)* to ATP. The additional phosphate bond so formed represents approximately 7,300 calories of stored energy. *The cytochrome electron-transfer system capable of fixing the energy obtained from the oxidations of the Krebs cycle into ATP lies in mitochondria.* The source of energy for virtually every energy-requiring activity of the cell is ATP. It is translocated from mitochondria into surrounding cytoplasm and its energy is released by ATPases, which lie at different locations in the cell. One depot rich in ATPase is the cell membrane. Here the energy obtained from the conversion of ATP to ADP is used in the active transport of compounds across the cell membrane.

Mitochondria may be observed in living cells by phase-contrast microscopy (Fig. 1–1). They are quite pliant and appear to be carried passively in cytoplasmic streams, twisted, bent, and changing shape. On occasion they appear contractile or motile. They are subject to swelling in certain physiological states.

Mitochondria may be vitally stained with Janus green B, pinacyanole, or other vital dyes that exist in either a colored oxidized form or a colorless reduced form. Because of their oxidative enzymes, mitochondria are able to maintain the dye in its oxidized form (a green or blue in the case of Janus green B), whereas the rest of the cytoplasm is usually unable to do so. Mitochondria stand out clearly as stained linear or punctate structures (Figure 11–5).

In fixed and stained light-microscopic preparations, mitochondria are usually demonstrated by virtue of the phospholipid contained in their membranes. Iron hematoxylin is an excellent stain for mitochondria that is used in the Regaud, Baker, and other methods, because it stains phospholipid. Sudan black B or other dyes that dissolve in lipid stain mitochondria faintly.

Mitochondria may also be demonstrated under the light microscope by cytochemical staining of the activity of their enzymes (Fig. 1–29). Thus stains that reveal the activity of succinic dehydrogenase, malic dehydrogenase, isocitrate dehydrogenase, fumaric dehydrogenase, and other oxidative enzymes effectively stain mitochondria. The cells must be carefully fixed to limit diffusion of enzymes and to retain structural clarity. Even slightly prolonged fixation destroys enzyme activity and renders the methods ineffective. Cytochemical methods provide valuable physiological information. For example, mitochondria may appear identical by methods that depend on phospholipid staining or by supravital staining or phase microscopy. Yet in such mitochondria, Krebs-cycle enzymes may have different activity, and by staining for a variety of these enzymes different functional classes of mitochondria may be recognized.

By electron microscopy, mitochondria may be recognized as distinctive tubular or, occasionally, spherical structures made of inner and outer membranes (Figs. 1–30 and 1–31). The outer membrane is unfolded. The inner membrane is folded to form *cristae,* which extend into the center of the mitochondrion. The space enclosed by the inner membrane is the *inner chamber.* It contains a finely granular material, the *matrix.* The space between outer and inner membrane is the *outer chamber.* In most mammalian cells the cristae are plates or shelves that extend partway across the inner chamber. In cardiac muscle and in kidney tubular cells there may be many cristae that reach across the mitochrondrion, whereas in macrophages there are usually few cristae, and they are short. In the testis, ovary, and adrenal gland, the mitochondria of cells secreting steroid hormones have tubular rather than shelflike cristae.

The unit membrane is modified in the cristae. The surface exposed to the inner chamber possesses knoblike repeating units attached to a basal membrane by slender stalks (Fig. 1–32). These units, called *elementary particles,* are best revealed at high magnification with negative staining after osmotic shock. Elementary particles contain a mitochondrial ATPase complex that appears to provide a channel for proton translocation. Normally the particles may be embedded in the membrane rather than project from it.

Mitochondria are subject to conformational change (Figs. 1–30 and 1–31). The *orthodox form,* described above, is typical of mitochondria in tissue section, since the methods of preparation usually result in low levels of ADP with the mitochondria inactive in oxidative phosphorylation. If, however, oxidative phosporylation is induced in isolated mitochondria by adding ADP or if measures are taken to maintain a high level of oxidative phosphorylation in tissue sections, a *condensed mitochrondrial conformation* is revealed. In this form the volume of the outer chamber is increased to approximately 50% of the organelle, and the inner chamber is reduced in volume.

Mitochondria may be isolated relatively easily by a technique that requires disruption of cells and centrifugation of the fragments. In density-gradient centrifugation, the mitochondria form a tan colored stratum lying above the nuclei and below the lysosomes and ribosomes.

Isolated mitochondria exhibit the reactions described above. In addition, they may be studied by standard chemical and microchemical methods. They may be dissociated by applying deoxycholate and other surface-active agents; in this way it has been shown that the electron-transfer system of cytochromes is firmly bound to membranes, whereas the enzymes of the Krebs tricarboxylic acid cycle are not. Electron-microscopic cytochemistry demonstrates the presence of cytochrome oxidase and other oxidative enzymes in sections of mitochondria.

Freeze-fracture-etch methods reveal particles in mitochondrial membranes (Fig. 1–33). The particles on the inner membrane are numerous and may constitute the enzymes of the electron-transfer chain of cytochrome enzymes.

The number and size of mitochondria are, in general, correlated with the level of oxidative phosphorylation. Hepatocytes may each contain about 1,000 to 1,500 mitochondria. Mature erythrocytes, totally dependent for energy on glycolysis, contain none.

Mitochondria may bear characteristic relationships to other organelles and cell structures. Their relationship is often of functional significance, as the mitochondrion is the primary source of energy. Thus in cells synthesizing protein, mitochondria may occur close to ribosomes. In cells engaged in large-scale active transport of materials across a cell membrane, such as the parietal cell of the stomach (which pumps protons across the plasma membrane in the production of hydrochloric acid), the plasma membrane dips into the cell in many folds and mitochondria are closely held in them. In striated muscle cells, which contain myofilaments that slide on one another to effect contraction, mitochondria are present close to the myofilaments. In the development of fat cells, the minute fat droplets that form and then coalesce are intimately associated with mitochondria.

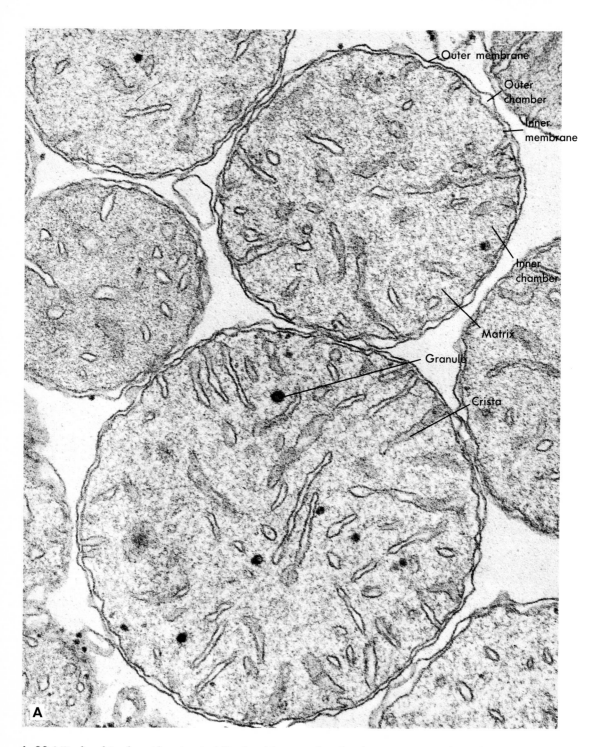

1–30 Mitochondria of a rat hepatocyte. Mitochondria undergo reversible ultrastructural transformations between a condensed and an orthodox conformation in relationship to the level on oxidative phosphorylation (see text). These changes may be observed in isolated mitochondria and in tissue section. Mitochondria are isolated from disrupted hepatocytes and sectioned. **A.** The conventional

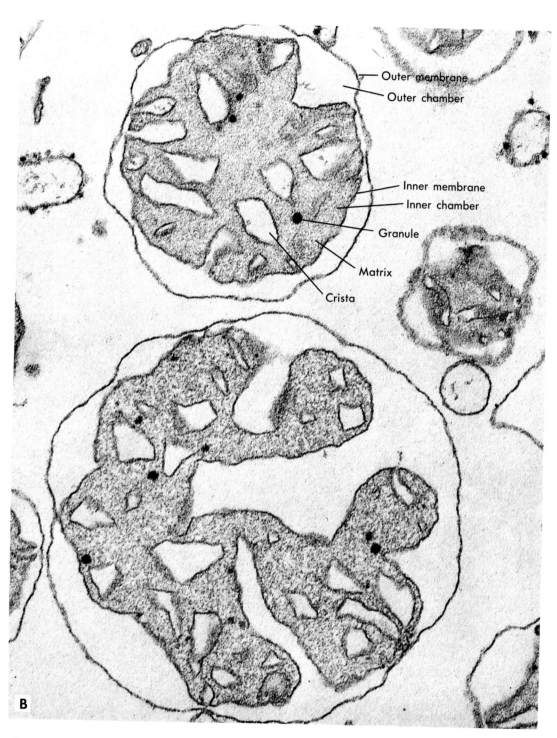

conformation, the outer membrane, outer chamber, inner membrane with cristae, and inner chamber containing matrix and granules may be seen. **B.** The condensed state: the outer chamber is considerably enlarged and the inner membrane and matrix thereby condensed. Each × 110,000. (From Hackenbrock, C. R., 1968. J. Cell Biol. 37:345.)

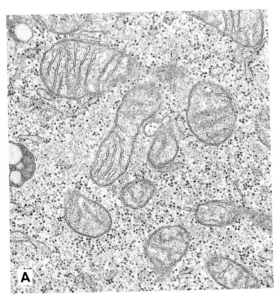

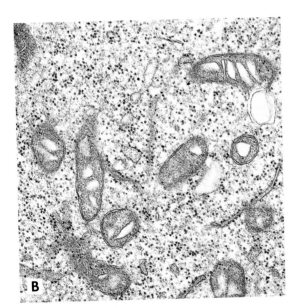

1–31 Mitochondria of an ascites tumor cell. **A.**
△   Mitochondria are present in the orthodox
conformation. A mitochondrion is enclosed in an
outer membrane. The inner membrane is folded into
cristae that extend into the matrix of inner chamber.
× 26,800. **B.** The condensed form, wherein the outer
chamber is expanded, is evident. The cytoplasm also
contains polyribosomes and rough ER. × 26,800.
(From Hackenbrock, C. R., Rehn, T. G., Weinbach,
E. C., and Lemasters, J. J. 1971. J. Cell Biol. 51:123.)

1–32 Mitochondrion from beef heart; negatively
▽   stained electron micrograph. **A.** The cristae of
the mitochondrion are outlined at a magnification of
62,000. Note that small bodies **(arrow)** appear on the
outer cristal membrane facing the interior of the
mitochondrion. **B.** Under 420,000 magnification these
small bodies, the elementary particles **(EP),** are seen
attached to the cristal membrane by a slender
stalk. (From Fernandez-Moran, H., Oda, T., Blair,
P. V., and Green, D. E. 1964. J. Cell Biol. 22:63.)

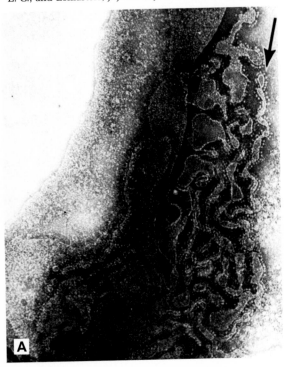

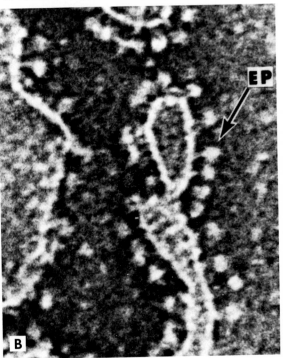

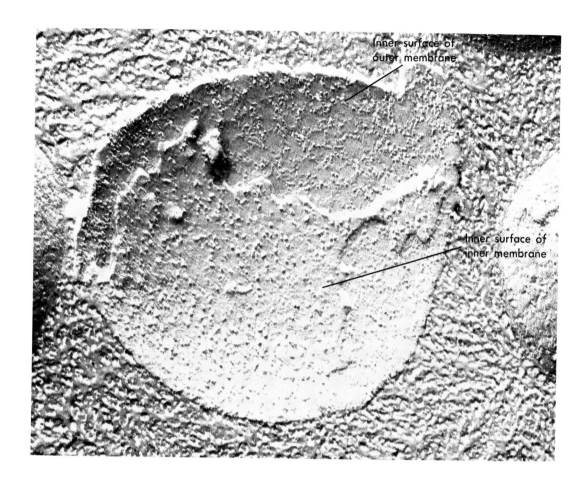

Inner surface of
outer membrane

Inner surface of
inner membrane

The primary function of mitochondria is respiratory, as has been described. They may display other activities as well, notably the concentration of cations. The dense granules of the mitochondrial matrix in the inner chamber may represent concentrations of Ca^{++}.

Mitochondria contain circular DNA typical of prokaryotes, and mitochondrial ribosomes are similar to bacterial ribosomes in several respects. There is evidence, moreover, that existing mitochondria produce new mitochondria. It is possible that in the evolution of eukaryotes, ancestral prokaryote structures established a felicitous symbiotic relationship and permitted the highly successful evolution of eukaryotes. Alternatively, the prokaryotic character of mitochondrial nucleoproteins may be the result of later eukaryotic evolution (convergent evolution) without any contribution of symbiotic prokaryotic organisms.

Endoplasmic Reticulum. The endoplasmic reticulum (ER) is a cytoplasmic system of tubules,

1–33 Mitochondria of a rat hepatocyte. Freeze-fracture-etch of isolated mitochondria. The fracture line exposed the inner surface of the outer membrane and the inner surface of the inner membrane. Note the rather regularly arranged system of granules on the inner surface of the outer membrane. The granules are the size of certain enzymes and may represent membrane-associated enzymes. × 110,000. (From the work of C. R. Hackenbrock.)

vesicles, and sacs or cisternae fashioned of membranes. It is continuous with the outer membrane of the nuclear envelope (Fig. 1–34). The development of ER varies with cell type and function.

The ER has been defined by electron microscopy, although it has been observed by light microscopy in some cells, notably as the sarcoplasmic reticulum, the specialized ER of striated muscle (Chap. 7). The ER was first described in fibroblasts in tissue culture examined in electron micrographs of whole mounts, i.e., without sec-

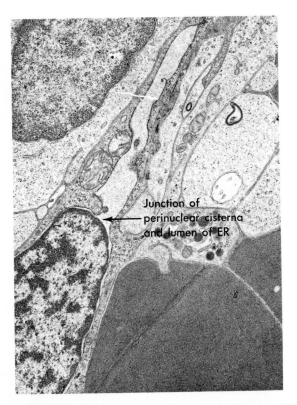

1–34 Connective tissue cell from human embryo spleen. Here the continuity of the outer nuclear membrane and the smooth ER is evident. Thus the perinuclear space and the lumen of the ER are continuous. × 12,000.

◁

Junction of perinuclear cisterna and lumen of ER

1–35 Fibroblast, tissue culture. The preparation in this electron micrograph has not been sectioned. It is a whole mount of the cell, and only the peripheral region is sufficiently thin to permit passage of the electron beam. (From the work of K. R. Porter.) ▽

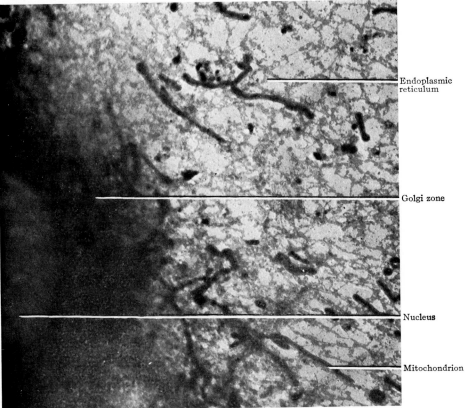

Endoplasmic reticulum

Golgi zone

Nucleus

Mitochondrion

tioning. Ordinarily, whole cells are too thick for electron-microscopic study, but cells in culture may put out cytoplasmic processes thin enough to pass an electron beam. In such preparations the ER may be seen as a cytoplasmic network (Fig. 1–35).

Two major forms of ER occur. They are *rough* or *granular* ER (Fig. 1–36), which has ribosomes on its outside surface, and *smooth* or *agranular* ER, whose surface is free of ribosomes. Ribosomes synthesize protein (see below) and need not be associated with ER. The association of ER and ribosomes occurs in cells that bind the protein they produce in membranous sacs. For example, erythroblasts synthesize the protein hemoglobin, which remains dispersed through the cytoplasm; thus, ribosomes are plentiful but little ER is present. In plasma cells, on the other hand, which synthesize large volumes of antibody, confine it by membranes, and then secrete it, rough ER is abundant. Peptide chains are synthesized in the ribosomes and sent across the ER membrane into the lumen of the ER. The ER thereby isolates synthesized material from the rest of the cytoplasm, permits further assembly of peptides into larger molecules, and conveys the material by means of *transport vesicles* to the Golgi complex where further synthesis and pro-

cessing occur. The Golgi then release the secretion enclosed in membranous sacs, the *condensing vacuoles*, which mature into secretory vacuoles. (See discussion of the Golgi complex, page 48.) Rough ER, well developed in secretory cells, is also abundant in cells that synthesize protein and hold it membrane-bounded within their cytoplasm, as in leukocytes and macrophages. These cells contain enzyme-rich membrane-bounded granules, the *lysosomes*. The formation of these granules parallels the formation of secretory vacuoles, except that the granules tend to be retained rather than released (secreted). The process of secretion is fully discussed in Chap. 21. See, particularly, Figs. 21–9 to 21–13.

In nerve cells rough ER exists as large, flattened sacs lying on one another in lamellated fashion to form masses, *Nissl bodies*, identifiable by light microscopy. Hepatic parenchymal

1–36 Hepatocyte of a rat. In this portion of the cytoplasm most of the cisternae of the rough ER were cut transversely and others tangentially. In the latter (**arrow**) the membrane of the ER and the attached polysomes are seen *en face*. A section of a mitochondrion (**mit**) is present. × 64,000. (From the work of G. E. Palade.)

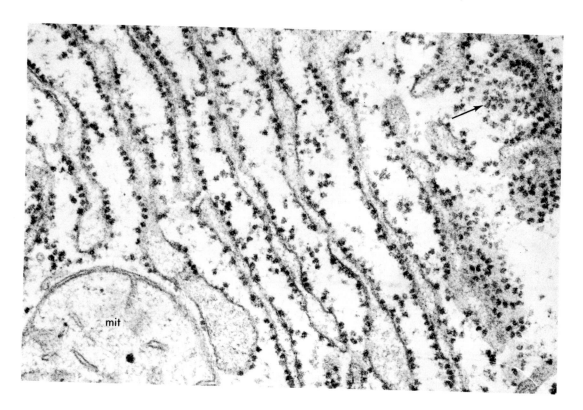

cells contain smaller blocks of rough ER. In plasma cells the rough ER is rather uniformly distributed through the cytoplasm except in the region of the cytocentrum. It may be tubular, vesicular, or flattened, depending on the phase of antibody secretion. Rough ER occupies the base of the pancreatic acinar cell. This rough ER, recognizable by light microscopy as basophilic material (because of the affinity of its ribosomes for cationic dye) is termed *ergastoplasm* (Figs. 1–3 and 1–4).

Smooth ER, free of ribosomes, occurs in a number of cell types and may have diverse functions. It has a role in the production of steroid hormones and it is abundant in such cells as the Leydig cells of the testis, which produce the steroid testosterone. Smooth ER synthesizes complex lipids from fatty acids. It also detoxifies certain drugs and becomes very prominent in hepatocytes during the inactivation of phenobarbital. In striated muscle, smooth ER is distinctly organized as the sarcoplasmic reticulum whose functions include delivering high concentrations of Ca^{++} and other ions to critical places in the sarcomere for muscular contraction and relaxation. Smooth ER in megakaryocytes delimits platelet zones in the cytoplasm and, by fusing, frees platelets from the megakaryocyte. Appropriately, this ER is termed "*demarcation membrane*". Carbohydrate synthesis is associated with smooth ER and the Golgi apparatus. The reformation of the nuclear membrane in telophase is accomplished by smooth ER.

The membranes of the ER possess a self-healing capacity after disruption. When fractions rich in ER are recovered from disrupted ultracentrifuged cells, the ER is found as small vesicles (*microsomes*) (Fig. 1–37). Evidently the tubular system is fragmented, but the membranes reunite or "heal" to form small vesicles. After fixation with osmium tetroxide (but not gluteraldehyde) the tubular T system of sarcoplasmic reticulum is revealed as an artifactual system of vesicles— another example of the readiness with which the tubules of ER may be broken up and reformed as small vesicles.

Ribosomes. A single ribosome is below the limit of resolution of the light microscope, but in aggregate, the presence of ribosomes can be recognized. Owing, in all likelihood, to their PO_4^{3-} groups, they have a pronounced affinity for cationic or basic dyes such as methylene blue⁺. As a result, cells rich in ribosomes are basophilic;

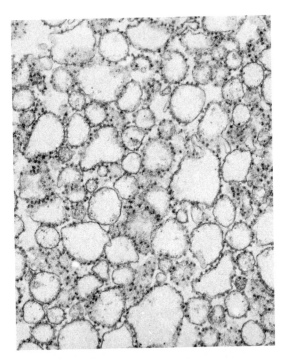

1–37 Microsomes of rat liver. The liver was disrupted and various fractions recovered by ultracentrifugation. This is the microsome fraction. It consists almost entirely of rough ER that had been disrupted and "healed" as vesicles. Ribosomes remain attached to the outer surface. × 40,000. (From the work of D. Sabatini and M. Adelman.)

this basophilia may be abolished by pretreating the tissue with ribonuclease. The intensity and disposition of the basophilia are highly characteristic of cell type. Basophilic material visualized by light microscopy has been designated *chromidial substance*. Consult the description of pancreatic islet cells (Chap. 22), lymphocytes (Chap. 11), and erythroblasts (Chap. 12) for patterns of chromidial substance.

Ribosomes are flattened, spheroidal, complex cytoplasmic particles measuring approximately 150 × 250 Å that synthesize protein (Figs. 1–38 to 1–41). They consist of RNA and protein. Their RNA is classed as rRNA, which accounts for 85% of the RNA of the cell. In addition to this form of RNA, there is mRNA and tRNA. The instruction for protein synthesis is encoded in DNA. This information is transcribed to mRNA, which is about 300 to 600 nm long, depending on the protein. Messenger RNA is produced in the nucleus, on a template of uncoiled DNA. It moves to the

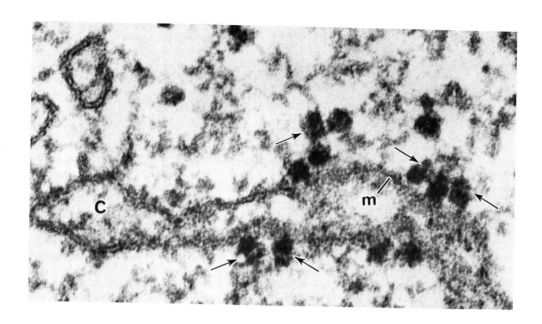

cytoplasm where it associates itself with ribosomes that lie along the mRNA like beads on a necklace. Ribosomes occurring singly in the cytoplasm are not active; only when they are linked by mRNA to form polyribosomes do they engage in protein synthesis. The ribosomes are the small machines that receive the amino acid constituents of protein, assemble them into peptide chains, and release these chains into the cytoplasm or into the lumen of the ER where they continue to aggregate to form protein. Each amino acid is brought to the ribosome by its distinctive tRNA, a low molecular-weight nucleic acid (see below) that may be produced in the nucleolar region of the nucleus (as is rRNA) and passes out of the nucleus into the cytoplasm. In protein synthesis, a ribosome moves along mRNA and reads the genetic message that has been transcribed from DNA. As the ribosome translates the message, it binds on its surface the particular activated amino acyl-tRNA specified by the codon being read and synthesizes the peptide linkage of this amino acid to the earlier ones.

The peptide chain grows larger as the ribosome moves along the mRNA, and as the ribosomes slides off the mRNA, it releases the peptide chain. As one ribosome slides off one end of the mRNA, another slides onto the other end and several ribosomes "read" or translate the mRNA at any time. The ribosomes lie on the mRNA approximately 340 Å apart (Fig. 1–40). For a poly-

1–38 Ribosomes, hepatocyte, of a guinea pig.
Ribosomes at high magnification show a larger and smaller component. When associated with the ER, the larger component lies upon the membrane. In this field a single cisterna (c) of the ER is present. The arrows indicate the position and orientation of the partitions separating the large from the small subunits of the ribosomes. Note that these partitions lie generally parallel to the surface of the membranes (m). This specimen was fixed in osmium tetroxide, embedded, sectioned, and stained with uranyl acetate. × 270,000. (From the work of D. Sabatini, Y. Toshiro, and G. E. Palade.)

peptide chain of hemoglobin 150 amino acids long, 60 to 90 sec are required for the ribosome to run the length of mRNA.

The ribosome is composed of two unequal subunits, one large and the other small (Fig. 1–42). Both are highly organized macromolecular assemblies consisting of one or more RNA molecules and numerous different proteins. In humans, as in most eukaryotes, the smaller subunit has a molecular weight of 1.5×10^6 and is composed of a single molecule of RNA with a sedimentation constant of 18S and approximately 30 different, rather small proteins (10,000 to 40,000 daltons). The small subunit functions to bind the mRNA to the ribosome and forms part of the tRNA binding site as the codon is being read by the anticodon of the tRNA. The larger subunit with a molecular weight of 3.0 ×

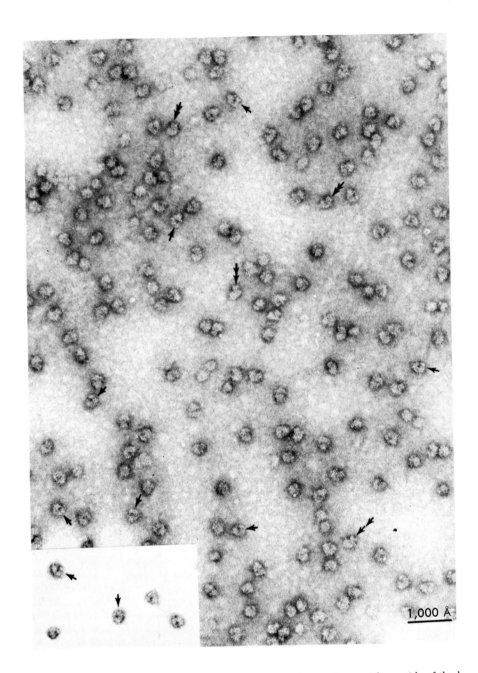

1–39 Ribosomes of a guinea pig. General view of a field of native monomeric ribosomes. Several image types are predominant. Frontal images **(arrows)** have an elongated small subunit profile and a dense spot toward the side of the separation between subunits. All frontal images in the field have this spot to the left of the observer if the particle image is oriented with the elongated small subunit horizontally and toward the top. In lateral images **(double arrows)** the small subunit produces a small rounded or rectangular profile toward one side of the large subunit profile. The inset shows images of monomeric ribosomes, reconstituted in vitro from the isolated large and small subunits. This preparation was made from ribosomes isolated by differential centrifugation of disrupted cells. The ribosomes were then floated on a membrane-covered electron-microscopic grid, dried, and negatively stained with phosphotungstic acid. × 125,000. (From the work of D. Sabatini, Y. Nonomura, and G. Blobel.)

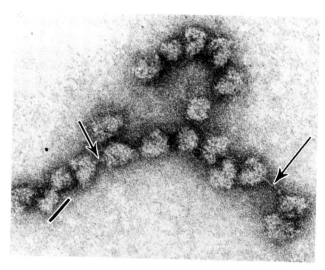

1–40 Ribosomes of a guinea pig. Here a strand of messenger RNA **(arrows)** links ribosomes into a polyribosomal unit. The mRNA runs between the small and large subunits. × 240,000. (From the work of D. Sabatini, Y. Nonomura, and G. Blobel.)

◁

1–41 An electron micrograph of *E. coli* small ribosomal subunits reacted with antibodies directed against ribosomal protein S14. The antibodies attach at only a single region in the upper one-third of the subunit, and are indicated by arrows. The centrally located pairs of subunits are connected by single IgG molecules, while the pair of subunits on the left is connected by two different IgG molecules, both attached to the same region of the subunit surface. (From the work of J. Lake, M. Pendergast, L. Kahan, and M. Nomura.)

◁

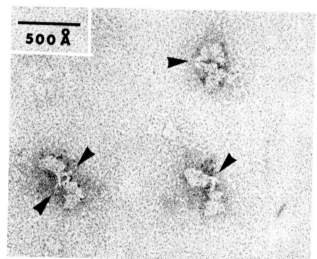

1–42 Model of the *E. coli* ribosome showing the relationship of the large and the small subunits. The view on the left shows the interface between the small subunit **(light)** and the large subunit **(dark)**. This interface is an important region where the tRNAs, the mRNA, and factors involved in protein synthesis are located. In the view at the right showing the ribosome viewed from above, a prominent feature of the large subunit is the elongated projection extending from the subunit. At present, the function of this feature of the large subunit is not well understood. (From the work of J. Lake.) ▽

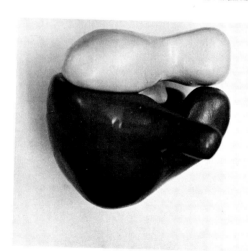

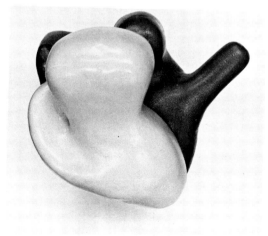

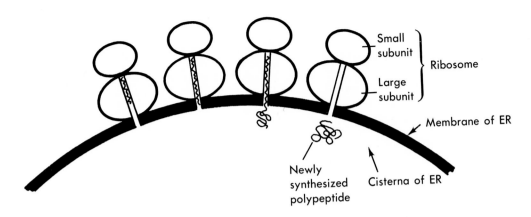

1–43 Model of the relationship between ribosomes and ER membrane. Attachment by the large subunits and orientation of the partition separating the two ribosomal subunits are strongly suggested by the evidence presented. The central channel in the large subunit and the discontinuity in the subjacent ER membrane are tentative features of the model, included only to indicate a possible pathway for the release of the newly synthesized protein in the cisternal space. (From the work of D. Sabatini and G. Blobel.)

10^6 has a sedimentation constant of 60S and contains two RNA molecules (5S and 28S) and probably a third (5.8S). The approximately 40 different proteins contained in the large subunit are on the average slightly larger than those in the small subunit. The large subunit functions in protein synthesis by forming part of the tRNA binding sites, catalyzing peptidyl transfer, and holding the growing polypeptide chain. Ribosomes bound to the rough ER are attached through the large subunit (Fig. 1–43). In bacteria, and prokaryotes in general, ribosomes (70S) and their subunits (30S and 50S) are somewhat smaller. Bacterial ribosomes differ from eukaryotic ribosomes in their responses to antibiotics affecting protein synthesis. Some antibiotics, such as puromycin, inhibit protein synthesis on both prokaryotic and eukaryotic ribosomes; others, such as cycloheximide, affect only eukaryotic ribosomes. (The ribosomes found in the mitochondria of eukaryotes differ from others in eukaryotic cytoplasm by resembling bacterial ribosomes in their responses to antibiotics.) Eukaryotic and prokaryotic ribosomes have important similarities despite their differences. The sequence of events that occur during the protein synthesis cycle is the same in both eukaryotic and prokaryotic ribosomes, and although there

are differences in size, these ribosomes greatly resemble each other in gross morphology as observed in the electron microscope.

The three-dimensional locations of specific ribosomal proteins are being mapped by using antibodies directed against individual ribosomal proteins (Figs. 1–41 and 1–44).

Polyribosomes may lie free in the cytoplasm, releasing their peptide chains into the cytoplasm for further combination and complexing. This is how hemoglobin is synthesized. Where the ribosomes attach to the outer surface of ER, the larger unit maintains attachment. The mRNA and the ER membranes are parallel. Furthermore, there may be a canal running through the larger ribosomal component at right angles to the mRNA and the ER. This canal has been postulated to run through the membranous wall of the ER, with the result that the amino acids, in peptide linkage, are "spun out" by the ribosomes directly into the lumen of the ER (Fig. 1–43). This peptide is "led" across the wall of the ER into its lumen by a signal peptide produced by the large ribosomal subunit and linked to the amino terminal of the peptide. See Chap. 21 for further discussion of secretion.

Ribosomes have a short life span. When protein synthesis ceases, they are quickly metabolized and disappear.

Golgi Complex. The Golgi apparatus or complex is a membranous system of cisternae and vesicles, usually located in or around the cytocentrum. It is involved in intracellular transport of secretory proteins, membrane proteins, and proteins that remain membrane-bounded within the cell, in distinction to proteins such as hemoglobin and keratin that lie free in the cytoplasm.

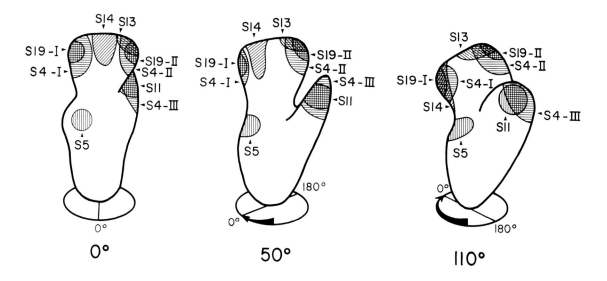

0°   50°   110°

The Golgi complex has a characteristic appearance by light microscopy. It may be a small compact structure; it may be a cluster of small structures (termed dictyosomes in earlier literature); or it may be a large netlike structure, the *internal reticular apparatus* as initially defined by C. Golgi in nerve cells. The Golgi complex is often juxtanuclear and may partially enclose the centrioles. Its size fluctuates with cell type and secretory activity. It is well developed in secretory cells, for example, in the mucus-producing intestinal epithelial cells, in plasma cells, and cells of the pituitary gland. The Golgi complex has the capacity to reduce metal salts, such as salts of osmium and of silver (Figs. 1–4 and 1–45), and may therefore be stained with these compounds. Such staining methods were responsible for the discovery of the Golgi complex.

By electron microscopy, the Golgi complex consists of 3 to 15 large flat sacs or cisternae apposed to one another. They are relatively compressed at their centers and somewhat dilated peripherally. The sacs tend to be bowed, presenting a convex *proximal face* (toward the nucleus) and concave *distal face* (away from the nucleus (Figs 1–35 to 1–37, 21–9, and 22–8). These stacked cisternae thus form bowl-shaped structures, and the Golgi complex as a whole looks like a stack of shallow bowls with the concavity directed away from the nucleus. The cisternae may communicate with one another by slender channels at places along their contiguous surfaces. The proximal membranes (those near the nucleus) are thinner than the distal membranes.

1–44 A diagrammatic representation of three views of the *E. coli* smaller ribosomal subunit illustrating the locations of some of the ribosomal proteins. The views from left to right represent rotations of the subunit about its long axis of 0°, 50°, and 110°, respectively. The cleft formed between the vertically oriented platform and the upper one-third of the subunit is best seen in the +50° view. The platform itself is attached to the lower two-thirds of the subunit. The vertical axis of the subunit is approximately 250 Å long. Many of the proteins are located at only a single region of the subunit but some, such as S4 and S19, are elongated and extend through the subunit. Three different regions of S4 are exposed and indicate that this protein must be at least 170 Å long. Protein S4 is required for the proper self-assembly of subunits and its extended nature may be related to its role in subunit assembly. (From the work of J. Lake, M. Nomura, and L. Kahan.)

branes (facing out toward the bulk of the cytoplasm), which are more like those of plasmalemma. At the edge of the lamellated sacs, near their expanded peripheries, vesicles 400 to 800 Å in diameter are typically present. Similar vesicles may also be abundant at the distal face. The vesicles vary in size and probably fuse to form larger vesicles. They, like the lateral vesicles, may contain a dense material. The proximal face is relatively free of vesicles and has been termed the *forming face* (also known as the *cis* face). The distal face, which is typically engaged in granule formation, has been termed the *maturation face* (also known as the *trans* face) (Figs. 1–46 to 1–49).

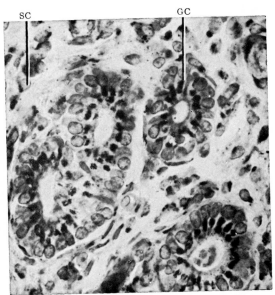

1–45 Golgi material in cells of guinea pig uterus.
The Golgi material was blackened with silver by the method of Da Fano. Large quantities of it lie above the nuclei of the glandular cells **(GC)**; smaller amounts lie next to the nuclei of the stromal cells **(SC)**. × 500.

◁

1–46 Human myelocyte. In this developing blood cell (see Chap. 11), the nucleus is lobed. Nuclear pores **(np)** are present. The cytoplasm contains granules, vesicles, rough and smooth ER, mitochondria, and free ribosomes. A Golgi apparatus is present, partially surrounding a centriole. × 26,000. (From the work of G. A. Ackerman.) ▽

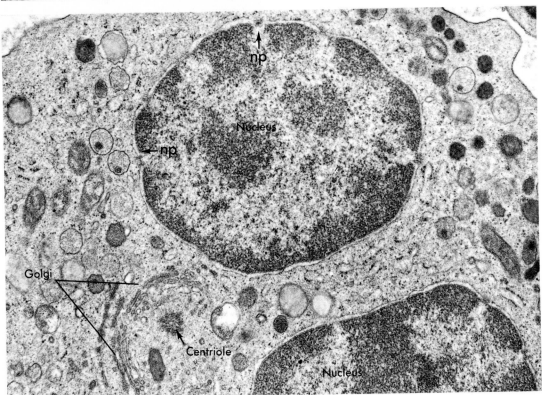

Proteins destined to be secreted or stored in lysosomes or other membrane-bounded granules are synthesized by polysomes attached to the outer surface of ER. Newly synthesized proteins collect within the lumen of the rough ER and move into contiguous ER free of ribosomes.

These elements are called "transitional elements" because they lie between the rough ER and the Golgi complex. It is thought that they bud off as *transport vesicles*, which carry quanta of ER content to the Golgi complex. The Golgi complex not only serves as a way station for pro-

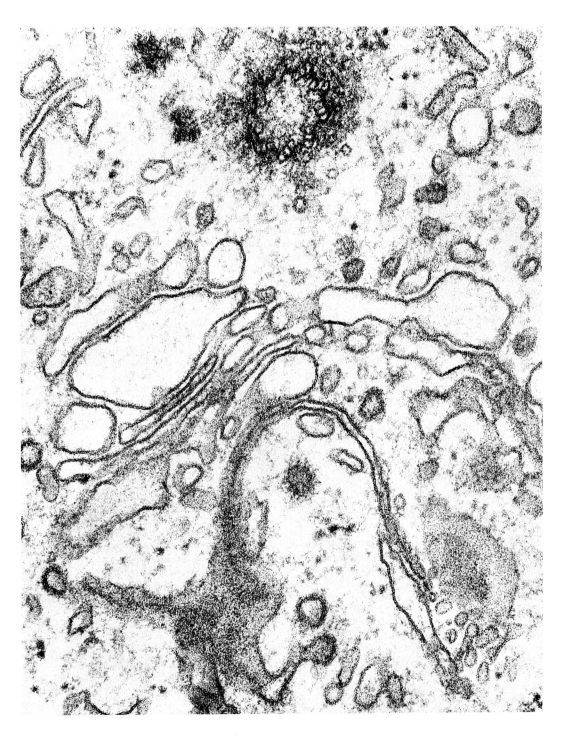

tein intracellular transport, but several covalent modifications of proteins may occur as they pass through it. For example, a portion of the carbo-hydrate moiety of many glycoproteins is added in the Golgi complex (e.g., immunoglobulins and pancreatic enzymes). The high concentration of

1–47 Golgi complex. It is evident, in this field, that the Golgi membranes and vesicles are made of the trilaminar unit membrane. A centriole is also present. (From the work of E. D. Hay and J. P. Revel.)

the *glycosyl transferase* enzymes on the inner surface of Golgi membranes reflects this function.

There are several patterns of secretion. In "nonregulated" secretory cells (e.g., plasma cells and fibroblasts), secretion is continuous and is effected by small Golgi-derived secretory vesicles, perhaps 50 nm in diameter. In "regulated" secretory cells (e.g., pancreatic acinar cells), on the other hand, secretion is intermittent and depends on hormonal stimuli. In this case, the secretory granules accumulate in the apical cytoplasm and may become rather large, up to 1,500 nm in diameter. In such cells, the ability of the Golgi complex to concentrate secretory protein is especially evident. Distal to the stacked cisternae are "condensing vacuoles" of irregular shape. These organelles further concentrate their content to become zymogen or storage granules. Upon hormonally triggered secretion, the granule membrane fuses with the plasma membrane. At the site of fusion the membranes break down and the contents of the secretory granule are released from the cell. See Figs. 21–9, 21–12, 21–13, and 22–8.

The Golgi complex also functions in lipoprotein synthesis. Lipids enter the Golgi cisternae from smooth ER and in the Golgi apparatus they are complexed to protein produced in rough ER. Membrane-bounded lipoprotein granules are then released from the Golgi (Figs. 1–48 and 1–49).

A major technique for delineating the sequence of protein intracellular transport is *pulse-chase electron-microscopic autoradiography*. With this method, a radioactive metabolite, such as an amino acid or sugar that will be incorporated into the macromolecular product undergoing synthesis, is injected rapidly in a single dose into an experimental animal. As a result, a short, sharply delineated "pulse" of radioactively labeled metabolite enters the synthetic process and is carried through it. By sampling tissue at appropriate times for autoradiography, the "pulse labeled" radioactive macromolecules (e.g., proteins) can be visualized at their site of synthesis and followed during transport to the site of discharge.

The Golgi complex has been isolated by differential centrifugation and has been partially characterized chemically. It consists of approximately equal parts of lipid and protein and tends to be unusually rich in nucleoside diphosphatases. These phosphatases serve as cytochemical and biochemical markers for Golgi membranes. After a short time an identical but now radioactive compound is digested rapidly. This "chases" the radioactive amino acid, diluting it out.

Smooth Vesicles and Coated Vesicles. The cytoplasm contains several kinds of membrane-bounded vesicles that enclose diverse materials and carry them from place to place within the cytoplasm and to and from the cell surfaces. These vesicles include phagosomes, macropinosomes, micropinosomes, condensing vesicles, transport vesicles and secretory vesicles. Lysosomes, peroxisomes, and microbodies may also be included and are discussed in the next section. The movement and destination of vesicles within the cell may be rather specific. For example, vesicles originating at the cell surface may selectively take in immunoglobulin, transport it across the cell using well-defined cytoplasmic streams, and release it at the lateral or basal surfaces of the cell. In addition, protein, partially synthesized in the ER, may be delivered for further synthesis to the Golgi complex by a system of transport vesicles that bud off the ER, travel to the Golgi sacs, and fuse with them.

The cytoplasm of virtually every cell contains membrane-bounded vesicles originating at the cell surface from invaginations of plasma membrane that pinch off. Because such vesicles carry material from outside into the cell, the process that results in their formation has been called *endocytosis*. In the reverse process, *exocytosis*, intracellular material is conveyed within vesicles to the cell surface where the membrane of the vesicle fuses with the plasma membrane and then breaks down, releasing the material to the extracellular compartment. In the process, the vesicle disappears and its membrane is translocated into the plasma membrane.

In endocytosis, the endocytotic vesicles may contain particulate material, such as bacteria or cell fragments. These vesicles are called *phagocytic* vesicles or *phagosomes*. Phagosomes typically flow toward lysosomes and fuse with them, forming *phagolysosomes, heterolysosomes,* or *secondary lysosomes* (Chap. 4). The hydrolytic enzymes of the lysosomes mix and digest the particulate material of the phagosome, and the resulting low molecular-weight compounds diffuse from the phagolysome into the hyaloplasm. Phagocytic vesicles tend to be large, visible by light microscopy. Certain cell types such as macrophages (Chap. 4) and leukocytes (Chap. 11) are

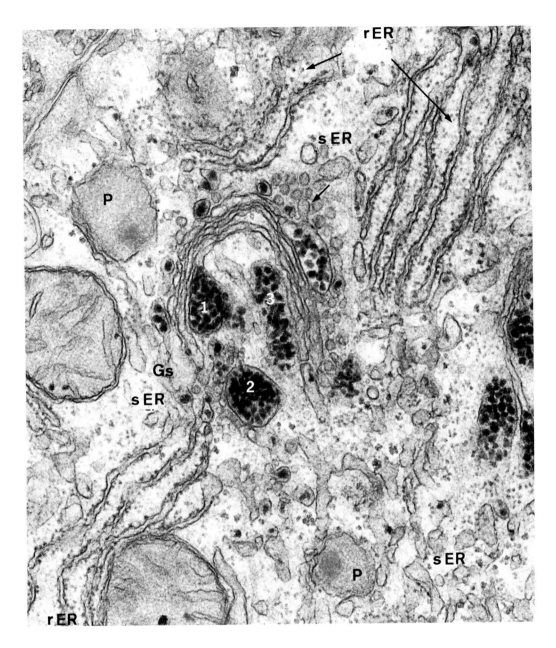

1–48 Golgi complex from a rat hepatocyte. The complex lies near the center of this field. The forming face of the Golgi, where the development of secretory product is initiated, is at the convex side of the apparatus, with extensions from the smooth ER network **(sER)** piling up from below and above, along the curved structure. This smooth ER is probably produced by the rough ER **(rER)** that surrounds the Golgi. The smooth ER may be continuous with the Golgi saccules or may break up into transport vesicles that move to the Golgi and fuse with it. A cluster of small vesicles, on top of the Golgi structure and next to a concentrating or secretory vesicle, is interpreted as representing cross sections of tubular, smooth ER extensions, with one of them **(arrow)** connecting with the concentrating vesicle. At the concave or maturing face of the Golgi three concentrating or secretory vesicles (1 to 3) are present. Each contains many small granules. At P, there are two peroxisomes (see text). Compare this process of lipoprotein granule formation with that of the formation of granules within leukocytes, described in Chap. 11. × 56,500. (From Claude, A. 1970. J. Cell Biol. 47:745.)

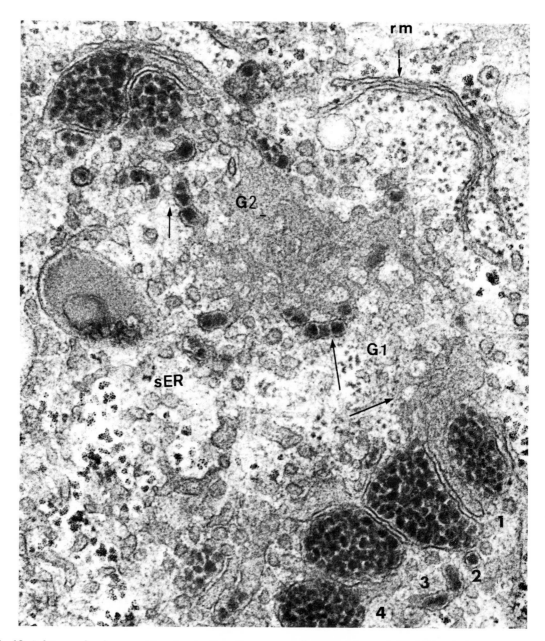

1–49 Golgi complex from a rat hepatocyte. Smooth-surfaced membranes **(rm)** similar to those in Fig. 1–48 are cut in cross section. As they are traced to the right, they are continuous with rough ER. At G2 Golgi membranes at the forming surface are cut in a plane parallel to their surface. These membranes are fenestrated and, in all probability, are formed by coalescence of smooth ER (**sER**) tubules **(arrows)** carrying rows of dense lipoprotein granules. Four large concentrating or secretory vesicles are present (numbered 1 to 4). These would develop from the maturing face of the Golgi, corresponding to the concave portion in Fig. 1–48. × 67,800. (From Claude, A. 1970. J. Cell Biol. 47:745.)

quite proficient or "professional" phagocytes. Other cell types, however, can be phagocytic, such as the endothelium of the vascular sinuses of bone marrow and spleen (Chap. 13), and phagocytosis must be regarded as a general property of cells.

Another class of endocytotic vesicles may contain fluids imbibed from the extracellular fluid at the cell surface. These are *pinocytotic vesicles* or *pinosomes* (*pino*, drinking). Pinosomes may bring fluid in unselectively or they may depend on receptors to bring material into the cell selectively, which is called *receptor mediated pinocytosis*. A type of pinosome is greater than 0.2 μm in diameter. This type is large enough to be visible by light microscopy, and in fact, was first described more than 50 years ago in living cells in tissue culture. These *macropinosomes* characteristically move in cytoplasmic streams toward the center of the cell, becoming smaller and denser as they travel, their contents presumably becoming more concentrated owing to loss of water. Macropinosomes, like phagosomes, may fuse with lysosomes.

A variety of pinocytosis undertaken by virtually every cell of the body, *micropinocytosis*, is distinguished by vesicles visible only by electron microscopy (70 to 100 nm in diameter).

The endocytic vesicular systems function to bring material into a cell, to segregate that material, and to transport it to selective destinations within the cell. In endothelium, for example, vesicles originate at the luminal surface, cross the cell and release their contents at the basal surface. Vesicles may also move in the opposite direction. This type of transit, *transcytosis*, is discussed more fully in Chap. 9. In the epithelial cells lining the gut, materials are taken up at the luminal or apical surface and transported to the lateral cell surface by vesicles and discharged into the intercellular space (Chap. 19). In addition to the discharge of immunoglobulin, the many instances of secretion are examples of exocytosis. Secretory vesicles typically derive from the Golgi complex as *condensing* or *storage vesicles*, and become secretory vesicles, which collect in the apical or secretory pole of the cell. They then move to the cell surface, fuse with the plasma membrane, open to the extracellular space, and discharge their secretion (Figs. 21–9, 21–12, 21–13, and 22–8). Secretion is discussed throughout this book, but major presentations are in the chapters on epithelium (Chap. 3), salivary glands (Chap. 7), mammary glands (Chap. 26), pancreas (Chaps. 21 and 22), and hypophysis

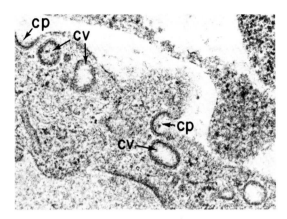

1–50 Endothelium, mouse bone marrow. Coated pits **(cp)** and coated vesicles **(cv)** are present.
× 25,000. See also Figs. 3–15, and 8–36.

(Chap. 29), as well as in the earlier sections of this chapter on the endoplasmic reticulum (page 41) and the Golgi complex (page 49).

Cytoplasmic vesicles can be smooth or coated. Smooth vesicles are bounded by membrane similar to the plasma membrane. Coated vesicles are coated on their outside (cytoplasmic) surface by a protein, *clathrin*, of molecular weight 180,000. Clathrin invests the vesicle and appears in sections as radiating spikes, each about 15 nm long and about 5 nm apart, which gives the vesicle a fuzzy look. On surface view the clathrin forms a lattice of hexagons, the side of the polygons being the projections or spikes seen in sections. Coated pinosomes originate as invaginations from coated invaginations of the cell surface, *coated pits* (Figs. 1–50 and 1–51).

Coated and smooth vesicles have similar and complementary functions. Any type of vesicle may be smooth, but coated vesicles are almost always of small diameter (70–10 nm) and only in a few instances are larger. The nature and special functions of coated vesicles are being sorted out. Coated endocytotic vesicles transport immunoglobulin across the placenta from mother to fetus, thereby conferring passive immunity on the fetus. Coated vesicles also transport yolk proteins into the cytoplasm of oocytes. As the yolk-containing coated vesicles move centrally, they lose their clathrin coat and fuse with other yolk-containing vesicles to form rather large yolk vesicles. They, in turn, fuse with lysosomes, and the yolk is digested into low molecular-weight nutrients that diffuse out of the lysosome-yolk vesicle to be metabolized by the oocyte. Casein, as noted above, is carried in exocytotic coated ves-

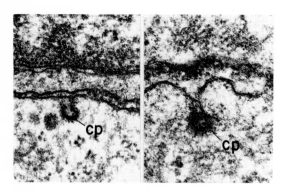

1–51 Leukocytes, mouse bone marrow. Varieties of coated pit **(cp)**. left panel × 42,000, right × 70,000. See also Figs. 3–15 and 8–36. Courtesy Joyce S. Knoll

icles that may be rather large. The liver produces a very low density lipoprotein (VLDL) which it releases to the blood through exocytotic coated vesicles. VLDL is a component of blood serum that controls the dispersment of serum lipids, a factor important in the development of athero-sclerosis in the walls of the blood vessels. The clathrin coat may play a distinctive role in recy-cling exocytic membrane. In the synaptic bulb at the end of certain nerves, a number of synaptic vesicles are present. These vesicles are bounded by smooth membrane and contain neurotrans-mitter substances. When the nerve is stimulated the synaptic vesicles move to the plasma mem-brane at the synapse, fuse with it, and discharge their contents. After discharge, the membrane of the synaptic vesicle is intercalated into the plasma membrane. It appears that this interca-lated membrane may be translocated a short dis-tance away from the synapse and then recycled into the cell where it again forms synaptic vesi-cles. Clathrin seems to play an essential role in this recycling by moving beneath the translo-cated synaptic membrane intercalated in the plasma membrane and inducing it to invaginate and pinch off in the cytoplasm as a coated vesi-cle. When the clathrin first moves beneath the plasma membrane, its latticework is entirely hexagonal. Then pentagons appear in the lattice, and with this change the clathrin assumes a cur-vilinear form, bringing in the membrane as an in-vaginated coated pit that proceeds to form a coated vesicle. The coated vesicle next loses its clathrin coat and becomes, once again, a smooth synaptic vesicle. Its clathrin coat appears to pre-vent a coated vesicle from fusing with other membranous structures. When material is endo-cytized by a coated vesicle, therefore, that mate-

rial remains within that vesicle as long as it re-mains coated. When the coat drops away, the membrane of the vesicle may fuse with similar vesicles forming larger vesicles, with lysosomes forming heterolysosomes, with plasma mem-brane resulting in exocytosis, or with such other membranous structures as the Golgi complex to facilitate transport and synthesis.

Lysosomes, Peroxisomes and Multivesicular Bodies. Lysosomes are membrane-bounded cy-toplasmic vesicles containing 50 or more hydro-lytic enzymes, virtually all of which are glyco-proteins active at acid pH (Figs. 1–52 and 1–53). Lysosomes may become quite large but in their primary state usually measure 50 to 80 Å in di-ameter. They may be isolated by differential cen-trifugation of disrupted cells, where they lie cen-tripetal to mitochondria. They may be identified

1–52 Lysosomes of the epithelioid cell of chicken. In this cell, derived from a macrophage, the cytoplasm is filled with lysosomes. They crowd out the centrosome. From the centriole, rays of gelated cytoplasm free of organelles radiate. At one place a small pocket of Golgi membranes is present. (From Sutton, J., and Weiss, L. 1966. J. Cell Biol. 28:303.)

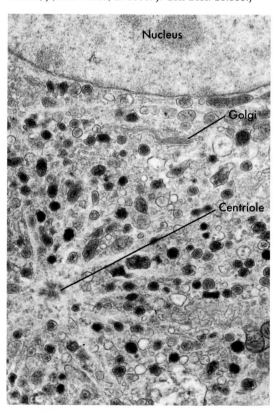

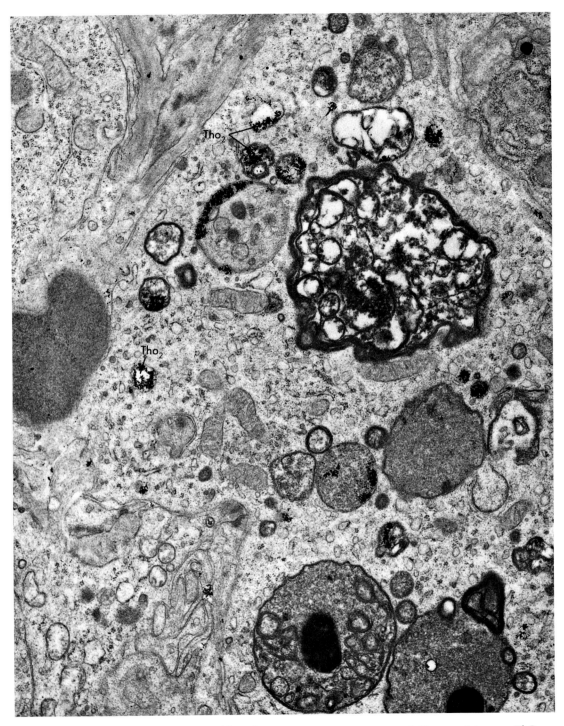

1–53 Lysosomes of a macrophage from a rabbit. This animal was given thorium dioxide (ThO$_2$), an electron-dense heavy metal, shortly before this cell was fixed. Heterolysosomes, considerably different in appearance, are present. Many contain some ThO$_2$. × 40,000. (From Weiss, L. 1964. Bull. Hopkins Hosp. 115:99.)

Table 1–3 Major Enzymatic Activities
of Lysosomes

Acid phosphatase
lipase and esterase
phospholipases
ribo- and deoxyribo-nucleases
galactos- and glucos-aminidases
fuco- and gluco-sidases
glucuronidase and hyaluronidase
aryl- and chondro-sulfatases
cathepsins and other peptidases

cytochemically by reactions for acid phosphatase, a commonly used marker, or by reactions for other enzymes they contain. In such cytochemical preparations lysosomes appear as punctate structures by light microscopy. In electron micrographs they are oval or round and contain variably dense granular material. Most cells contain lysosomes. Hepatocytes and macrophages, cell types rich in lysosomes, contain approximately 200. Their large complement of hydrolytic enzymes (Table 1–3) endows lysosomes with the capacity to hydrolyze or digest a great many substrates. The activity of these enzymes is controlled by their bounding membrane. This membrane selectively admits substrates into the lysosome and protects the cells against indiscriminate digestion by its own lysosomal enzymes.

The digestive capacities of lysosomes have been adapted to the functions of disparate cell types. In phagocytic cells, for example, lysosomes digest microbes or other phagosomal contents brought into the cell (heterophagy). In almost any cell of the body, moreover, organelles that have become worn out or exhausted and need to be replaced may be incorporated into lysosomes and digested (autophagy). Furthermore, secretory substances synthesized by endocrine cells may be digested by lysosomal enzymes and the level of secretion thereby regulated (crinophagy). In fact, lysosomes may participate in the destruction and recycling of many cell components, such as receptors and membrane.

The life cycle of lysosomes is complex and accounts for their marked structural heterogeneity (polymorphism). The primary lysosome or storage body is produced at the Golgi complex. Its genesis parallels that of secretory granules (Chaps. 3 and 21) in that its protein is synthesized in rough ER, is conveyed to the Golgi complex by transport vesicles, and in the Golgi complex it is cross-linked and aggregated, and

carbohydrate is added (see preceding section on Golgi Complex). Novikoff and his colleagues believe that lysosomes may also be produced in Golgi-associated ER, bypassing the Golgi complex proper, and they have coined the acronym "GERL complex" to encompass these cooperating structures. Primary lysosomes move to phagosomes and pinosomes and fuse with them to form secondary lysosomes, heterolysosomes, heterophagosomes, or heteropinosomes (Fig. 1–53), as described in the preceding section on smooth and coated vesicles. After fusion, the lysosomal enzymes mix with and digest the contents of the pinosomes or phagosomes. The low molecular-weight digestion products diffuse out of the lysosome into the surrounding cytoplasm where they are metabolized. Heterolysosomes may be long-lived and new endocytized material added over time. Heterolysosomes, moreover, may fuse with one another and form rather large, irregular complexes. Lysosomes finally reach a state in which the material they contain is not further degradable and their enzymatic capacity declines. They become residual bodies or telolysosomes. They may contain pigments, myelin bodies, crystals, lipids, and assorted materials. Residual bodies may be expelled from macrophages and from invertebrate cells, as amebocytes (exocytosis). Alternatively, they may accumulate in the cytoplasm as indices of "wear and tear" of aging, as exemplified by lipofuscin granules. Residual bodies, as expected, are notable in long-lived metabolically active cells, such as nerve cells and muscle cells.

Another group of secondary lysosomes consists of autophagocytic vacuoles or cytolysosomes. These vacuoles are heterolysosomes that contain some organelles of the cell such as mitochondria and ribosomes. They may originate from segments of smooth ER that curve around some cytoplasm and fuse to enclose it in a vacuole. These vacuoles may then fuse with primary lysosomes just as phagosomes do. Another mechanism accounting for their origin may be the incorporation of some cytoplasm directly into a lysosome. The formation of autophagosomes is a mechanism of "internal policing" of a cell that removes damaged or senescent cell substance. Autophagocytic vacuoles increase in starvation and aging and after tissue injury. They participate in the normal turnover of cell organelles by destroying the aged ones. Thus, mitochondria have a half-life of only 10 days in rat hepatocytes. They are removed by autophagy. Autophagocytic vacuoles form residual bodies.

Lysosomes have other metabolic functions. They may function in the degradation of glycogen. Evidence for this role comes from a type of glycogen storage disease, an illness of children characterized by a marked increase in liver size (hepatomegaly) due to the accumulation of glycogen. In this disease, lysosomes are deficient in *glycosidase*, the enzyme responsible for glycogen breakdown. Lysosomes function to regulate hormone production by *crinophagy*. The thyroid hormone *thyroxin* is produced as a conjugate of globulin. Its separation or hydrolysis from globulin seems to depend on incorporation of the thyroglobulin into lysosomes and hydrolysis by their hydrolytic enzymes. The destruction of excess mammotrophic hormone in the secretory cells of the pituitary gland and of parathyroid hormone in the secretory cells of the parathyroid gland is accomplished by autophagy of secretory granules (crinography).

Unlike secretory granules, lysosomes are typically not released but remain within the cytoplasm. Their genesis is parallel to that of secretory granules, however. In their synthesis in rough ER and Golgi complex, lysosomal enzymes retain phosphorylated mannose residues which interact with membrane receptors in the Golgi complex to induce the formation of membrane-bounded lysosomes which remain within the cytoplasm indefinitely (See discussion in Chapter 21). In the case of secretory proteins, on the other hand, the phosphorylated mannose residues are cleaved off in the ER or Golgi, leading to the formation of membrane-bounded secretory granules which do not remain within the cytoplasm but move to the cell surface and are secreted. In some instances, however, lysosomes may be secreted. Thus, transformed platelets plugging a tear in a blood vessel secrete lysosomes (lambda granules) and lysosome-related vesicles (alpha granules), which intensify blood coagulation. Osteoclasts lying on bone that is undergoing lysis seal off an area by sheetlike cytoplasmic processes whose edges attach to the bone. They then secrete their bone-dissolving lysosomal enzymes into this sealed pouch and thereby remove bone with great precision. A number of lysosome-associated diseases have been identified. The lysosomal membrane in leukocytes in Chediak-Higashi disease is abnormally resistant to fusion with phagosomes. Phagocytized bacteria are therefore not exposed to the lysosome's lytic enzymes; the cell's capacity to destroy bacteria is impaired, and affected individuals die of infection. More than 20 *storage diseases* due to deficient activity of lysosomal enzymes have been identified. In *Hurler's syndrome* connective tissue matrix accumulates because lysosomes fail to degrade acid mucopolysaccharides. The enlarged spleen (splenomegaly) and other pathology of *Gaucher's disease* seem to be due to a defect in lysosomal β-glucosidase. In glycogen-storage disease type II, α-glycosidase is absent from lysosomes so that hepatocytes (and the whole liver) become enlarged by stored glycogen-filled vesicles that cannot be metabolized. A contrasting group of lysosomal diseases is due to intracellular breakup of lysosomes. In gout, as a result of genetically induced high levels of uric acid in the body fluids, urate crystals form in the synovial cavities and other connective tissue spaces. Leukocytes engulf these crystals. As the crystals become incorporated into secondary lysosomes they disrupt the lysosomes, loosing the hydrolytic enzymes. The leukocytes are destroyed and the enzymes, released to the tissue, induce inflammation characteristic of gouty arthritis. This sequence may occur in asbestos intoxication, in experimentally induced methylcellulose disease, and in other instances in which lysosomes are confronted with irritating materials that they are unable to degrade.

Peroxisomes, or *microbodies of Rouiller* are involved in H_2O_2 metabolism. They are membrane-bounded organelles, somewhat larger than primary lysosomes (Fig. 1–48) and may be continuous with tubules of smooth ER. Peroxisomes are relatively numerous in hepatocytes (Chap. 20), in renal tubular cells (Chap. 24), and in macrophages. They contain flavin enzymes, such as *urate oxidase* and D-*amino acid oxidase*, which produce H_2O_2 by using molecular oxygen as an oxidizing agent. Peroxisomes have a variegated granular internum and, in the hepatocyte and some other cell types, contain a crystalline component that represents urate oxidase. However, H_2O_2, although necessary in a number of cellular reactions and capable of killing microorganisms, is tolerated in only low concentration by cells. In a sequential action to their generation of H_2O_2, peroxisomes, because they contain the enzyme *catalase*, convert H_2O_2 to water. Peroxisomes are also associated with α-keto acid formation and thereby participate in forming glucose from lipids and other noncarbohydrate precursors, a process termed *gluconeogenesis*.

Multivesicular bodies (MVB) are membrane-bounded vesicles 0.5 to 1.0 μm in diameter that contain a number of small vesicles with a diameter of 50 to 75 nm. They may be found in most

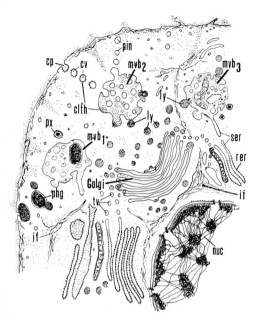

1–54 Multivesicular bodies **(mvb)** are prominent in this drawing. **mvb₁** contains a phagosome **(phg)**. **mvb₂** receives smooth **(pin)** and coated **(cv)** pinocytotic vesicles, the latter originating as coated pits **(cp)**. Plaques of clathrin **(clth)** lie on the surface of mvb₂ and mvb₃. Lysosomes fuse with mvb. **mvb₃**, containing mitochondria and rough ER **(rer)**, is autophagocytic. It is continuous with smooth ER **(ser)**. The Golgi complex is engaged in lysosome production and receives material from the ER in transport vesicles **(tv)**. Vimentin, a class of intermediate filament **(if)** surrounds the nucleus **(nuc)** and radiates in the cytoplasm.

cell types and are more numerous in cells rich in lysosomes. The membranes bounding MVB are usually smooth, but patches of their surface may be coated (see discussion of coated vesicles above). The MVB bounding membrane itself may invaginate and form some of the smaller vesicular structures and, like peroxisomes, may be continuous with short segments of smooth ER. Multivesicular bodies appear to represent reaction vats, receiving the contents of the endocytic vesicles and lysosomes that fuse with them. As a result, MVB possess the functions of a large heterolysosome. They may also receive the contents of secretory granules by crinophagy. They incorporate peroxisomes, partaking of their functions. Indeed, peroxisomes and other cellular structures may be autophagocytized in MVB (Fig. 1–54).

Microfilaments and Intermediate (100 Å) Filaments. There are two major groups of fine filaments in virtually every cell type. One group is approximately 50 Å in diameter (Fig. 1–55) and is made of *actin*. These filaments, called *microfilaments*, are contractile and are believed to underlie the locomotion of cells, the ruffling and invagination of cell membranes, contraction, and other aspects of contractility. They form the terminal web of epithelial cells and enter microvilli. They also form the contractile ring in dividing cells (Fig. 1–55). They are best developed in muscle cells (Chap. 7). A second group of fine intracellular filaments is stouter, approximately 90 to 120 Å in diameter. They represent a more diverse population of filaments than the microfilaments and are referred to as *intermediate filaments* or *100-Å filaments*. They possess mechanical functions in supporting or stiffening cells and in organizing intracellular organelles for coordinated activity.

Microfilaments are part of the actin–myosin system and become contractile by sliding over myosin filaments, as occurs in muscle cells. In nonmuscle cells actin, in the form of microfilaments, is visible by electron microscopy whereas myosin is not. Yet myosin is also present, as shown in a number of cell types by immunocytochemistry (Chap. 2). Thus, in the mitotic contractile ring in which actin microfilaments have been demonstrated by electron microscopy, the presence of myosin has been shown by fluorescence immunocytochemistry. It is likely that myosin is not visible in electron micrographs because it occurs in short segments representing oligomers, which aggregate into filaments only transiently or form filaments that our preparative methods fail to preserve. Furthermore, myosin is present in much lower concentration in most cells than actin. Its high concentration and layout in cells suggest that actin, in addition to its major contractile functions, has a cytoskeletal role. Actin can be detected by an excellent cytochemical test: its specific reaction with the S-1 subfraction of heavy meromyosin (HMM) (Fig. 1–55). The tissue is first extracted with glycerol to increase permeability and permit the penetrance of HMM. After irrigation with HMM, microfilaments become "decorated" with HMM, which gives them a characteristic fuzzy appearance resembling arrowheads. Actin may also be detected by more conventional immunocytochemical methods. Microfilaments are often concentrated at the surface of nonmuscle cells and, by high-resolution electron microscopy, appear to be attached to the cytoplasmic surface of the plasma membrane. Whether the microfilaments

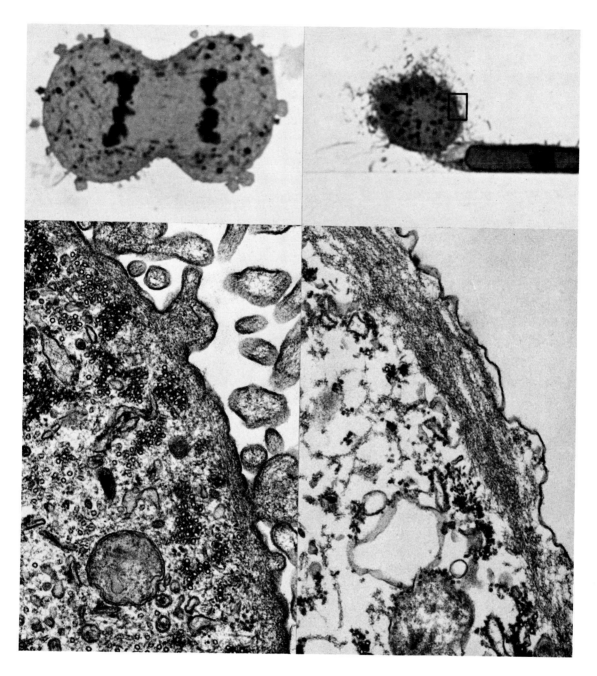

1–55 Cytoplasmic microfilaments in many cells are composed of actin. These micrographs illustrate this point for the contractile ring in dividing HeLa cells. The upper figures are light micrographs (× 2000) of 1 μm Epon sections of cells midway through cleavage: at the left parallel to the plane of the monolayer and at the right perpendicular to it at the level of the furrow constriction; hence the cell's circular profile. Electron micrographs below (× 50,000) illustrate portions of perpendicular sections, as indicated by the black rectangle. In standard preparations (lower left) the contractile ring appears as a layer of thin microfilament encircling the cell just beneath its membrane. After extraction in glycerol and irrigation with heavy meromyosin these same microfilaments appear "fuzzy" (lower right) in a way that is characteristic of actin filaments. Small circles in the electron micrographs are transverse profiles of microtubules of the mitotic apparatus. (From Shroeder, T. E. 1973. Proc. Natl. Acad. Sci. U.S.A. 20:1, 688.)

are directly linked to certain intrinsic proteins of the plasma membrane or connected through a set of anchoring proteins is not known. Microfilaments may be disaggregated and rendered functionless by the antibiotic *cytochalasin* B. (Refer to Chap. 7 for further discussion of actin and contractile filaments.)

Intermediate filaments may be divided into a number of classes, each with a distinctive cytoskeletal function. *Keratin filaments* occur in epithelial cells as *tonofilaments* and are particularly well developed in such stratified squamous epithelia as the epidermis (Chap. 17). They are tough filaments that serve to strengthen and stiffen cells, particularly at intercellular junctions, where they are closely associated with desmosomes (Chap. 3). When present in very high concentration, as in the keratinocytes of epidermis, keratin filaments laminate to form dense, strong, impermeable protective layers. Keratins are quite diverse, displaying somewhat different properties in different locations, as, for example, in the skin, snout, hoof, and feather. *Desmin filaments* hold myofibrils in place in muscle cells. In striated muscle they have distinctive locations on the myofibrils (Z, N, and M lines), and connect them to plasma membrane, mitochondria, and other elements of the cell. Desmin filaments are particularly abundant in smooth muscle cells, forming networks linking plaques of microfilaments to the cell surface. By these links desmin mechanically organizes muscle cells and coordinates the whole process of contraction. The protein *vimentin* forms intermediate filaments that enmesh the nucleus, in some cases forming a nuclear cap. They appear to control the location of the nucleus. Vimentin probably plays a role in such nuclear activities as mitosis and in maintaining nuclear–cytoplasmic passageways. *Neurofilaments* and *glial filaments* are, with microtubules, major structural elements in nervous tissue. These intermediate filaments are present in patterns and quantities distinctive to a given neural cell type. Their roles include maintaining the extraordinary asymmetry and cytoplasmic processes characteristic of neural cells (see Chap. 8). Spectrin is a tetramer found in erythrocytes where, as an intermediate filament, it forms a subplasmalemmal lattice anchored into the plasma membrane. As discussed in Chap. 11, spectrin protects the erythrocytic plasma membrane from shearing forces of flow, it stabilizes the intrinsic proteins of the cell membrane that penetrate its subplasmalemmal lattice, and it maintains the shape of the erythrocyte. Portions of the spectrin molecule occur as components of intermediate filaments in other cell types, such as macrophages and sea urchin epithelium, but the complete spectrin molecule appears restricted to erythrocytes. Spectrin, like other intermediate filaments, is conserved in evolution, being present in the red blood cells of many species with little variance in amino acids.

Microtubules. Microtubules are major structures in prokaryotic and eukaryotic cells. They function as a cytoskeleton and permit the asymmetry in shape necessary for cellular movement and differentiation. For example, the development of axons appears to depend on alignment of microtubules in the axonal processes. Dispersal of the microtubules prevents formation. Microtubules are important in intracellular transport. Particles and organelles such as mitochondria move along microtubules. The motility of cilia seems to depend on microtubules sliding upon one another.

Microtubules appear as hollow, nonbranching cylinders 210 to 240 Å in diameter and many micrometers long (Figs. 1–56 and 1–57; see also succeeding figures on centrioles and mitosis). Their dense wall is made of globular subunits 40 Å in diameter, arranged in helix with 13 subunits per turn. The center zone is lucent in most microtubules and is 160 Å in diameter. The major biochemical component of microtubules is the 110,000 dalton protein *heterodimer* tubulin, composed of α and β polypeptide subunits. Microtubules often appear in groups of 30 or 40 or more and may be connected by slender bridges.

Microtubules are the basis of such complex and well-defined structures as centrioles, cilia, and the achromatic mitotic apparatus. In addition, there are bands of microtubules in the axons of nerve cells (neurotubules), beneath the plasma membrane of many cylindrical or asymmetric cells, and within the endoplasm of such cells as macrophages. Microtubules may originate from a nucleating or initiating site in the cell. The centriole is a nucleating site for microtubular structures such as cilia and the achromatic apparatus. Most groups of microtubules are less stable than those in cilia and centrioles. They disappear with many fixatives, including osmium tetroxide, and on fixation in the cold. Microtubules are relatively easily dispersed by colchicine, vinblastine, or high hydrostatic pressure. When such dispersing factors are removed, the subunits quickly reassociate to reform microtubules.

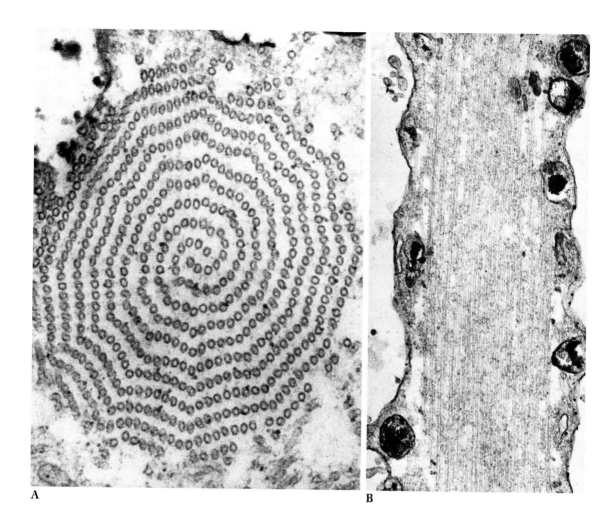

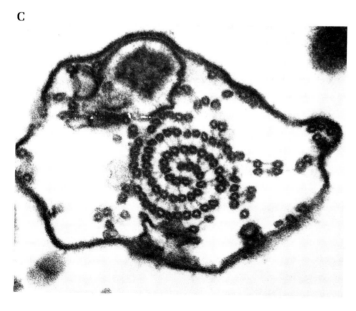

1–56 Microtubules in axoplasm of *Echinoshaerium*. Much correlative morphologic work in chemistry, physiology, and morphology has been done on invertebrates. **A.** Tranverse section of an axoneme at the base of an axopodium. There are 12 sections of microtubules in cross section. × 70,000. **B.** Longitudinal section of an axoneme. Peripheral to the parallel array of microtubules constituting the axoneme are dense granules that undergo saltations. × 40,000. **C.** Transverse section of an axoneme heavily stained with MnO_4 to emphasize the bridges that connect the microtubules. × 110,000. (From Tilney, L. G., and Porter, K. R. 1965. Protoplasma 60:317.

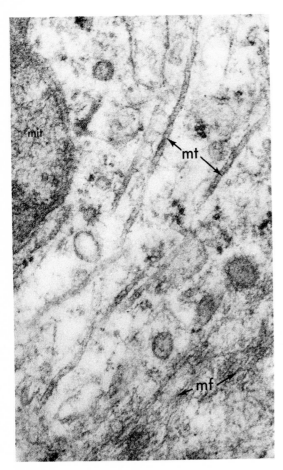

1–57 Microtubules of a human splenic reticular cell.
△   This field is from the peripheral cytoplasm and
contains sections of microtubules **(mt)**, microfilaments
(mf), and a mitochondrion **(mit)**. × 90,000. (From
Chen, L. T. and Weiss, L. 1972. Am. J. Anat. 134:425.)

Centrioles. Centrioles are cylinders, 0.25 to 2
μm in length and 0.1 to 0.2 μm in diameter,
whose walls are composed primarily of microtubules. Centrioles lie in the cytocentrum and may
be surrounded by microtubules radiating out into
the cytoplasm. Diploid metazoan cells contain
two centrioles. Multinucleate cells may contain
centrioles: in osteoclasts and foreign-body giant
cells, which may have 25 or more nuclei, the
central regions of the cells are composed of fused
cytocentra strewn with centrioles. Higher plants
lack centrioles.

Centrioles function in mitosis, in the genesis
of cilia, microtubules, mitochondria, and new
centrioles. Unlike other cytoplasmic structures,
centrioles are duplicated before mitosis.

By light microscopy, centrioles are minute
rods, well stained with a number of dyes, of
which iron hematoxylin is the most commonly
used (Fig. 1–4).

By electron microscopy, the centriolar wall is
made up of nine vanes or blades each consisting
of three fused microtubules (Figs. 1–58 to 1–60).
The nine blades are set next to one another, their
long axes parallel; the edge of one is slightly
shingled beneath the edge of its neighbor, curv-
ing around to form the cylinder that is the outer
wall of the centriole. In cross section, this array
resembles a pinwheel.

The fused microtubules making up each of the
blades extend the length of the centriole and lie
almost in a plane, with the result that the long

1–58 Centrioles of a Chinese hamster fibroblast. **A.**
▽   The centriole is cut in cross section (from an
interphase cell). **B.** The centriole is cut in longitudinal
section (from a metaphase cell). × 100,000. (From the
work of B. R. Brinkley.)

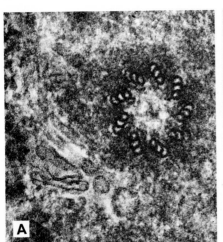

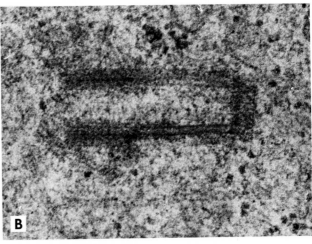

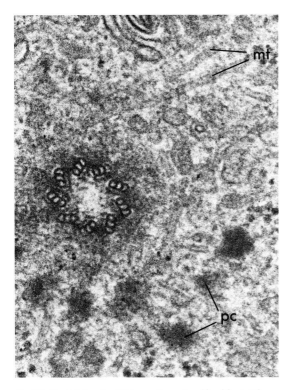

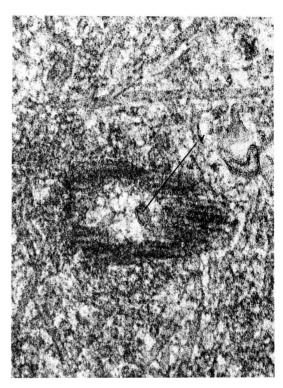

1–59 Centriole of a Chinese hamster fibroblast. The centriole is cut in cross section. Paracentriolar material **(pc)** is evident around the lower half of the centriole. Microtubules **(mt)** are also present, particularly in the upper half of the field. × 92,000. [From Brinkley, B. R., and Stubblefield, E., 1970. *In* D. M. Prescott, L. Goldstein, and E. McConkey (eds.), Advances in Cell Biology, vol. 1. New York: Appleton-Century-Crofts.]

1–60 Centriole of a melanoma cell. The centriole is cut in oblique section. It contains a small vesicle **(v).** The field surrounding the vesicle abounds in microtubules. × 120,000. (From the work of G. G. Maul.)

blades they form are slightly curved from side to side. In addition, each of the blades is subject to a slight twist about its long axis.

The principal structure within the lumen of the centriole is a 75-Å filament wound into a helix that curves against the inside surface of the wall, apparently held in place by small spurs. The lumen of the centriole may also contain a large clear vesicle. An end of the centriolar cylinder may show spokes radiating out from the wall.

Satellites are amorphous masses about 750 Å in diameter that lie close to the surface of centrioles, near an end; they may be aggregates of microtubular subunits.

A new centriole is assembled at an end of each extant centriole a few hours before DNA replication. It is oriented at right angles to the parent centriole and requires several hours to

form. A mature centriole is preceded by a *procentriole,* a cylinder 150 nm in diameter with nine single microtubules in its wall. These singlets develop into the triplets of the centriole. The procentrioles are themselves preceded by small, dense procentriolar precursor bodies, which are apparently transformed into procentrioles by the stimulation of "procentriole organizers," dense amorphous surrounding masses.

Centrioles induce microtubule formation. In mitosis they separate, move to opposite poles, and become foci for the development of the achromatic mitotic apparatus. Centrioles move beneath the cell surface and, as basal bodies, initiate the formation of cilia. Flagella are similarly related to centrioles. Basal bodies are structurally different from centrioles, primarily in possessing a basal plate that closes the end directed toward the cell membrane. The other end, directed toward the nucleus, is open and may display spokes. In spermatocytes one centriole may be associated with both the mitotic apparatus and the flagellum. Microtubular formations other

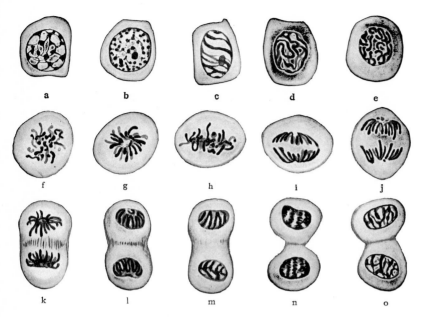

a   b   c   d   e

f   g   h   i   j

k   l   m   n   o

1-61 Mitosis. Epidermal cells of a mouse. These drawings are arranged in sequence from early prophase into telophase. **a** to **f**, prophase; **g** and **h**, metaphase; **i**, anaphase; **k** to **o**, telophase. Bouin fixation: iron–hematoxylin. (From the work of Ortiz-Picon.)

than those of the mitotic apparatus, cilia, and flagella may extend into the cytocentrum in characteristic alignment with centrioles.

Cell Division

The division of one cell into two is the basis of the continuity of life and underlies the complexity of metazoan organisms. The life of an individual protozoan is limited, but by cell division the line of Protozoa goes on. In Metazoa, division provides the cells that constitute these organisms and the replacement of lost cells, underlies the phenomena of cellular differentiation and specialization, and permits the continuity of the species despite the death of individuals. Several types of cell division exist. We shall consider *mitosis*, *amitosis*, and *meiosis*. Cell division may be separated into two events: *karyokinesis*, or nuclear division, and *cytokinesis*, or cytoplasmic division. As indicated above, karyokinesis may occur without cytokinesis, resulting in binucleate or multinucleate cells.

Mitosis. DNA is capable of precise replication, ensuring constancy of genetic information from generation to generation and, thereby, maintenance of the characteristics of the species. Mitosis is a complex, highly ordered process wherein the original and replicated molecules of DNA are separated from one another and distributed to two nuclei. Cytokinesis typically follows karyokinesis and two cells result. The DNA with

associated protein is organized as chromosomes, whose number is highly characteristic for a species. These chromosomes are typically matched in pairs or homologs.

The human nucleus contains 46 chromosomes, paired as 23 homologs. The partners in 22 of these pairs, the *autosomes*, are morphologically alike. The remaining two chromosomes are sex chromosomes. In the female they are matched and alike; they are the X chromosomes. In the male, however, these two chromosomes are morphologically different from one another; they are the X and Y chromosomes. Chromosomes in the interphase nucleus are so long and thin that it is not possible to recognize 46 of them.

The first phase of mitosis is *prophase* (Figs. 1–61, 1–62, 1–65, and 1–66). During prophase the extended chromosomes characteristic of the interphase become progressively thicker and

1-62 Mitosis. Human leukocytes. Only the chromosomes are stained. Each chromosome is seen to consist of two chromatids joined at the kinetochore. Note the secondary constrictions in several of the chromosomes and the presence of satellites **(arrows)**. Note, too, the coiling evident in several of the chromatids. In anaphase, two chromosomes lie near the equatorial plane, lagging behind the others in joining the two diverging masses of chromosomes. This happens frequently. Note the sharp separation furrow in telophase. Aceto-orcein stain. × 4,000. (From the work of B. Reuben Migeon.)

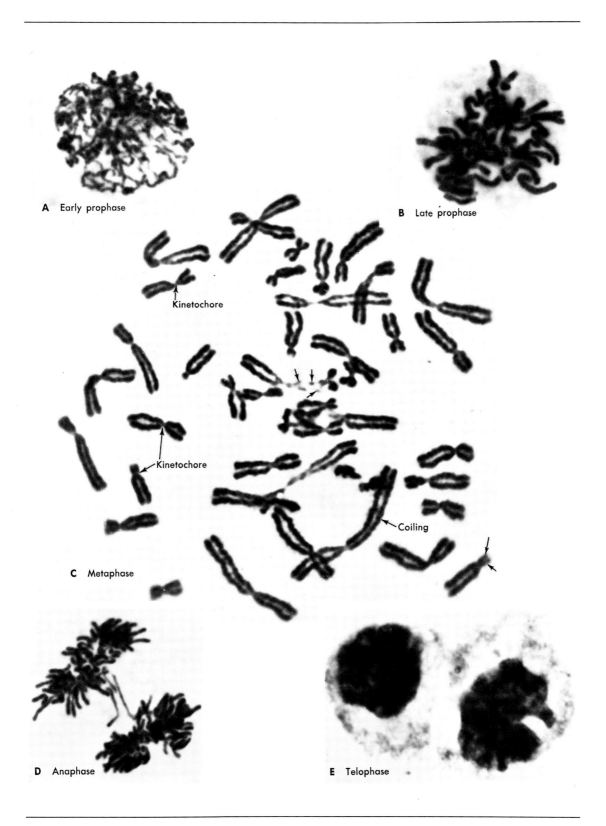

A Early prophase

B Late prophase

Kinetochore

Kinetochore

Coiling

C Metaphase

D Anaphase

E Telophase

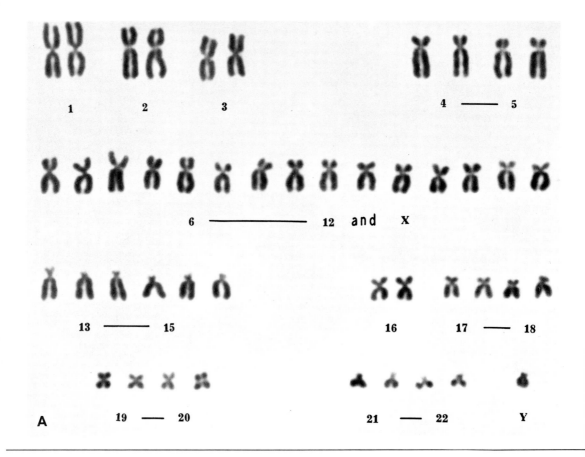

1   2   3   4 ——— 5

6 ————————— 12 and X

13 ——— 15   16   17 ——— 18

A   19 ——— 20   21 ——— 22   Y

more tightly coiled. The coils may undergo secondary coiling. As perceived by light microscopy, the individual chromosomes emerge from the nuclear substance as strands that appear progressively shorter, thicker, and more intensely stained. Moreover, as prophase goes on, one can see that each of the chromosomes is split longitudinally into precisely equal halves, or *chromatids*. This longitudinal splitting of the chromosome actually occurs in the S and G_2 phases just preceding mitosis but becomes apparent only in late prophase.[1] Through most of prophase the individually emerging chromosomes remain confined within the nuclear envelope and are too bunched together to be clearly characterized as to size and shape. Near the end of prophase, when the chromosomes are maximally contracted, the nuclear membrane disappears.

[1]The centrioles duplicate in late G or early S and remain close together until prophase. See discussion of cell cycle, page 82.

The centrioles diverge from one another and move to opposite poles of the cell. From the polar centrioles, radiating toward the center of the cell, into and around the mass of chromosomes, is a system of poorly stained fibers, the *spindle.* Some of them, the discontinuous fibers, attach to chromosomes. Others, the continuous fibers, pass around the chromosomes, going from one centriole to the other. In addition, a set of fibers radiates around each centriole, forming an *aster.* The fibers of the spindle and of the asters are preponderantly microtubules. They are called the *achromatic apparatus* because they lack affinity for dyes and are thus distinguished from the deeply stained ensemble of chromosomes, termed the *chromatic apparatus* (Figs. 1–61 to 1–69).

In the next phase of mitosis, *metaphase*, the chromosomes arrange themselves in an equatorial plane, forming an *equatorial plate* (Figs. 1–61, 1–62, and 1–67 to 1–69). Viewed from the side, this plate appears as a somewhat irregular,

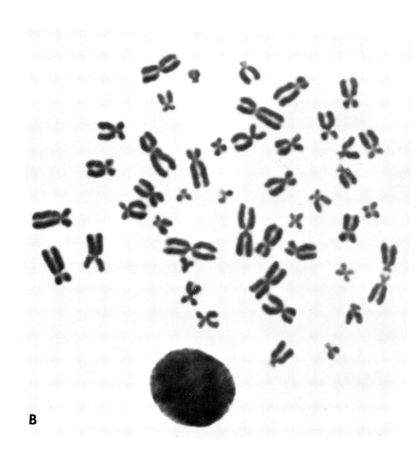

B

1–63 **A.** Human karyotype. Metaphase chromosomes have been arranged into morphologically similar groups of paired chromosomes and numbered. Pairs 1, 2, 3, and 16 can be identified as different from other chromosomes. It is impossible to separate 4 from 5, but 4 and 5 may be separated from the remainder. Similarly it is impossible to separate 6, 7, 8, 9, 10, 11, 12, and the X chromosome as different from one another, but this large group may be recognized as different from the other chromosomes. Chromosomes 13, 14, and 15, 17 and 18; 19 and 20 form similar groups. This individual is male, having an X and Y chromosome. **B.** The metaphase from which the karyotype was prepared. An interphase nucleus is present for comparison of size. Aceto-orcein stain. × 2,400. (From the work of B. Reuben Migeon.)

dense line transecting the cell. Viewed from one of the poles, the chromosomes form a circlet. Metaphase chromosomes are linear, densely stained structures. Each chromosome is constricted at one place along its length, an unstained zone called the *centromere* or *kinetochore*. The two chromatids of the chromosomes are free of one another except at the centromere, and the spindle fibers also attach there. Chromosomes may be divided into three groups, depending on the location of the centromere. If the centromere divides a chromosome into segments of equal length, the chromosome is *metacentric*. Those chromosomes separated into larger and smaller limbs by the centromere are *submedian*. Chromosomes in which the centromere is almost at the end, so that there is virtually only one limb, are *telocentric*.

The chromatic material of the chromosome may have another *secondary constriction* in one of the limbs. This constriction may have some length, and so it isolates the chromatic material

at the end of the chromosome into a *satellite*. Typically, nucleoli develop in certain zones of constriction in satellited chromosomes on reconstitution of daughter nuclei.

Metaphase chromosomes of each species may be classified on the basis of the location of the centromere, the size and shape of the limbs, and the presence of secondary constrictions and satellites. These characteristics make up the *karyotype*, or the morphology of the metaphase chromosomes. The karyotype of the human male is presented in Fig. 1–63A. The metaphase plate from which the karyotype was prepared is shown in Fig. 1–63B. The karyotype is prepared by cutting out the chromosome pairs from a photograph of a squash preparation of a metaphase cell selectively stained with a dye such as aceto-orcein. The cut-out chromosomes are then arranged in clusters of similar chromosomes. It is not possible to differentiate chromosomes occurring within a cluster by the standard aceto-orcein procedure. Thus, in the human male karyotype

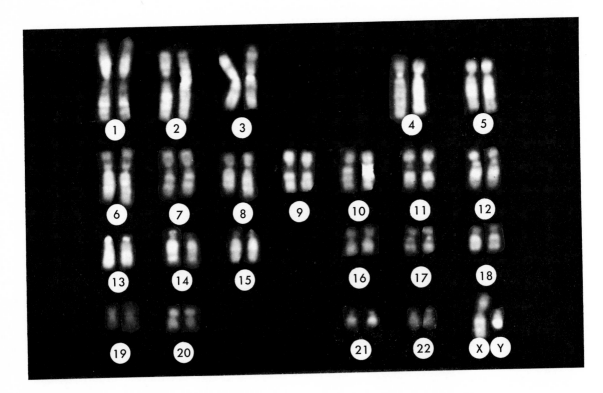

1–64 Karyotype of normal male (XY) cultured human leukocyte, showing quinacrine fluorescence patterns. Note the bandings present in each of the chromosomes. Although the significance of this banding is not understood, it has proved useful in differentiating chromosomes that are morphologically alike. Compare with the conventional karyotype in Fig. 1–63A and B. × 2,500. (From the work of W. R. Breg.) It has proved possible to obtain a similar banding pattern by staining a chromosomal preparation with a giemsa stain at a pH of about 6.8. The latter is a relatively easy procedure and may become more widely used than fluorescence staining.

one cannot separate chromosomes 6, 7, 8, 9, 10, 11, 12, and the X chromosome from one another. Certain fluorochromes produce a banded staining pattern in each of the chromosomes (Fig. 1–64). The banding pattern can also be shown in a more stable preparation by staining a squash preparation of a metaphase cell with dilute giemsa stain at pH 6.8. By this means it has proved possible to identify chromosomes not differentiable otherwise. Correlations of genetic diseases such as Down's syndrome (mongolism) and leukemia with abnormal karyotypes are being made in increasing number.

At the beginning of metaphase, the chroma-tids of a chromosome are connected only at the centromere. At the end of metaphase the centromeres divide and each of the chromatids, now a daughter chromosome and attached to the spindle by its own centromere, moves outward from the metaphase plate toward one pole of the cell. Thus, in human somatic cells, one set of 46 chromosomes moves to one centriole and the other set to the other. This divergent movement constitutes the *anaphase* of mitosis (Figs. 1–61, 1–62, and 1–65C). The spindle fibers attached to the centromeres are responsible for the characteristic orderly diverging movement of the chromosomes in anaphase. The drug colchicine interferes with the spindle by breaking up microtubules, leaving dividing cells suspended in metaphase and unable to complete the cell division.

Anaphase is concluded when the two chromosomal masses have moved to opposite poles of the cell. There now begins the final stage of nuclear division, *telophase* (Figs. 1–61, 1–62, and 1–65), during which two daughter nuclei are formed. Nuclear membranes form around each of the chromosomal masses, nucleoli appear at the satellite-bearing chromosomes, and segments of the chromosomes uncoil to become euchromatin.

Although primary attention must be accorded

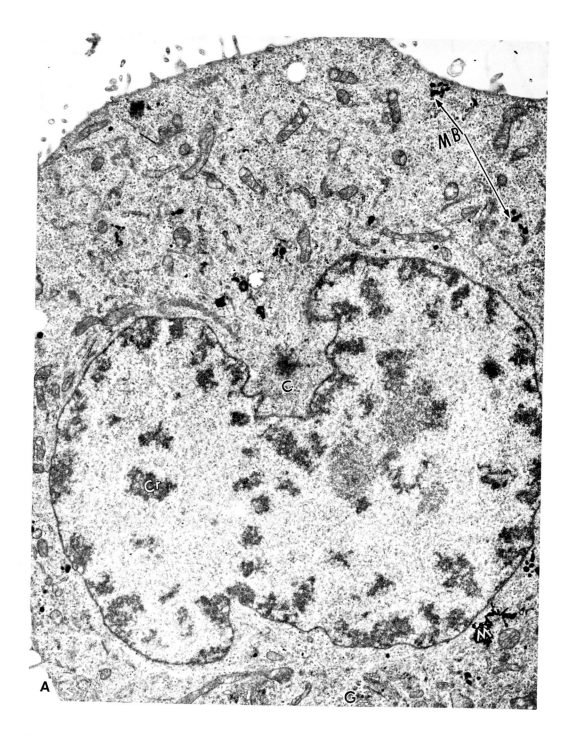

1–65 A–D Electron micrograph of mitosis in a human HeLa cell in tissue culture. These cells, originally derived from a carcinoma of the uterine cervix, form a strain of cells maintained in tissue culture. **A.** In early prophase, the chromatin becomes clumped because of the condensation of chromosomes **(Cr).** The nuclear membrane is still intact, and the centriole **(C)** and multivesicular bodies **(MB)** are prominent. Approximately × 3,850. (From Robbins, E., and Gonatas, N. K. 1964. J. Cell Biol. 21:429.)

(continued)

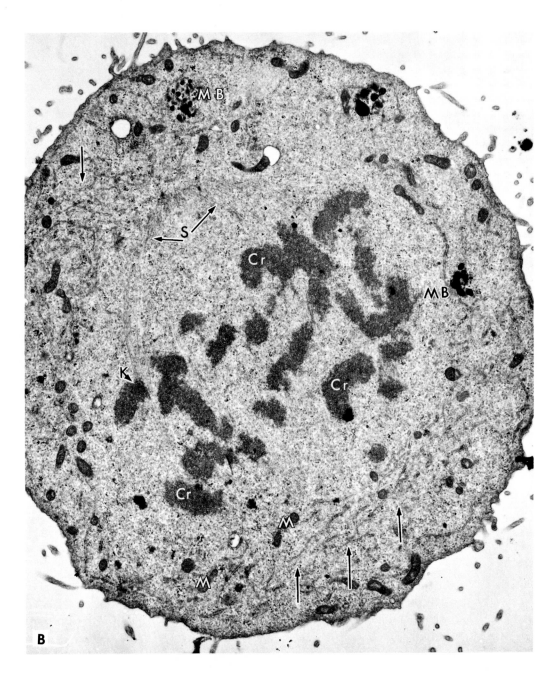

Figure 1–65 B △ and C ▷

B. In later prophase the chromosomes are close to the equatorial plate and metaphase. The spindle fibers **(S)** are seen radiating from the centriole and attached to a chromosome at the kinetochore **(K).** Approximately × 5,640. (From Robbins, E., and Gonatas, N. K. 1964. J. Cell Biol. 21:429.)

C. In late anaphase, the two chromosomal masses have moved apart. They are already surrounded by a double nuclear membrane. At the lower pole, a portion of a centriole and spindle fibers may be seen. Note how the spindle fibers are present, together with some mitochondria, in the constriction between what will be the two daughter cells. Note, too, the blebs of cytoplasm **(BL)** about the periphery of the se cells, indicating the frothing that occurs in this phase. Approximately × 5,225. (From Robbins, E., and Gonatas, N. K. 1964. J. Cell Biol. 21:429.)

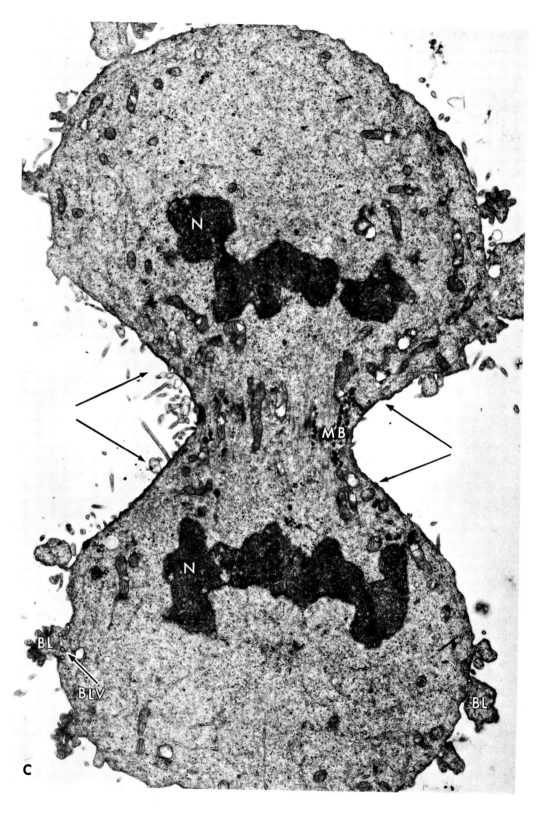

C

(continued)

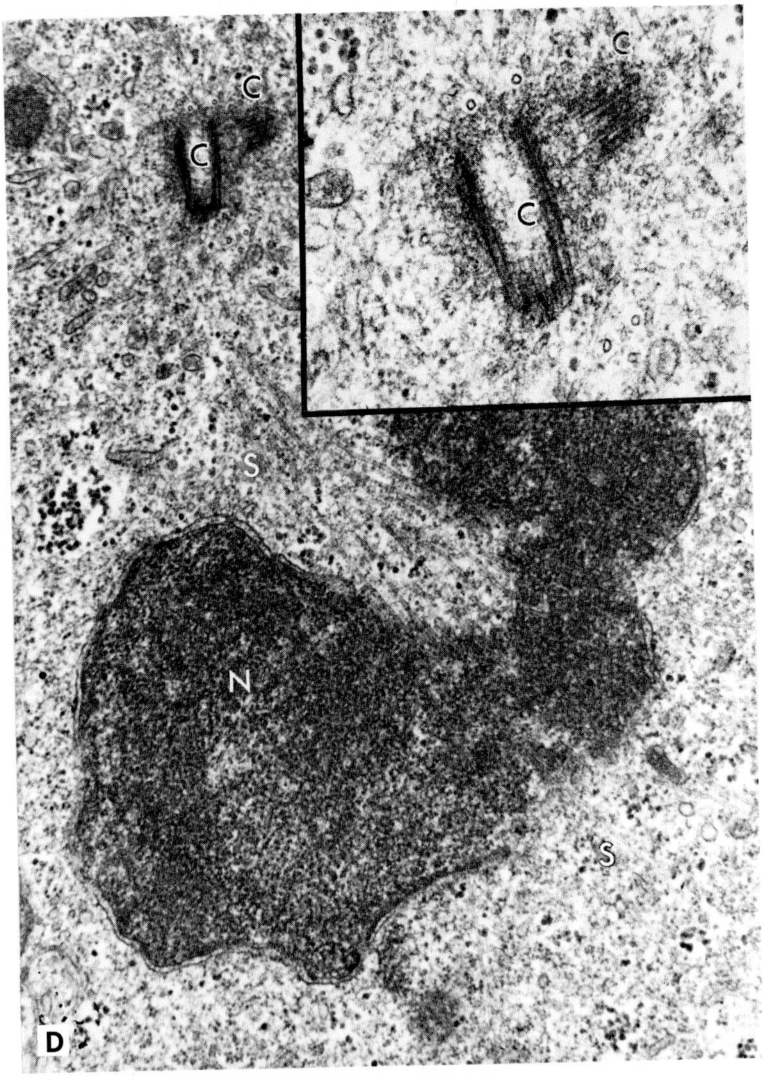

Figure 1–65D

D. Telophase. Note the presence of a double nuclear membrane about a daughter nucleus. The centriole (at higher magnification in the inset) has already been duplicated. Approximately × 13,750 (inset × 30,800). (From Robbins, E., and Gonatas, N. K. 1964. J. Cell Biol. 21:429.)

the nucleus in mitosis, characteristic changes occur in the cytoplasm. The division of the centrioles and the formation of the achromatic apparatus in prophase have already been discussed. Frothing or bubbling of the cytoplasm occurs in anaphase. During this bubbling phase, the cell surfaces are covered with microvilli. Indeed, microvilli occur throughout mitosis, being most prominent in anaphase. They also occur during G, but are usually absent or scanty in the rest of the cell cycle (Fig. 1–70). With the separation of the nuclear masses in anaphase, a partition of cytoplasmic constituents occurs. Mitochondria, lysosomes, ribosomes, and cytoplasmic membranes become distributed in approximately equal amounts about the two newly formed nuclei. As the nuclear membrane is reconstructed, the cytoplasm becomes deeply constricted in a *constriction ring* (Figs. 1–55 and 1–65C) between the two masses of chromosomes. The cytoplasm divides, forming two equal daughter cells. For a short time, the spindle may persist as a transient bridge between daughter cells.

Amitosis. Amitosis may occur in terminal or highly transient cell types such as certain cells of the placenta or of the blood. It may also occur in some multinucleated cells, as the giant cells of the connective tissue. In amitosis the nuclear

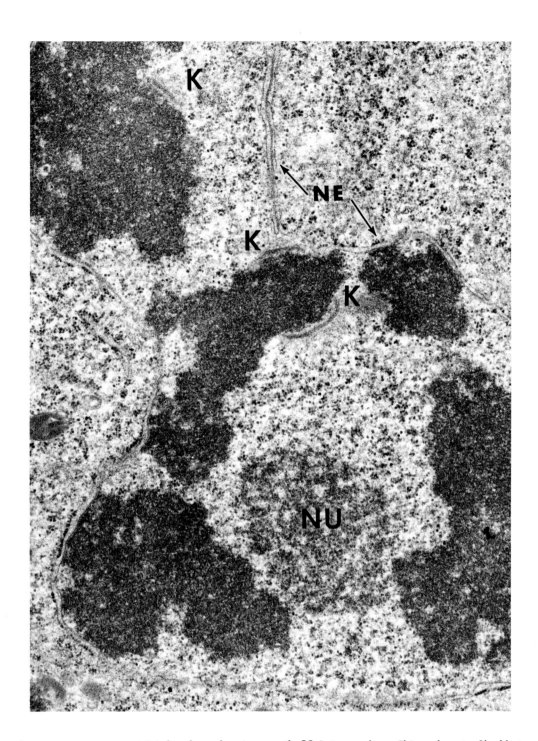

membrane appears to constrict deeply and a single nucleus becomes pinched into two. Although equal-sized daughter nuclei may sometimes result, it is impossible that a precise separation of chromosomal material can be achieved (Fig. 1–71).

1–66 Later prophase. Chinese hamster fibroblast.
Fully formed kinetochores **(K)** and a nucleus **(NU)** are present. The nuclear envelope **(NE)** is almost completely intact. [From Brinkley, B. R., and Stubblefield, E. 1970. *In* D. M. Prescott, L. Goldstein, and E. McConkey (eds.)]

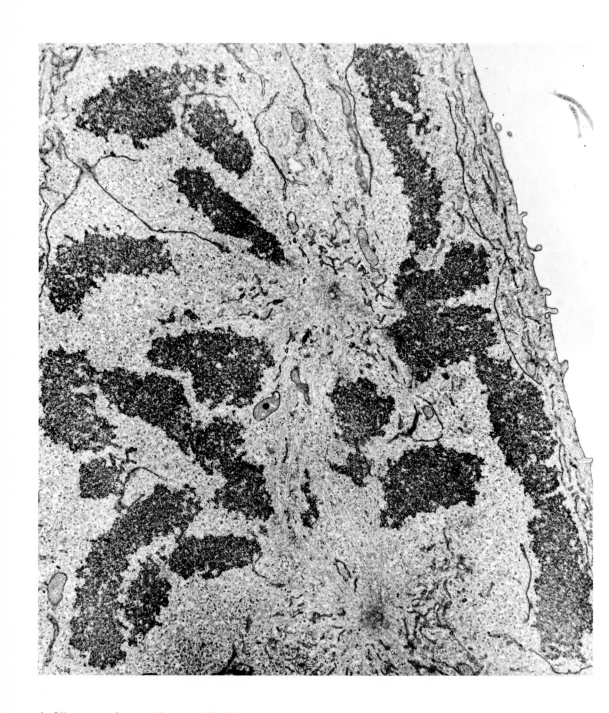

1–67 Prometaphase, rat kangaroo fibroblast. Here each of the chromosomes is tightly coiled and, although not evident, split into two chromatids. The chromosomes are moving to take positions on the metaphase plate. A centriole and microtubules are present in the cytoplasm. × 14,000. (From the work of B. R. Brinkley.)

Polyteny and Poliploidy. DNA replication may occur without nuclear division. It is characteristic of certain cell types, such as the salivary gland cells of diptera, that DNA replication occurs without subsequent chromosomal division, resulting in *polytene* chromosomes. These chromosomes replicate themselves many times over. However, the replicates remain together

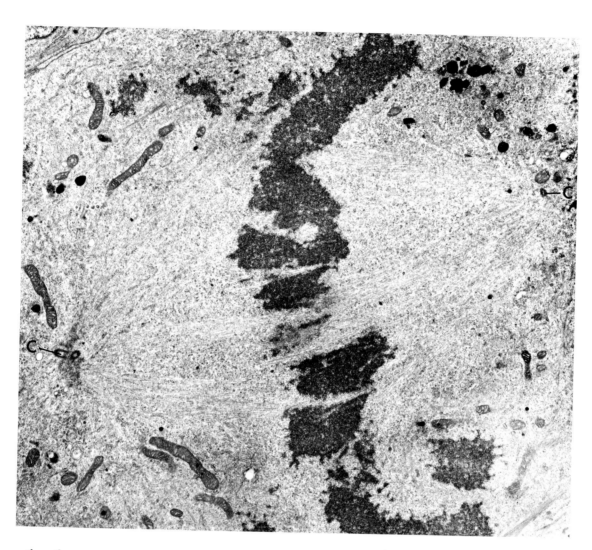

rather than move apart into separate chromosomes and thereby form giant chromosomes. Polytenic chromosomes readily show a type of banding that requires fluorochromes or special giemsa staining (Fig. 1–64) to demonstrate in other chromosomes.

DNA replication may occur with subsequent chromosomal duplication but without loss of nuclear membranes or karyokinesis, resulting in polyploid nuclei. The process has been termed *endomitosis*. Polyploid nuclei thus contain multiples of the diploid number of chromosomes. They are typically larger than diploid nuclei, as in some hepatocytes and megakaryocytes.

Meiosis. Meiosis is a type of nuclear division, restricted to gametes (i.e., spermatocytes and

1–68 Metaphase, rat kangaroo fibroblast. The metaphase plate is present in edge-on view. On the left, two centrioles **(C)** may be observed; on the right, one centriole. The microtubules of the spindle radiate from the centrioles. Both chromosomal (attached to kinetochore) and continuous (pole to pole) microtubules are present. × 10,350. (From Brinkley, B. R., and Cartwright, J., Jr. 1971. J. Cell Biol. 50:416.)

oocytes) wherein the number of chromosomes characteristic of somatic cells, the *diploid* number (2n), is halved to the *haploid* number (1n). This halving occurs because the homologs in each chromosome pair separate from one another. Each daughter nucleus in meiosis contains a set of homologs. For this reason, meiosis is called *reduction division*. The haploid nuclei of

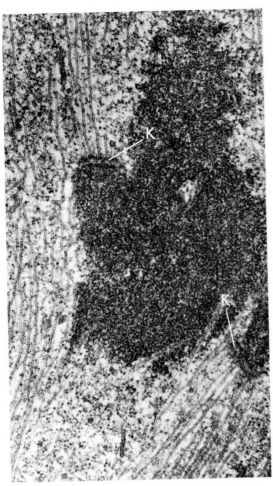

1–69 Metaphase, rat kangaroo fibroblast.
Chromosomal microtubules are inserted into
kinetochores **(K)**. Note the double nature of the
kinetochore. Continuous microtubules pass between
the chromosomes running from pole to pole without
insertion into kinetochores. × 30,800. (From Brinkley,
B. R., and Cartwright, J., Jr. 1971. J. Cell Biol. 50:416.)

the gametes unite and the diploid number of
chromosomes is restored in the process of fertilization. The fertilized ovum and all its somatic
descendants divide by mitotic division, and the
diploid number is thereby maintained in somatic
cells. But meiosis has the second major function
of providing genetic variation by the exchange of
segments between homologous chromosomes
and the random selection of one of the two homologs during the reduction division into a given
daughter nucleus.

Meiosis involves two successive nuclear divisions with only one division of chromosomes
(Figs. 1–72 and 1–73). The first meiotic division
is characterized by a prolonged prophase. In this
prophase the homologous chromosomes come to
lie together, closely and exactly paired in a
point-for-point correspondence along their entire
length (synapsis). During the process the chromosomes shorten by coiling, but not as much as
in the prophase of mitosis. Moreover, each of the
chromosomes is observed to be longitudinally
split into two chromatids. The homologous
paired chromosomes, termed a bivalent, therefore consist of four chromatids. A spindle forms
and the bivalents arrange themselves on a metaphase plate. The divergent movement of anaphase begins as the homologs, consisting of two
chromatids each, move apart to opposite poles
and are then separated into daughter cells at telophase. Thenceforth, after the first meiotic division, each of the daughter cells contains one of
the homologous chromosomes split into two
chromatids. It is of great significance that in the
first meiotic division the kinetochore does not
divide, as it does in mitosis, and so the chromatids remain together. A second meiotic division
ensues in which the chromosomes become arranged in a metaphase plate and the kinetochores divide. The chromatids that make up each
of the chromosomes are now free of one another
and diverge from the metaphase plate in an anaphase movement. Later in telophase they are
grouped into daughter nuclei and then daughter
cells. The two meiotic divisions have thus sorted
the four homologous chromatids present in prophase of the first meiotic division into four separate gametes, each of which has the haploid
number of chromosomes. In a male, four functional spermatozoa will result from the two
meiotic divisions. Curiously, the completion of
cytokinesis in the spermatozoa is delayed so that
four otherwise mature spermatozoa may remain
linked in Siamese-quadruplet style. In a female
four ova are produced as well, but the cytoplasmic division leaves virtually all the cytoplasm with one nucleus. The remaining nuclei,
surrounded by minimal cytoplasm, cannot survive. They are called polar bodies. This unequal
cytoplasmic division provides one nucleus with
sufficient cytoplasm to support fertilization and
embryogenesis. Each of the gamete nuclei contains 23 chromosomes. In female gametes one of
these is an X chromosome, whereas in male ga-

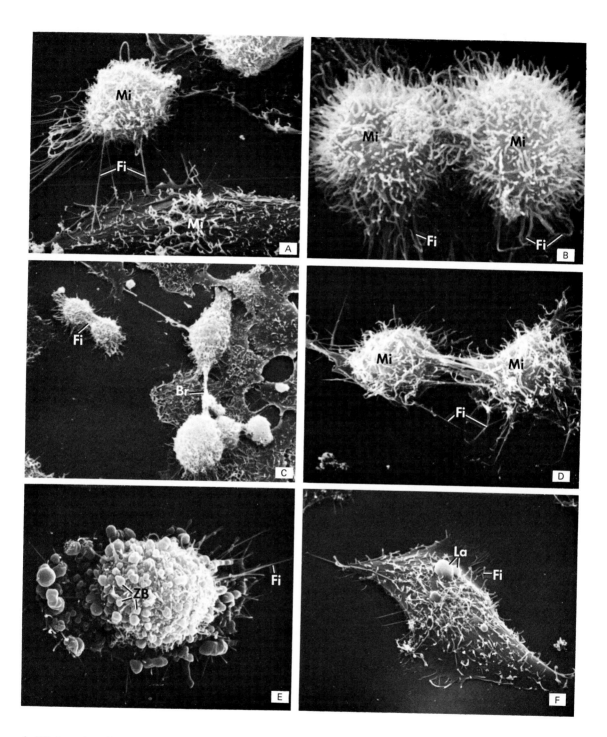

1–70 Scanning electron microscopy of cultured HeLa (**A, C, and F**) and KB cells (**B, D, and E**) in mitosis. Late stages in cell division are illustrated in B to D; interphase cells are illustrated in C, E, and F. Note the long bridge (**Br**) connecting the daughter cells in C. Other surface specializations identified are microvilli (**Mi**), filopodia (**Fi**), lamellapodia (**La**), and blebs (**ZB**). A, × 1,664; B, × 3,600; C, × 684; D, × 2,040; E, × 1,889; F, × 1,680. (From Beams, H. W., and Kessel, R. G. 1976. Am. Sci. 64:279.)

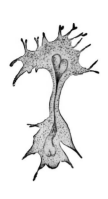
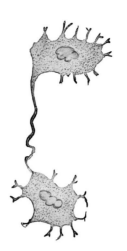
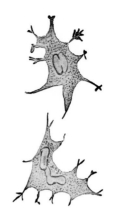

1-71 Amitosis in a histiocyte of a frog. The drawing is prepared from a cell in tissue culture. (From the work of Arnold.)

metes one is either an X or a Y. During fetal life in a human female, oocytes migrate into the ovary, proliferate by mitosis a short time, and then undergo meiosis, entering the prophase of the first meiotic division. They remain in that state until shortly before ovulation. Because a woman may ovulate until about 45 years of age, oocytes may remain in meiosis for more than 45 years. It may well be that the first meiotic prophase constitutes a particularly stable state for DNA.

Another essential function of meiosis is to provide genetic variation. It will be recalled that in diploid cells one chromosome in a homologous pair is contributed by the spermatozoon and the other by the oocyte. When the homologous chromosomes are arranged on the first meiotic metaphase plate, it is a matter of chance whether the homolog contributed by the sperm or the homolog contributed by the ovum faces a given pole. As a result, in each cell produced in the first meiotic division, the proportion of chromosomes derived from the sperm and that from

the egg are a matter of chance. This chance separation is one mechanism of genetic mixture. A second mechanism is the exchange, by homologous chromosomes, of corresponding segments. This exchange occurs when the homologs are in synapsis during the early phases of meiotic prophase I (Fig. 1–73). The extent of the exchange becomes apparent as the homologs pull away from their synaptic union. It is then seen that they frequently remain attached in one or more places. This persistent link between diverging chromosomes is termed a *chiasma*. The exchange of segments is termed *crossing over*.

The stages in meiosis are as follows (Fig. 1–72):

1. The first prophase, prophase I, is long and may be divided into five stages. In *leptotene* the chromosomes are long and thin. In *zygotene* the homologous chromosomes move toward one another and pair, lying in close touch in a point-for-point correspondence along their length (synapsis). In *pachytene* the

1-72 The stages of meiosis I and II shown schematically. A pair of homologous chromosomes, one dark and the other light, is followed through meiosis I. Then chromatids of a daughter cell are traced through meiosis II. The events are as follows:

Prophase I. Leptotene: The chromosomes become apparent as thin linear structures. Zygotene: Homologous chromosomes line up and pair with one another point to point (synapsis). Pachytene: With pairing completed, the chromosomes become shorter and thicker and each longitudinally splits into chromatids, the centromere remaining single. The four

chromatids of the two chromosomes constitute a bivalent. Chromatids from each of the homologous chromosomes may cross over one another forming a chiasma. Diplotene: The chromosomes further shorten and broaden; they also coil. Homologous chromosomes begin to move apart but are held together at the chiasma. Diakinesis: The chromosomes become broader, thicker, more tightly coiled; they move further apart.

- Metaphase I. The chromosomes are on the equatorial plate.
- Anaphase I. The chromosomes diverge, exchanging chromosomal segments at the site of the chiasma.

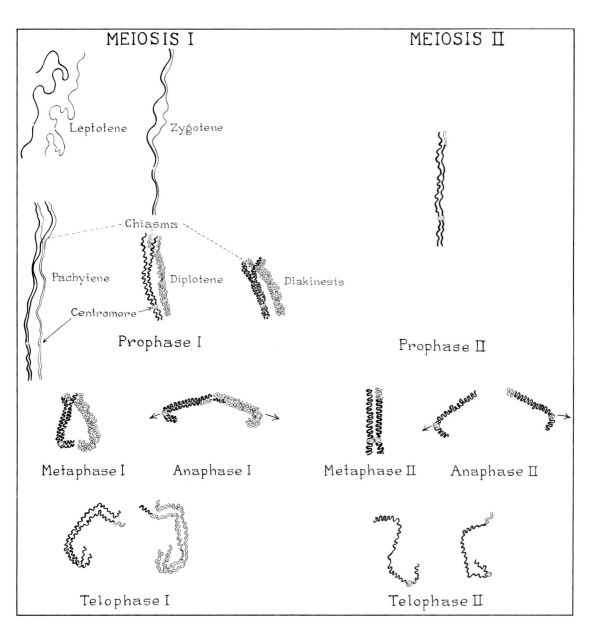

MEIOSIS I — MEIOSIS II

Leptotene — Zygotene

Chiasma

Pachytene — Diplotene — Diakinesis

Centromere

Prophase I — Prophase II

Metaphase I — Anaphase I — Metaphase II — Anaphase II

Telophase I — Telophase II

- Telophase I. Each chromatid pair joined by a single centromere, lies in a daughter cell. The chromatids uncoil and lengthen to some extent.
- Chromatids in the left-hand daughter cell pass through the following stages in meiosis II.
- Prophase II. This stage is transient and possibly absent since the chromatids may move directly to metaphase II.
- Metaphase II. Chromatids become shorter, broader, and coiled. The centromere divides.
- Anaphase II. Chromatids separate and move to opposite poles.

- Telophase II. Each of the chromatids is now a daughter cell.

Thus in the course of these two divisions the four chromatids forming the bivalent of prophase I are separated, first into two daughter cells of telophase I, each containing two chromatids ($4n \rightarrow 2n$), and then into two daughter cells again in telophase II, each containing one chromatid ($2n \rightarrow 1n$). A total of four daughter cells is produced each having the haploid ($1n$) number of chromosomes. In a male individual four sperms are produced; in a female, one ovum and three polar bodies. On fertilization the diploid ($2n$) number is restored.

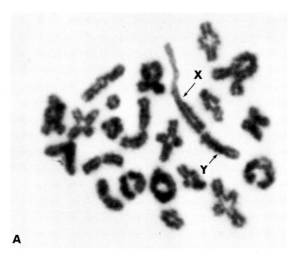

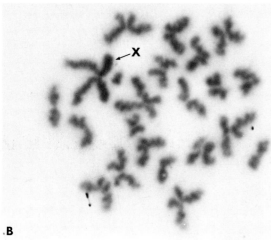

1–73 Meiosis in the golden hamster *Mesocricetus
auratus*. **A.** Primary spermatocyte showing the
22 bivalents at the first meiotic metaphase. The X and
Y chromosomes are associated terminally, the X being
distinguished by its length. The autosomal bivalents
demonstrate chiasmata in various stages. Note the
coiling of the chromatids. **B.** Secondary spermatocyte
at the second meiotic metaphase, containing the
haploid number of 22 chromosomes. This cell has
received the Y chromosome. At this stage, the
chromosomes show "relic" spirals, which are probably
remnants of coiling from the first meiotic division.
Aceto-orcein stain. × 2,200. (From the work of
M. Fergusen-Smith.)

chromosomes coil considerably, appearing
shorter and thicker. At about this time it becomes apparent that each of the chromosomes
of the bivalent contains four chromatids. The
centromere does not split. In *diplotene* the
chromosomes begin to separate from one an-

other, but the separation is incomplete, with
chiasmata forming. The separation continues
into the *diakinesis*, a stage that shows the
chiasmata and the thickened, coiled, partially
separated chromosomes to good advantage.
The nuclear membrane disappears.

2. In metaphase I the bivalent chromosomes are
   arranged on an equatorial plate. There are two
   centromeres, one for each of the chromosomes, and the centromeres are attached to
   spindle fibers.
3. In anaphase I the chromosomes, each of
   which consists of two chromatids, move to
   opposite poles.
4. Telophase I follows, but the chromosomes
   may remain in a shortened form.

In the first meiotic division, therefore, the
diploid number of chromosomes has been reduced to the haploid number; an exchange of genetic information may have occurred between
the chromosomes; the distribution of chromosomes of a given bivalent to each pole has been
a matter of chance, further increasing genetic
variation; and each of the chromosomes is longitudinally split to form two chromatids.

5. Interphase, or *interkinesis,* is brief.
6. In prophase II a spindle forms, the nuclear
   membrane breaks down, and the chromosomes move equatorially.
7. In metaphase II the chromatids are arranged
   on an equatorial plate and their centromeres
   divide and become attached to spindle fibers.
8. In anaphase II the chromatids, now daughter
   chromosomes, move to opposite poles.
9. Telophase II is marked by the appearance of a
   nuclear membrane uncoiling of the chromosomes, and the development of daughter cells.

The Life Cycle of Cells

Two major types of cell may be recognized: *somatic cells,* which are the diverse cells making
up the somatic structure of the body, fated to die
with or before the individual they constitute;
and *germ cells,* which are the gametes capable
of uniting sexually with those of another individual to form a new individual.

A somatic cell begins its life span as one of
the daughter cells of a mitotic division. Directly
after this division the cell may undergo a period
of intense protein synthesis, resulting in the
emergence of the granules, filaments, or other
specific structures that mark the cell as mature

and specialized. As the cell matures and morphological signs of specialization occur, it is differentiated from an unspecialized, perhaps multipotential, cell into a highly specialized unit of limited cellular potency. Although a cell may appear undifferentiated, its direction of maturation may be fixed and limited genetically, only time being required to disclose the nature of the differentiation by the appearance of morphological specializations. In short, a cell that appears morphologically undifferentiated may, in fact, be quite specifically determined.

The frequency of mitotic division varies with the cell type and tissue. Tissues may be classified as showing no mitotic division, resulting in no renewal (nervous tissue); little division, resulting in slow renewal (liver and thyroid); and active division, resulting in fast renewal (gastrointestinal tract and hematopoietic tissue). Some slowly renewed tissues may be termed "conditional renewal" systems because their renewal rate can be considerably increased under certain circumstances. After partial hepatectomy, for example, the remaining hepatocytes divide very actively, providing fast renewal until the mass of the liver is restored. Even some cells showing no mitotic division may, with appropriate stimulation, proliferate and differentiate. Certain small lymphocytes (T cells) may circulate and recirculate for many years in humans without dividing, but when stimulated by the appropriate antigen, or with certain mitogens, such as phytohemagglutinin or pokeweed, they may divide rapidly, producing clones of immunologically competent cells. In neurons, mitosis occurs only prenatally and neonatally until the full number of neurons is reached. Thereafter, no replacement occurs; a cell lost diminishes the total number, and its absence may cause functional impairment. The cells in tissues undergoing slow renewal tend to be long-lived. The relatively low levels of mitotic division provide new cells to replace those dying off or to permit the growth and increased functional capacity of the tissue. Rapidly renewing tissues are characterized by short-lived cells replaced by cell division, so that a rather stable number of cells results. In the intestinal epithelium, new cells formed in the depths of the intestinal glands appear to move up the wall of the gland replacing the topmost cells, which fall into the gut lumen. As a result, the entire intestinal epithelium is renewed in a span of days. The kinetics of hematopoietic tissues, particularly of the granular leukocytes, follows this pattern.

It is possible to define a *generation time* for a population of similar cells, relating the interphase state, the period of DNA replication, and the process of mitotic division. A series of three periods follows mitosis: G_1, S, G_2, then M. G_1 is an interval or gap that follows cell division; S is the period of DNA replication; G_2 is the gap between replication of DNA and the start of mitosis; and M is mitosis.

The duration of G_1 varies greatly with cell types and mitotic turnover. In rapidly dividing cells it may be a matter of several hours. In nonrenewing tissues it may last the life of the organism. Such prolonged G_1 periods may be designated G_0. S is demonstrated by autoradiography. Thymidine is a base distinctive to DNA. Therefore, replicating DNA specifically and selectively takes up thymidine. If the thymidine is radioactive, accomplished by the incorporation of tritium (^{3}H) in the molecule, and is administered during DNA replication, it is taken up by the replicating DNA and can mark it in autoradiographs. Indeed, the ability to delineate the S period by this means makes it possible to determine the entire generation time. In a rapidly renewing tissue, S is approximately 7 h. It is a matter of great interest that the DNA in a given chromosome does not all replicate at the same time. Instead, different segments of the chromosome replicate at different times in the S period, and in a characteristic sequence. G_2 is very short—about an hour—in rapidly renewing tissues. In cells destined to be polytenic, G_2 may last indefinitely. The whole of the cycle in such rapidly dividing rodent tissues as germinal centers or thymus may be about 12 h. In the epithelium of the gastrointestinal tract in humans G_2 is 1 to 7 h.; the S phase, 10 to 20 h; G_1, 10 to 20 h; and the whole of the cycle, 1 to 2 days. In rodents this cycle may take only a third of this time.

The sequences in the generation cycle may be illustrated as follows[2]:

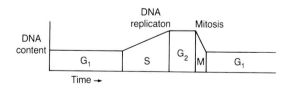

[2]After Lamerton, L. F., 1969, In Fry, R. J. M., Griem, M. L., and Kirsten, W. H. (eds.), Normal and Malignant Cell Growth. New York: Springer-Verlag.

After functioning as a mature cell for varying lengths of time, a cell dies, its death often presaged by a period of senescence. Perhaps the best-studied case is that of the erythrocyte, whose life span in the circulation of humans is approximately 120 days. Near the end of its life span, the activity of glucose-6-phosphatase and certain other enzymes declines, and the cell becomes mechanically more fragile. There are, however, no morphological concomitants of erythrocyte senescence.

In other cell types, however, morphological changes may signify senescence and coming cell death. In muscle cells, these changes include attenuation, decrease in specific functional elements such as contractile filaments, and accumulation of pigment. Other changes include diminution in mitochondria, accumulation of fat, and vacuolization of cytoplasm and nucleus. Dead cells may disappear by lysis, by phagocytosis, or by displacement from the tissue, seen in desquamated skin cells and intestinal cells.

References and Selected Bibliography

General

Baker, J. R. 1958. Principles of Biological Microtechnique: A Study of Fixation and Dyeing. New York: John Wiley and Sons, Inc.

Baker, J. R. The cell-theory: A restatement, history and critique. Q. J. Microbiol. Sci. 89:103 (1948); 90:87 (1949); 93:157 (1952).

Bensley, R. R., and Gersh I. 1933. Studies on cell structure by the freezing-drying method. I. Introduction. II. The nature of the mitochondria in the hepatic cell of amblystoma. III. The distribution in cells of the basophil substances, in particular the Nissl substance of the nerve cell. Anat. Rec. 57:205, 217, 369.

Bensley, R. R., and Hoerr, N. L. 1935. Studies on cell structure by the freezing-drying method. VI. The preparation and properties of mitochondria. Anat. Rec. 60:449.

Bodmer, W. F. 1981. The HLA system: Introduction. Brit. Med. Bull. 34:213.

Brachet, J., and Mirsky, A. E. (eds.). 1961. The cell. I. Biochemistry, physiology, morphology. II. Cells and their component parts. III. Mitosis and meiosis. IV. Specialized cells, pt. 1. V. Specialized cells, pt. 2. New York: Adademic Press, Inc.

Busch, H. B. (ed.). 1974. The Cell Nucleus. 3 vols. New York: Academic Press.

De Robertis, E. D. F., Saez, F. A., and De Robertis, E. M. F., Jr. 1975. Cell Biology, 6th ed. Philadelphia: W. B. Saunders Co.

Freeman, J. A., and Spurlock, B. O. 1962. A new epoxy embedment for electron microscopy. J. Cell Biol. 13:437.

Fuks, A., Kaufman, J. F., Orr, H. T., Parham, P., Robb, R. R., Terhorst, C., and Strominger, J. L. 1980. Structural aspects of the products of the human histocompatibility complex. Transplant. Proc. 9:1685.

Harris, H. 1974. Nucleus and Cytoplasm, 3rd ed. New York: Oxford University Press.

Karp, G. 1979. Cell Biology. New York: McGraw-Hill Book Co., Inc.

Organization of the Cytoplasm. 1982. Cold Spring Harbor Symp. Quant. Biol. Vol. 46.

Pretlow, T. G. II., Weir, E. E., and Zettergren, J. G. 1975. Problems connected with the separation of different kinds of cells. Int. Rev. Exp. Pathol. 14:91.

Siegel, B. M. (ed.). 1964. Modern developments in electron microscopy. In The Physics of the Electron Microscope: Techniques: Applications. New York: Academic Press, Inc.

Watson, D. D. 1976. Molecular Biology of the Gene, 3rd ed. New York: Benjamin.

Cell Cycle, Mitosis, and Centrioles

Ackerman, G. A. 1961. Histochemistry of the centrioles and centrosomes of the leukemic cells from human myeloblastic leukemia. J. Biophys. Biochem. Cytol. 11:717.

Bajer, A., and Mole-Bajer, 1971. Architecture and function of the mitotic spindle. Adv. Cell Mol. Biol. 1:213.

Baserga, R. (ed.). 1976. Multiplication and Division in Mammalian Cells. New York: Marcel Dekker.

Beams, W. H., and Kessel, R. G. 1976. Cytokinesis: A comparative study of cytoplasmic division in animal cells. Am. Sci. 64:279.

Brinkley, B. R., and Porter, K. R. (eds.). 1977. Symposium on "The Eukarocyte Cell Cycle." Inter. Cell Biol. New York: The Rockefeller Press, p. 409.

Brinkley, B. R., and Stubblefield, E. 1970. Ultrastructure and interaction of the kinetochore and centriole in mitosis and meiosis. In D. M. Prescott, L. Goldstein, and E. McConkey (eds.), Advances in Cell Biology, vol. I. New York: Appleton-Century-Crofts.

Bullough, W. S. 1975. Mitotic control in adult mammalian tissues. Biol. Rev. 50:99.

Edenberg, J., and Huberman, J. A. 1975. Eukaryotic chromosome replication. Ann. Rev. Genet. 9:245.

Fuge, H. 1974. Ultrastructure and function of the spindle apparatus and chromosomes during nuclear division. Protoplasm 82:299.

Gall, J. G., Porter, K. R., and Siekevitz, P. (eds.). 1981. Discovery in cell biology. J. Cell Biol. 91 (3, part 2):35.

Goss, R. T. 1970. Turnover in cells and tissues. In D. M. Prescott, L. Goldstein, and E. McConkey (eds.), Advances in Cell Biology, vol. 1. New York: Appleton-Century-Crofts, Inc.

Kornberg, A. DNA Synthesis. 1974. W. H. Freeman.

Lajtha, L. 1969. Proliferative capacity of hemopoietic stem cells. In R. J. M. Fry, M. G. Griem, and W. H. Kirsten (eds.), Normal and Malignant Cell Growth. New York: Springer-Verlag.

LeBlond, C. P., and Walker, B. E. 1956. Renewal of cell populations. Physiol. Rev. 36:255.

Lesher, S., and Bauman, J. 1969. Cell proliferation in the intestinal epithelium. *In* R. J. M. Fry, M. L. Griem, and W. H. Kirsten (eds.), Normal and Malignant Cell Growth. New York: Springer-Verlag.

Mazia, D. 1961. Mitosis and the physiology of cell division. *In* J. Brachet and A. E. Mirsky (eds.)., The Cell, vol. 3. New York: New Academic Press, Inc.

Mazia, D. 1964. The cell cycle. Sci Am. 230:54.

Mitchison, J. M. 1971. The Biology of the Cell Cycle. New York: Cambridge University Press.

Pelc, S. R. 1964. Labelling of DNA and cell division in so-called non-dividing tissues. J. Cell Biol. 22:21.

Prescott, D. M. 1970. Structure and Replication of Eukaryotic Chromosomes. 1970. *In* D. M. Prescott, L. Goldstein, and E. McConkey (eds.). Advances in Biology, vol. 1. New York: Appleton-Century-Crofts.

Prescott, D. M. 1976. The cell cycle and the control of cellular reproduction. Adv. Genet. 18:99.

Robbins, E., and Gonatas, N. K. 1964. The ultrastructures of a mammalian cell during the mitotic cycle. J. Cell Biol. 21:429.

Taylor, J. H. 1974. Units of DNA replication in chromosomes of eukaryocytes. Int. Rev. Cytol. 37:1.

Wheatley, D. N. 1982. The Centriole: A Central Enigma of Cell Biology. Amsterdam: Elsevier Biomedical Press.

Chromatin

Back, F. 1976. The variable condition of heterochromatin and euchromatin. Int. Rev. Cytol. 45:25.

Barr, M. L. 1966. The Significance of the Sex Chromatin. Int. Rev. Cytol. 19:35.

Barr, M. L. 1959. Sex chromatin and phenotype in man. Science 130:679.

Baserga, R., and Nicolina, C. 1976. Chromatin structure and function in proliferating cells. Biochem. Biophys. Acta 458:109.

Berendes, H. D. 1973. Synthetic activity of polytene chromosome. Int. Rev. Cytol. 35:61.

Elgin, S. C. R., and Weintraub, H. 1975. Chromosomal proteins and chromatin structure. Ann. Rev. Biochem. 44:725.

Fitzsimmons, D. W., and Wolstenholme, G. E. (eds.). 1975. The Structure and Function of Chromatin. Ciba Foundation Symposium 28 (new series). Amsterdam: Elsevier North-Holland.

Kornberg, R. D. 1977. Structure of chromatin. Ann. Rev. Biochem. 46:931.

Endocytosis—Cytoplasmic Vesicles

Brandt, P. W., and Pappas, G. D. 1960. An electron microscopic study of pinocytosis in ameba. I. The surface attachment phase. J. Biophys. Biochem. Cytol. 8:675.

Silverstein, S. C., Steinman, R. M., and Cohn, Z. A. 1977. Endocytosis. Ann. Rev. Biochem 46:669.

Stossel, T. P. 1974. Phagocytosis. N. Engl. J. Med. 290:717.

Straus, W. 1964. Occurrence of phagosomes and phagolysosomes in different segments of the nephron in relation to the reabsorption, transport, digestion, and extrusion of intravenously injected horseradish peroxidase. J. Cell Biol. 21:295.

Ockleford, C. D., and Whyte, A. (eds.). 1980. Coated Vesicles. Cambridge, England: Cambridge University Press.

Endoplasmic Reticulum

Brinkley, R. R., and Porter, K. R. (eds.). 1977. Symposium on "Endoplasmic Reticulum. Golgi Apparatus and Cell Secretion." Int. Cell Biol. New York: Rockefeller University Press, pp. 267-340.

Cardell, R. R., Jr. 1979. Smooth endoplasmic reticulum in rat hepatocytes during glycogen deposition and depletion. Int. Rev. Cytol. 48:221.

Depierre, J. W., and Dallner, G. 1975. Structural aspects of the membrane of the endoplasmic reticulum. Biochem. Biophys. Acta 415:411.

Porter, K. R., and Palade, G. E. 1957. Studies on the endoplasmic reticulum. V. Its form and differentiation in striated muscle cells. J. Biophys. Biochem. Cytol. 3:269.

Porter, K. R., and Yamada, E. 1960. Studies on the endoplasmic reticulum. V. Its form and differentiation in pigment epithelial cells of the frog retina. J. Biophys. Biochem. Cytol. 8:181.

Golgi Complex

Bennett, G., LeBlond, C. P., and Haddad, A. J. 1974. Migration of glycoproteins from Golgi apparatus to the surface of various cell types as shown by radioautography after labelled fucose injection into rats. J. Cell Biol. 60:258.

Dalton, E. J., and Felix, M. D. 1956. A comparative study of the Golgi complex. J. Biophys. Biochem. Cytol. 2:79.

Jamieson, J. D. 1971. Role of the Golgi complex in the intracellular transport of secretory proteins. *In* F. Clementi and B. Ceccarelli (eds.), Advances in Cytopharmacology, vol. 1. New York: Raven Books, Abelard-Schuman, Inc., p. 83.

Morre, D. J., and Oltacht, L. 1977. Dynamics of the Golgi apparatus: Membrane differentiation and membrane flow. Int. Rev. Cytol. 5:61.

Palade, G. 1975. Intracellular aspects of the process of protein synthesis. Science 189:347.

Tartakoff, A. M. 1982. Simplifying the complex Golgi. Trends Bio. Sci. 7:174.

Whaley, W. G. 1975. The Golgi Apparatus. Vienna, New York: Springer-Verlag.

Intermediate Filaments

Lazarides, E., 1980. Review Article: Intermediate filaments as mechanical integrators of cellular space. Nature 283:249.

Lysosomes

Allison, A. 1967. Lysosomes and disease. Sci. Am. 217:62.

De Duve, C. 1958. Lysosomes, a new group of cytoplasmic particles. *In* T. Hayashi (ed.), Subcellular Particles. New York: The Ronald Press.

De Duve, C. 1963. The separation and characterization of subcellular particles. Harvey Lectures 59:49.

De Duve, C. 1975. Exploring cells with a centrifuge. Science 189:186.

Holtzman, E. 1976. Lysosomes: A Survey. Vienna, New York: Springer-Verlag.

Kolodny, E. H. 1976. Lysosomal storage diseases. N. Engl. J. Med. 294:1217.

Meiosis

Comings, D. E., and Okada, T. A. 1972. Architecture of meiotic cells and mechanisms of chromosome pairing. Adv. Cell Mol. Biol. 2:309.

Moens, P. B. 1973. Mechanisms of chromosome synapsis at meitoic prophase. Int. Rev. Cytol. 35:117.

Rhoades, M. M. 1960. Meiosis. *In* J. Brachet and A. Mirsky (eds.), Cell, vol. 3, New York: Academic Press, Inc., pp. 1–75.

Stern, H., and Hotta, Y. 1972. Biochemical controls of meiosis. Ann. Rev. Genet. 9:37.

Mitochondria

Fernandez-Moran, H., Oda, T., Blair, P. V., and Green, D. E. 1964. A macromolecular repeating unit of mitochondrial structure and function: Correlated electron microscopic and biochemical studies of isolated mitochondria and submitochondrial particles of beef heart muscle. J. Cell Biol. 22:71.

Munn, E. 1975. The Structure of Mitochondria. New York: Academic Press.

Palmer, J. M., and Hall, D. O. 1972. The mitochondrial membrane system. Prog. Mol. Biol. 24:125.

Tedeschi, H. 1976. Mitochondria: Structure, Biogenesis and Transducing Function. Cell Biology Monographs, vol. 4. Vienna: Springer-Verlag.

Nuclear Envelope

Feldherr, C. M. 1962. The nuclear annuli as pathways for nucleocytoplasmic exchanges. J. Cell Biol. 14:65.

Franke, W. W. 1974. Structure, biochemistry and functions of nuclear envelope. Int. Rev. Cytol (Suppl) 4:72.

Maul, G. G. 1970. On the relationship between the Golgi apparatus and annucleate lamellae. J. Ultrastruct. Res. 30:368.

Microfilaments

LeBlond, C. P., and Clermont, Y. 1960. The cell web, a fibrillar structure found in a variety of cells in animal tissues. Anat. Rec. 136:230.

Perry, S., Margreth, A., and Adelstein, R. (eds.). 1977. Contractile Systems in Non-Muscle Tissues. Amsterdam: Elsevier North-Holland.

Pollard, T. D. 1975. Functional implications of the biochemical and structural properties. *In* S. Inoue and R. E. Stephens (eds.), Molecules and Cell Movement. New York: Raven Books, Abelard-Schuman, Ltd.

Pollard, T. D. 1976. Cytoskeletal functions of cytoplasmic contractile proteins. J. Supramol. Struct. 5:317.

Schroeder, T. E. 1973. Actin in dividing cells: Contractile ring filaments bind heavy meromyosin. Proc. Natl. Acad. Sci. U.S.A. 70:1,688.

Schroeder, T. E. 1975. Dynamics of the contractile ring. 1975 *In* S. Inoue and R. E. Stephens (eds.), Molecules and Cell Movement. New York: Raven Books, Abelard-Schuman, Ltd.

Membranes

Ash, J. F., Louvard, and Singer, S. J. 1977. Antibody-induced linkages of plasma membrane proteins to intracellular actinomyosin-containing filaments in cultured fibroblasts. Proc. Natl. Acad. Sci. U.S.A. 74:5,584.

Branton, D. 1966. Fracture faces of frozen membranes. Proc. Natl. Acad. Sci. U.S.A. 55:1,048.

Branton, D. 1971. Freeze-etching studies of membrane structure. Trans. R. Soc. Lond. (Biol.) 261:133.

Branton, D. 1966. Fracture faces of frozen membranes. Proc. Natl. Acad. Sci. U.S.A. 55:1,048.

Brinkley, B. R., and Porter, K. R. (eds.). 1977. Symposium on "Plasma Membrane Organization." *In* Int. Cell Biol. New York: Rockefeller University Press, pp. 5–28.

Cuatrecasas, P., and Greaves, M. F. 1977. Receptors and Recognition. Halsted.

Essner, E., Novikoff, A. D., and Masek, B. 1958. Adenosine triphosphatase and 5-nucleotidease activities in the plasma membrane of liver cells as revealed by electron microscopy. J. Biophys. Biochem. Cytol. 4:711.

Hughes, R. C. 1975 The complex carbohydrate of mammalian cell surfaces and their biological roles. Essays Biochem. 11:1.

Marchesi, R. T., Furthmayer, H., and Tomita, M. 1976. The red cell membrane. Ann. Rev. Biochem. 45:667.

Nicolson, G. L., Poste, G., and Ji, T. H. 1977. The dynamics of cell membrane organization. *In* G. Poste and G. L. Nicolson (eds.), Dynamic Aspects of Cell Surface Organization, vol. 3, Cell Surface Reviews. Amsterdam: Elsevier North-Holland, pp. 1–73.

Pinto da Silva, P., and Braxton, D. J. 1970. Membrane splitting in freeze-etching. Cell Biol. 45:598.

Quinn, P. J. 1976. The Molecular Biology of Cell Membranes. Baltimore: University Park Press.

Raff, M. C., and De Petris, S. 1973. Movement of lymphocyte surface antigens and receptors: The fluid nature of the lymphocyte plasma membrane and its immunological significance. Fed. Proc. 32:48.

Singer, S. J., and Nicolson, G. L. 1972. The fluid mosaic model of the structure of cell membranes. Science 175:720.

Singer, S. J. 1974. Molecular organization of membranes. Ann. Rev. Biochem. 43:805.

Microtubules

Blake, J. R., and Sleigh, M. A. 1974. Mechanics of Ciliary Locomotion. Biol. Rev. 49:85.

Borgers, M., and DeBrabander, M. 1975. Microtubules and microtubule inhibitors. New York: Elsevier North-Holland.

Olmstead, J. B., and Borisey, G. G. 1973. Microtubules. Ann. Rev. Biochem. 42:507.

Osborn, M., and Weber, K. 1977. The display of microtubules in transformed cells. Cell 12:561.

Roberts, K. 1973. Cytoplasmic microtubules and their functions. Prog. Biophys. Mol. Biol. 28:273.

Satir, P. 1974. How Cilia Move. Sci. Am. 231 (4):44.

Spooner, B. S. 1975. Microfilaments, microtubules, and extracellular materials in morphogenesis. Bioscience 25:440.

Nucleolus

Brinkley, B. R. 1965. The fine structure of the nucleolus in mitotic divisions of Chinese hamster cells in vitro. J. Cell Biol. 27:411.

Brown, D. D., and Gurdon, J. B. 1965. Absence of ribosomal RNA synthesis in the anucleate mutant of *Xenopus laevis. In* E. Bell (ed.), Molecular and Cellular Aspects of Development. New York: Harper & Row.

Busch, H., and Smetana, K. 1972. The Nucleolus. New York: Academic Press, Inc.

Ghosh, S. 1976. The nucleolar structure. Int. Rev. Cytol. 44:1.

Peroxisomes

DeDuve, C. 1969. The peroxisome: A new cytoplasmic organelle. Proc. R. Soc. (London) 173:71.

Novikoff, A. B., and Allen, J. M. (eds.). 1973. Symposium on "Peroxisomes." J. Histochem. Cytochem. 21:941.

Tolbert, N. E. 1971. Microbodies—peroxisomes and glycosomes. Ann. Rev. Plant. Phys. 22:45.

Ribosomes

Palade, G. E. 1975. Intracellular aspects of the process of protein synthesis. Science 189:347.

Rich, A., Warner, J. R., and Goodman, H. M. 1963. The structure and function of polyribosomes. Cold Spring Harbor Symp. Quant. Biol. 28:269.

Shore, G. C., and Tata, J. R. 1977. Functions for polyribosomes membrane interactions in protein synthesis. Biochem. Biophys. Acta 472:197.

Smith, D. W. E. 1975. Reticulocyte transfer RNA and hemoglobin synthesis. Science 190:529.

Spitnik-Elson, P., and Elson, D. 1976. Studies on the ribosome and its components. *In* W. E. Cohn (ed.), Progress in Nucleic Acid Research and Molecular Biology. New York: Academic Press, Inc., 17:77.

Weiss, J. M. 1953. The ergastoplasm: Its fine structure and relation to protein synthesis as studied with the electron microscope in the pancreas of the Swiss albino mouse. J. Exp. Med. 98:607.

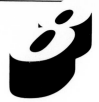

The Nervous Tissue

Edward G. Jones
and W. Maxwell Cowan

Development of Nervous Tissue

Neural Induction and the Formation of the Neural Tube

Except for the sensory epithelia and the associated ganglion cells of certain of the cranial nerves, all elements of the central and peripheral nervous systems are derived from a specialized region of ectoderm along the dorsal midline of the embryo. Initially, this zone is indistinguishable from the rest of the ectoderm, but under the inductive influence of the underlying notochord and the adjoining mesoderm, its cells become elongated and appear to be irreversibly determined to form neural tissue. In the human embryo, at about the 18-day stage, this specialized zone forms a slipper-shaped area immediately rostral to the *primitive knot*, or *Hensen's node*, and in transverse sections appears as a thickened and slightly depressed region dorsal to the notochord (Fig. 8–1). The central portion of this region is called the *neurectoderm*. Interposed between it and the nonspecialized or *somatic* ectoderm is a second specialized zone, the *neurosomatic junctional region*. The neurectoderm will form the *neural (or medullary) plate* from which the entire central nervous system is derived; the neurosomatic junctional region will give rise to the cells of the *neural crest* from which much of the peripheral nervous system (and a number of other tissues) will be formed.

As the epithelium of the neurectoderm thickens, the lateral edges of the neural plate become increasingly elevated to form a *neural groove* bounded on either side by raised *neural folds* (Fig. 8–1). Toward the end of the third embryonic week the lips of the neural groove fuse together in the upper cervical region. From this region the process of fusion extends rostrally and caudally, converting the original neural plate into a *neural tube* (Fig. 8–1). For a time, the tube remains open at its rostral and caudal ends (the openings are called the *anterior* and *posterior neuropores*), but with the closure of the neuropores (during the fourth embryonic week), it becomes completely closed. When the folds of the neural groove fuse, the cells of the neurosomatic junctional region are separated from both the somatic ectoderm and the neurectoderm and come to occupy a position along the dorsolateral aspect of the neural tube. This initially more or less continuous column of cells constitutes the *neural crest*. Subsequently, three vesicular swellings—called the *prosencephalic, mesencephalic,* and *rhombencephalic vesicles*—appear in the rostral part of the neural tube; respectively, they give rise to the forebrain, midbrain and hindbrain. The more caudal, unexpanded portion of the neural tube forms the spinal cord.

Histogenesis in the Neural Tube

Until shortly after its closure, the neural tube consists of a simple, columnar epithelium. However, as cell proliferation proceeds, the wall of the tube soon becomes converted into a *pseudostratified* epithelium, with nuclei at several levels but with each cell retaining a basal cytoplasmic process in contact with the *basement membrane,* or *basal lamina,* which surrounds the neural tube and separates it from the adjoining mesodermal tissues. The luminal processes of the cells are ciliated and joined to each other by a series of *junctional complexes* (or *terminal bars*). The epithelium as a whole is variously

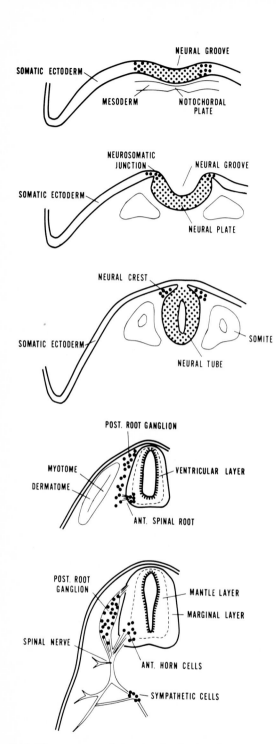

8–1 The sequence of changes that lead to the formation of the spinal cord and the associated nerve roots from the neural plate and the adjoining neurosomatic junctional region.

named the *germinal epithelium*, the *neuroepithelium*, and the *matrix* or *ventricular layer*; from it derive both the neuronal and supporting elements of the central nervous system.

As Figs. 8–2 and 8–3A show, all the readily identifiable mitotic figures in the neuroepithelium are found along its ventricular or luminal border. This unusual appearance results from the fact that although all the cells of the neuroepithelium are of the same type, their nuclei take different positions according to their stage in the cell cycle. This idea was initially formulated on cytological grounds in 1931 by Sauer, but it has been experimentally confirmed in several ways. Of these, the most convincing has been the analysis of cell proliferation in the neuroepithelium by tritiated [³H]thymidine autoradiography.

In autoradiographs of the neural tube taken within an hour or two after the administration of a small dose of [³H]thymidine to an animal, the label can be seen to have been incorporated into the DNA of cells whose nuclei lie in the basal or middle thirds of the neuroepithelium (Fig. 8–3B). At this time all other nuclei in the epithelium appear unlabeled. However, if the autoradiographs are prepared at a later time, say 8 to 12 h after administering the isotope, *most* of the nuclei in the epithelium (including those in the later stages of mitosis—metaphase, anaphase, and telophase) will be labeled. This type of experiment not only demonstrates that *all* the cells in the neuroepithelium are capable of DNA synthesis (and hence, of mitosis) but also suggests that cell proliferation in the epithelium proceeds in the following characteristic sequence. Interphase cells in the neuroepithelium (that is, those in the G_1 phase of the cell cycle—see Chap. 1) are elongated and their nuclei are in the upper or middle thirds of the epithelium (Fig. 8–2). As they enter the S phase of the next cycle, their nuclei first come to lie deeper within the epithelium; progressively later in this phase (which generally lasts about 8 to 12 h), the nuclei begin to migrate toward the luminal pole of the cell (Fig. 8–2). By the time the cell enters the G_2 phase of the cycle, its nucleus is close to the luminal margin, and the cell as a whole is beginning to round up by withdrawing its basal process from the basal lamina (Fig. 8–2). The G_2 phase lasts no more than 1 to 2 h and leads directly into the M phase, or mid- and late-mitotic phase of the cell cycle. Immediately before cytokinesis, the now more-or-less spherical cells appear to lose parts of their junctional complexes;

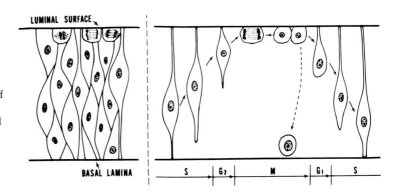

8–2 The pseudostratified character of the neuroepithelium and the pattern of interkinetic nuclear migration during the major phases of the cell cycle in the neuroepithelium.

this must be an extremely rapid process, because shortly after cytokinesis the two daughter cells resulting from telophase appear to have reconstituted the junctional complexes. The entire M phase lasts about 1 h and leads directly into the G_1 phase (which is of variable duration). During the G_1 phase the cells again become elongated, their nuclei descend, and their abluminal processes reestablish an association with the basal lamina (Fig. 8–2) before the next round of DNA synthesis. The changes in the structure of the cells at different phases of the cell cycle are strikingly demonstrated in scanning electron micrographs (Fig. 8–4).

The duration of each phase of the mitotic cycle varies somewhat from region to region in the neural tube and with the age of the embryo. (At late embryonic stages the G_1 phase becomes progressively longer and the entire cycle may take as long as 48 to 96 h.) However, the pattern of DNA synthesis and the interkinetic migration of the nuclei of the neuroepithelial cells remain the same. The process of cell proliferation continues in this manner for a variable period of time in

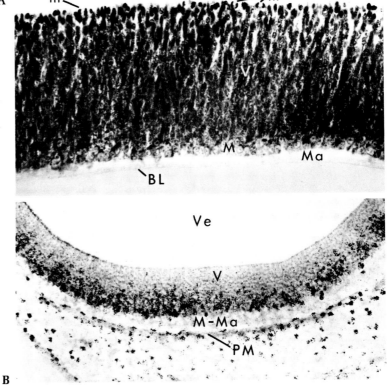

8–3 **A.** A photomicrograph of the neuroepithelium of the chick optic tectum with the mitotic figures **(m)** confined to the luminal surface. Postmitotic cells **(M)** form a mantle or intermediate zone immediately above the marginal zone **(Ma). BL,** basal lamina. Thionin stain. × 450.
B. An autoradiograph of the neuroepithelium a short time after the administration of [³H]thymidine. Only the nuclei in the deeper part of the ventricular zone **(V)** are labeled, together with cells in the surrounding pia mater **(PM). Ve,** ventricle. × 90.

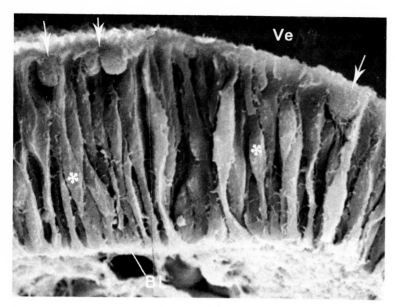

8–4 A scanning electron micrograph of the neuroepithelium to show the form of the interkinetic cells (marked by **asterisks**) and the dividing cells at the ventricular surface **(Ve)** marked by **arrows. BL:** basal lamina. × 1,300. (From Seymour, R. M., and Berry, M. 1976. J. Comp. Neurol. 160:5. Courtesy of Dr. M. Berry.)

different regions of the neural tube. However, at some point DNA synthesis ceases in certain of the neuroepithelial cells. The time at which the first postmitotic cells appear can also be readily determined by [³H]thymidine autoradiography, which has been used experimentally to establish the "dates of birth" of various classes of neurons. On completing their last mitotic division, one or both of the daughter cells become arrested in the G_1 phase of the cell cycle, and, in this state, the cells migrate out of the neuroepithelium and come to lie in a layer deep to the nuclei of the neuroepithelial cells. This newly formed layer of postmitotic cells is known as the *mantle* or *intermediate zone* (Fig. 8–3A and B); it is the growth of this layer that leads to the progressive expansion of the walls of the brain and spinal cord. The region of the neural tube between the developing mantle zone and the basal lamina is called the *marginal zone*. Initially this zone contains only the basal processes of the neuroepithelial cells, but it is soon invaded by the processes of the postmitotic cells in the mantle zone of the same area and by processes entering it from other parts of the nervous system.

We do not know what factor, or factors, bring about the cessation of DNA synthesis in certain cells while permitting it to continue for several further cell cycles in others. Nor is it known whether the two daughter cells of a terminal mitosis are both determined to form either nerve cells (or *neurons*) or supporting cells (*neuroglial*

cells), or if one cell may later differentiate into a neuron and the other into a glial cell. At present only three generalizations seem justifiable. First, in most regions of the nervous system the first neurons and the first glial cells *seem* to be formed at the same time. Second, glial cell proliferation generally continues for some time after all the neurons are formed, and indeed most glial cells retain the capacity for further division throughout the life of the organism. Third, the larger nerve cells are generated earlier than the smaller neurons in the same region. There is also some evidence that the positional information that determines where the larger (projection) neurons will send their axons becomes fixed at the time of the last mitotic division. In view of the importance of the changes that occur in the neuroepithelial cells when they become postmitotic, it is somewhat surprising that they show so little morphological evidence that the differentiated state has been established. In the light microscope, the only indications that the cells have made this transition are (1) their location in the mantle zone, and (2) the fact that they appear more rounded and have rather more cytoplasm. In the electron microscope they can be seen to have lost their junctional complexes, but otherwise they display the same cytoplasmic organelles as the neuroepithelial cells.

The cells of the mantle zone are customarily called *neuroblasts* (if they give rise to mature neurons) or *glioblasts* (if they form neuroglial changes that they undergo (including the growth and elaboration of their various processes and appendages) simply reflect their prior commitment to the neuronal or glial cell line.

The subsequent fate of these cells and their mature morphological appearance will be considered in a later section. With the notable exception of the last remaining neuroepithelial cells, which persist in the mature nervous system as the *ependymal cells* lining the ventricular system of the brain and spinal cord, all cells in the nervous system migrate, at least once, from the region in which they are generated to their definitive location. The details of the migratory process remain to be determined (at present it is thought to be similar to the migration of ameboid cells elsewhere), but one intriguing suggestion is that migrating neurons may be directed toward their terminal loci by the neighboring preformed neuroglial cell processes. Certainly, in many parts of the nervous system, the glial cells have long radially oriented processes (which may extend across most of the thickness of the expanding neural tube, or its derivatives), and the migrating neurons are nearly always found in close association with such processes (Fig. 8–5). In certain genetic disorders characterized by early degeneration or incomplete development of the glial cells, the neurons in the affected regions fail to migrate in the normal manner.

Some Less Common Histogenetic Patterns

The pattern of cell proliferation, differentiation, and migration just described is typical of most regions of the central nervous system, but in certain regions a different sequence of events occurs. In the cerebral hemispheres, a second proliferative zone appears immediately deep to the neuroepithelium. In this *subependymal* or *subventricular* layer (Fig. 8–6), cellular proliferation leading to the production of neurons and glial cells persists for some time after mitosis in the neuroepithelium has ceased. In the cerebellum, there is an early migration of a population of precursor cells (that is, true neuroblasts) from the neuroepithelium to form a second proliferative zone on the outer surface of the cerebellar cortex. In this layer (known as the *external granular layer*), cell proliferation continues for several weeks, the precursor cells giving rise to at least four different classes of neuron, including the enormous population of small granule cells whose later migration is illustrated in Fig. 8–6.

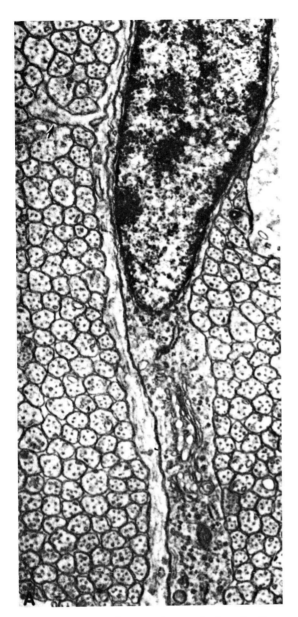

8–5 A low-power electron micrograph of a migrating granule cell (right) associated with a glial process (left) in the developing cerebellar cortex. × 21,300. (From Rakic, P. 1971. J. Comp. Neurol. 141:253. Courtesy of P. Rakic.)

cells). However, because the neuroblasts can no longer divide, the suffix *blast* (often used in cytology for a precursor cell) is inappropriate; *neuroblast* should be replaced by *young neuron*. In sum: the newly formed neurons and neuroglial cells are differentiated cells, and the further

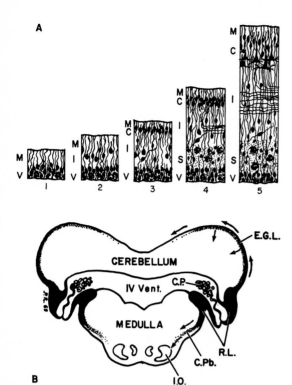

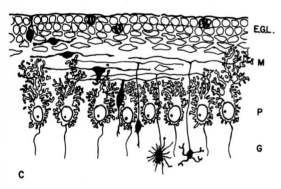

8–6 A. The progressive enlargement of the marginal and mantle or intermediate **(I)** zones of the neural tube at the expense of the neuroepithelial or ventricular **(V)** and subventricular **(S)** zones. **B.** The formation of the proliferative external granular layer **(EGL)** of the cerebellum from the rhombic lip **(RL)** of the developing brainstem. Several of the nuclei of the brainstem are also formed from the rhombic lip **(arrows). C.** Proliferation in the external granular layer and the migration of the granule cells **(G)** of the cerebellar cortex. (Drawings by P. Rakic to illustrate various of his publications, from Sidman, R. L. 1970. *In* The Neurosciences, Second Study Program. New York: Rockefeller University Press; courtesy of R. L. Sidman and P. Rakic.)

As they migrate from the neuroepithelium, or from one of the secondary proliferative zones in the central nervous system, the differentiated neuronal and glial cell precursors either are ellipsoidal in shape or have a single leading process. Such cells are said to be *apolar* and *unipolar*, respectively. A few neurons in the vertebrate central nervous system persist into adult life as *unipolar neurons*, but most pass through a *bipolar phase*. Several different classes of bipolar neurons are seen in the mature nervous system (Fig. 8–7), but the great majority develop a number of processes and are collectively called *multipolar neurons*. The development of the glioblasts is less well documented, and although it is formally convenient to divide them into two classes—astroblasts and oligodendroblasts (for the precursors of astrocytes and oligodendrocytes, which are the two main categories of supporting cell in the central nervous system)—there is little cytological distinction between them.

The Neural Crest and Its Derivatives

Whereas the neuroepithelium gives rise only to neurons, glial cells, and the modified columnar epithelium that forms the ependymal lining of the ventricles and the choroid plexuses (*see* below), the *neural crest* gives rise to an extremely diverse range of cells and tissues. Most of the nonneural derivatives are dealt with elsewhere in the appropriate chapters of this volume; they include:

1. The cells of the pia mater and arachnoid mater
2. Certain of the branchial cartilages and odontoblasts, and some of the cranial mesenchyme
3. Pigment-producing cells of the skin and subcutaneous tissues
4. Chromaffin tissue, including the chromaffin cells of the adrenal medulla

The neural derivatives include most of the sensory neurons of the cranial and spinal sensory ganglia, the postganglionic neurons of the sympathetic and parasympathetic ganglia, and the Schwann cells of the peripheral nervous system, including the sheath or satellite cells of the ganglia. At present we know little about the factors responsible for this morphogenetic diversity, but it is clear that many of the cells of the neural crest are determined, at a very early stage in development, to follow one or another line of dif-

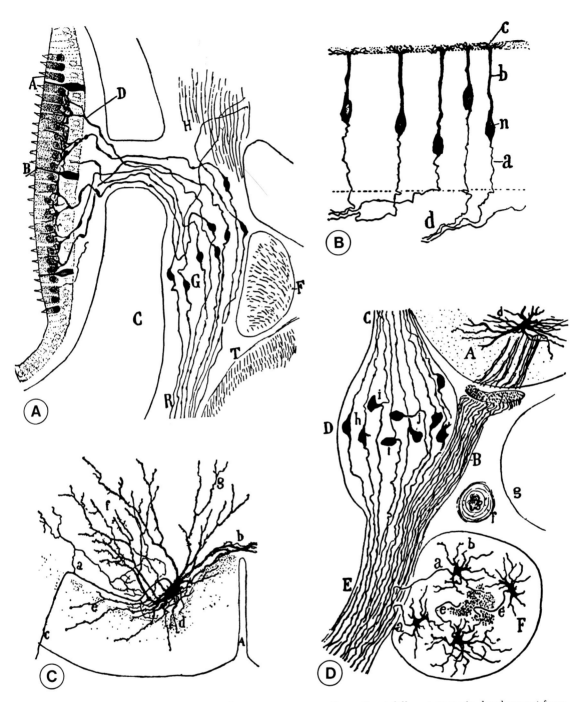

8–7 A variety of neurons stained by the Golgi method. **A.** Bipolar cells **(G)** of the vestibular ganglion in the mouse. Peripheral branches **(D)** innervate vestibular hair cells; central branches **(R)** pass to brain. **B.** Bipolar neurons in the olfactory mucosa with peripheral processes **(b)** and centrally projecting axons **(a). C.** A large multipolar neuron in the anterior horn of the spinal cord. **D.** Spinal ganglion cells at different stages in development from their early bipolar form **(h)** to the mature pseudounipolar form **(i).** (**A**, spinal cord; **B**, ventral root; **F**, sympathetic ganglion.) (From Cajal, S. Ramón y. 1909. Histologie du Système Nerveux de l'Homme et des Vertébrés, vol. 1. Republished 1952. Madrid: Consejo Superior de Investigaciones Cientificas.)

ferentiation. The neuronal derivatives of the crest show almost the same range of morphological specializations as do the cells in the central nervous system. Most of the cells begin as *apolar* neuroblasts; those in the sensory ganglia associated with cranial nerves V, VII, IX, X, and XI and with the dorsal roots of spinal nerves become *bipolar* and then, because the two processes come together and fuse, become *secondarily unipolar* (and for this reason are sometimes referred to as *pseudounipolar* neurons) (Fig. 8–7). The sympathetic and parasympathetic neuroblasts generally grow many processes and become *multipolar*.

Other Neural Derivatives

The sensory epithelia of certain of the cranial nerves, and the associated sensory ganglion cells, derive either wholly or in part from specialized ectodermal thickenings, or *placodes*. The first of these is the nasal placode, which gives rise to the olfactory epithelium in the upper part of the nose, including the olfactory receptors. The latter are modified bipolar neurons, with a shorter peripheral process or dendrite being specifically adapted to respond to the presence of odoriferous molecules in the overlying mucous layer, and with a longer central process (or axon) passing into the olfactory bulb. Parts of the trigeminal (Vth), facial (VIIth), glossopharyngeal (IXth), and vagal (Xth) ganglia are also formed from placodes. The thickened epithelial cells sink beneath the rest of the ectoderm and then proliferate and migrate toward clusters of neural crest cells that form the remaining parts of the ganglia. The *acousticovestibular placode* gives rise to the sensory epithelia of the internal ear and to the bipolar ganglion cells of the *acoustic* (or *spiral*) ganglion and on the *vestibular ganglion*. It is not known if the sheath cells in the trigeminal, facial, glossopharyngeal, or vagal ganglia are derived from the placodes or from the neural crest, but in the case of the acoustic and vestibular ganglia, it is quite clear that the placodal epithelium can form both neurons and sheath cells.

The Structure of Neurons and Neuroglial Cells

The result of the histogenetic sequence outlined above is the production of two classes of cells that together constitute the nervous tissue. They are the nerve cells, or *neurons*, and the supporting or *neuroglial* cells.

Neurons

Functionally, the most significant single feature of neurons is that they are surrounded by an *excitable membrane* which, under normal resting conditions, is capable of maintaining a differential distribution of ions on either side of it. This membrane in turn gives rise to the so-called resting membrane potential of about 90 mV (inside negative), which may be either partially or wholly depolarized or hyperpolarized by influences from other nerve cells. In addition, each neuron has a characteristic morphological structure. Different classes of neuron may have radically different appearances (see Figs. 8–7 to 8–9), but all neurons have an underlying similarity in form. The expanded part of the cell containing the nucleus is the *cell soma*; in certain types of preparations, this is the only part of the neuron stained (see Fig. 8–10). However, when the cell is stained in its entirety (for example, by means of the Golgi method; see Figs. 8–11 and 8–12), one or more slender processes, which may be of considerable length and highly branched, can be seen extending from the soma. All the neurons illustrated in Fig. 8–8 have two distinct types of processes: a number of *dendrites* and a single *axon*. The *dendrites* are drawn out of the soma in such a way that it is often difficult to define their exact point of origin; and they usually undergo several generations of branching that become progressively narrower in diameter. Together with the soma, the dendrites provide the main recipient surface of the nerve cell, and the processes of other nerve cells terminate on them at specialized regions of contact called *synapses*. The sum of the influences (excitatory and inhibitory) exerted by other nerve cells at any instant determines the state of excitability of the neuron, and the soma–dendritic membrane can be regarded as an integrating mechanism that adds these influences together.

Also arising from the soma (or less commonly from one of the dendrites) is a single process, the *axon*. The axon is usually thinner than the dendrites, and when it arises from the soma, it usually does so at a clearly recognizable elevation, the *axon hillock*. Just beyond this elevation, the axon narrows over a length of a few microns, forming what is known as the *initial segment* of the axon. Beyond the initial segment it may at first increase in diameter somewhat, but as it passes to its destination, its diameter tends to re-

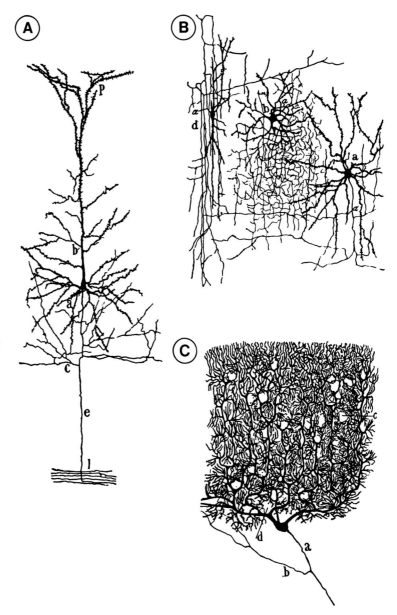

8–8 **A.** A pyramidal neuron from the cerebral cortex with a prominent apical dendrite **(b)**, several basal dendrites **(a)**, and a lengthy axon **(e)** which gives off a number of collateral branches **(c)** and enters the subcortical white matter. **B.** A variety of short-axon (Golgi type II) cells in the cerebral cortex. **a,** stellate; **b,** "spider-web"; **d,** "double bouquet." **C.** A cerebellar Purkinje cell with its extensive planar-arranged dendritic tree, axon **(a)** and recurrent axon collaterals **(b).** (From Cajal, S. Ramón y. 1911. Histologie du Système Nerveux de l'Homme et des Vertébrés, vol. 2. Republished 1952. Madrid: Consejo Superior de Investigaciones Científicas.)

main relatively uniform until it reaches its terminal arborizations. Although usually longer than the dendrites, the axon is of variable length and may terminate close to or at considerable distance from the soma. Along its course it may give off branches, the largest of which are termed *axon collaterals.* They may accompany the main axonal trunk or they may reenter the area containing the parent cell, in which case they are called *recurrent collaterals.* The axon and its branches are the main transmitting channels through which the neuron affects other nerve cells and other tissues such as muscles and glands, usually by the rapid conduction of nervous impulses.

The Shapes of Neurons. From the above it is apparent that neurons exhibit what has sometimes been called *dynamic polarization;* that is, they have a receiving surface—the synaptic sites on the dendrites and soma; an integrating mechanism—the somatic and dendritic membrane; an

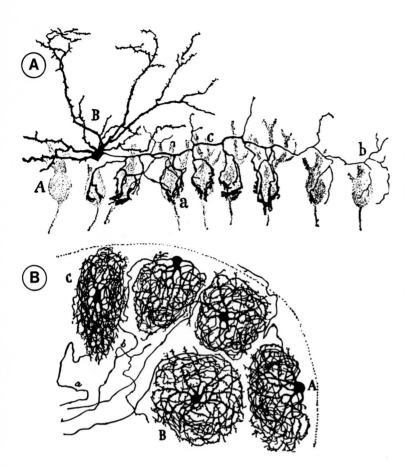

8–9 **A.** A basket neuron from the cerebellum with its axon **(c)** giving off characteristic axonal baskets **(a)** surrounding adjoining Purkinje cells **(A).**
B. Multipolar neurons with complex dendritic arborizations in the inferior olivary nucleus. (From Cajal, S. Ramón y. 1909. Histologie de Système Nerveux de l'Homme et des Vertébrés, vol. 1. Republished 1952. Madrid: Consejo Superior de Investigacions Cientificas.)

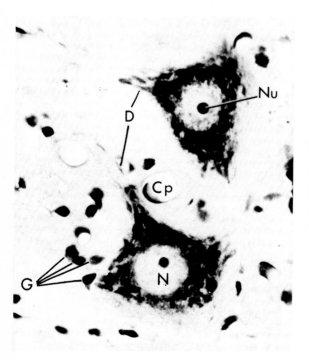

8–10 Two motoneurons from a Nissl-stained preparation of the spinal cord of a cat. Note the large, angular Nissl bodies in the cytoplasm, the pale nuclei **(N)**, the prominent nucleolus **(Nu)**, and the extension of the Nissl material into the large dendrites **(D).** Several small glial cells **(G)** are also shown, and a small capillary **(Cp).** × 480.

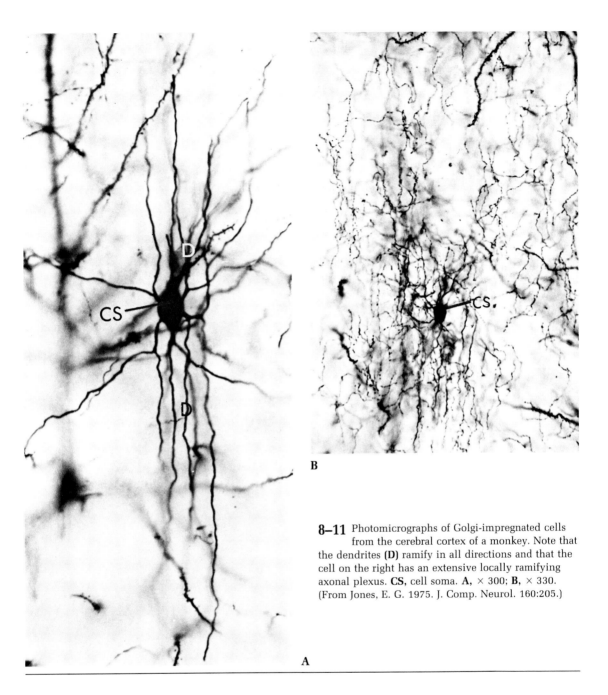

8–11 Photomicrographs of Golgi-impregnated cells from the cerebral cortex of a monkey. Note that the dendrites **(D)** ramify in all directions and that the cell on the right has an extensive locally ramifying axonal plexus. **CS**, cell soma. **A**, × 300; **B**, × 330. (From Jones, E. G. 1975. J. Comp. Neurol. 160:205.)

impulse initiating mechanism—the initial segment of the axon; and an impulse conducting process—the axon itself. Most neurons conform to this basic pattern of organization, although the overall shape of different nerve cells may vary considerably.

Perhaps the simplest class of neuron is that in which only a single process arises from the soma; such cells are commonly called *unipo-*

lar neurons. From the single process, several branches are usually given off, some of which are mainly receptive and function as dendrites; others are effectors and together they represent the branching axonal plexus of the cell. Unipolar neurons are particularly common in invertebrates. In vertebrates, true unipolar neurons are rare.

A second class of neuron that is also relatively

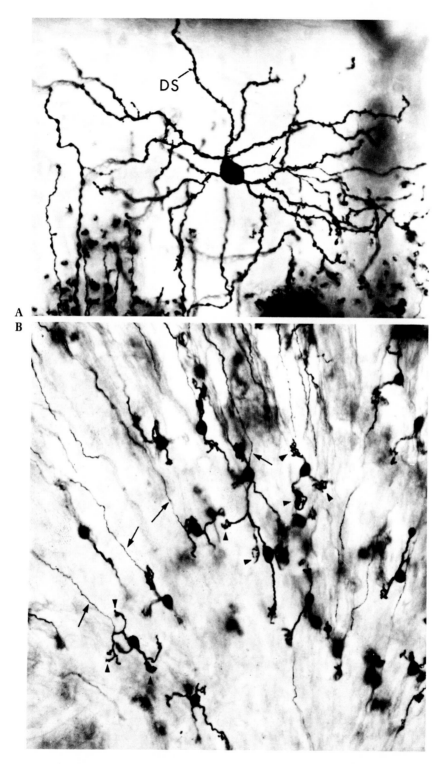

8–12 Photomicrographs of a stellate cell **(A)** and several granule cells **(B)** in Golgi-stained preparations of the cerebellar cortex of a monkey. **Arrows** indicate axons. **Arrowheads** in **B** indicate the terminal claws on the dendrites of the granule cells. Some of the axons of these cells arise from the dendrites. **DS,** dendritic spine. × 500.

uncommon in vertebrates, being found primarily in the retina and in the vestibular and acoustic ganglia, is the *bipolar neuron* (Fig. 8–7). Such neurons are relatively symmetrical, with the axon (or central process) and a single dendritic (or peripheral) process arising from opposite poles of the ovoid or elongated soma. The dendrite may or may not branch profusely, and the axon may be short (as in the retinal bipolar cells) or long (as in the vestibular and acoustic ganglion cells). A unique type of unipolar cell is found in the dorsal root ganglia of the spinal nerves and in the sensory ganglia of certain of the cranial nerves (Fig. 8–7). These cells, referred to above as *pseudounipolar neurons*, give rise to a single process that bifurcates into a peripheral process directed toward the skin and underlying tissues and a central process that enters the spinal cord or brainstem. It should be noted, however, that both the central and peripheral processes resemble axons in their structure and in their ability to conduct nerve impulses.

All other classes of neuron in the adult nervous system are *multipolar neurons*. That is, the parent soma gives rise to more than one dendritic trunk. Most neurons have only a single axon, although rare cases with multiple axons have been described. In a few special cases to be described later, the cell may lack an axon altogether. Within the general category of multipolar neurons, many types have characteristic shapes that are surprisingly constant from species to species and, within any one species, from individual to individual. These types have generally been given special names that either describe some aspect of their morphology or record the name of the investigator who first described them.

Perhaps the most typical multipolar neurons (Fig. 8–7) are the *motor cells*, or *motoneurons*, of the ventral horn of the spinal cord. The large somata of these cells customarily give rise to six or more large dendritic trunks that radiate in all directions from the perikaryon and branch into secondary and tertiary dendrites. The length of the primary dendrites is fairly uniform, so that the total *dendritic field*, (that is, the spatial volume occupied by all the dendrites together) is nearly symmetrical and, when viewed three-dimensionally, forms a round or ovoid figure enclosing the perikaryon.

In some cases the dendritic fields are particularly symmetrical, and because the dendrites radiate more or less uniformly in all directions, these cells are called *stellate neurons*. However,

few of the cells that are commonly termed stellate, such as those in the fourth layer of the cerebral cortex, have uniform dendrites or dendritic fields. More often, the field tends to be eccentric or flattened in one dimension, and then the cells are described as *spindle-shaped* or *fusiform*, for example.

Several types of multipolar neurons that have been given special names are shown in Figs. 8–8 and 8–9. Some of these neurons have long axons that leave the territory of the cell soma, and each has a highly characteristic dendritic field. The *Purkinje cells* of the cerebellar cortex have only ascending dendrites directed toward the surface of the cerebellum, but these dendrites and their branches are all oriented in the plane at right angles to the long axis of the cerebellar folia so that the dendritic field has a very narrow profile when viewed from the side. The *pyramidal cells* of the cerebral cortex are so named because of the pyramidal shape of their somata. From the base of the perikaryon, four or more branching *basal dendrites* extend laterally and downward; from its apex, an *apical dendrite* ascends toward the surface of the cortex giving off side branches along its course and commonly ending in a small spray of laterally directed branches. Another class of cells has a dendritic field in the shape of an inverted cone; these are the *mitral cells* of the olfactory bulb, so named because the shape of the cell soma was thought to resemble a bishop's miter.

In an unusual class of small multipolar cell, an axon is lacking altogether. These cells are most common in the retina, where they are called *amacrine cells* and in the olfactory bulb, where they are called *granule cells*. Although these cells lack an axon, they can influence the activity of other nerve cells by means of unusual specializations of their processes, which seem to have some of the characteristics of axons and dendrites (see Fig. 8–38).

In some instances the name given to a neuron is determined by the nature of its axonal ramifications. This is especially true of neurons with relatively short axons that break up into their terminal branches close to the parent cell soma. A well-known example is the *basket cell* of the cerebellar cortex, whose axons give sprays of small branches that enclose the somata of adjoining Purkinje cells as though in a series of baskets (Fig. 8–9 and 8–25). The small cell from the cerebral cortex illustrated in Figs. 8–7 and 8–11B with its highly branched and intensely intertwined axon, was called a spider-web cell by the

Spanish histologist Ramón y Cajal. Cajal referred to other cells of the type illustrated in Fig. 8–7 as double bouquet cells because of their long ascending and descending axonal systems. These latter two examples are of interest because they show that cells with essentially the same type of dendritic field (both would be called stellate cells) may give rise to quite different systems of axon branches.

The three examples given above show that the nature of a cell's axonal plexus may be just as characteristic as the shape of its dendritic field. And, as in the case of dendritic fields, certain basic types can be recognized. Very shortly after introducing the stain upon which so much of our knowledge of the shapes of nerve cells depends, the Italian histologist Camillo Golgi pointed out that most nerve cells fall into one of two classes. These two classes have come to be called Golgi type I and Golgi type II neurons. Golgi type I neurons have long axons that pass out of the region in which the parent cell soma is situated and terminate at some distance, either in some other part of the nervous system or in another tissue such as skin or muscle. The motoneurons of the spinal cord, the pyramidal cells of the cerebral cortex, and the Purkinje cells of the cerebellar cortex are all examples of Golgi type I cells. Golgi type II neurons, on the other hand, have short axons that ramify locally in the region of the parent cell soma and may not even extend much beyond the confines of its dendritic field (like the spider-web cell shown in Fig. 8–11B).

To get an idea of the significance of the Golgi classification, consider, for example, any of the ascending sensory pathways of the nervous system. The cells with long axons are the main transmission lines conveying information from the periphery through various synaptic relay centers (nuclei) to the cerebral cortex. Cells with short axons are situated at each synaptic station; they may influence cells with long axons that project up to the next level. The Golgi type II cells thus serve as modulators of synaptic transmission in the long pathways of the nervous system. A common alternative term for these cells is, therefore, *interneurons*, since they are, in a sense, intercalated between any two links in a long pathway.

The name applied to a particular type of nerve cell may vary depending on the nature of the histological preparation in which it is observed. The names of the examples cited above were derived from the *total* appearance of the nerve cell—soma, dendrites, and axon—as seen in the silver impregnation method of Golgi. Unfortunately, some names are based on the appearance of the cells when stained by more routine histological techniques that show only the cell somata. For example, the small stellate neurons of the cerebral cortex (Fig. 8–8) have been called granule cells, but the same term has also been applied to quite different cells in the cerebellar cortex (Fig. 8–12B), the dentate gyrus, the olfactory bulb, and certain other sites, even though their dendritic and axonal configurations are not at all comparable.

Factors Governing the Size and Shape of Neurons. Neurons differ greatly both in size and shape. Possibly the smallest neurons in the mammalian central nervous system are found in parts of the hypothalamus. Such neurons have somata measuring little more than 3 to 4 μm in diameter, and their axons and dendritic fields are comparably small. Among the largest cells are the giant pyramidal cells of the motor area of the cerebral cortex whose somata may measure as much as 120 μm in their largest dimension; and, in addition to giving rise to a long, thick apical dendrite, they have axons that may be 50 cm or more in length. Between these two extremes, all sizes can be found.

Two factors appear to determine the size of a cell: (1) the number, length, and diameter of its processes, and (2) the number of synapses that it receives on its surface. It is a useful generalization that neurons with the longest and thickest axons have the largest somata. In the case of one of the larger motoneurons in the lumbar or sacral parts of the spinal cord, for example, the axon may be almost a meter in length and 15 to 20 μm in diameter. Clearly, most of the volume of the cell is in the axon. As the axon itself appears to be incapable of synthesizing proteins and most other structural or functional constituents, the cell soma must maintain the appropriate amount of metabolic machinery to support the axon. Similarly, cells with long, thick, profusely branching dendrites also have large somata, and even though the dendrites have certain synthetic capabilities, there is evidence that they, too, are partly maintained by the soma.

The number and length of the dendrites possessed by a particular cell seem to be related to the number of synaptic contacts that it receives from the axons of other cells. The large motoneurons of the spinal cord, which integrate activity from many diverse sources, have been estimated to receive as many as 10,000 synaptic contacts, and the large Purkinje cells of the cerebellum may receive as many as 200,000. Small interneurons, on the other hand, have not only short axons of small diameter but also relatively few dendrites and ultimately few synaptic contacts.

The Structure of Nerve Cell Somata

Along with providing a large surface area of membrane that may receive synaptic contacts from other neurons, the cell soma, which contains the nucleus, is the trophic or nourishing center of the nerve cell. Chief among the functional characteristics of the nerve cell other than those concerned with the integration and transmission of nervous activity is the need to maintain itself and to supply various organelles and macromolecules to the terminals of its axon. This is achieved by the active synthesis in the soma of large amounts of proteins, lipids, etc., and a highly efficient somatofugal transport system that delivers these metabolic products and organelles to the cell's processes.

The Nucleus. The *nucleus* of most nerve cells is either spherical or ovoid, and is large relative to the size of the perikaryon.[1] Because a substantial part of the genome is continually being transcribed in keeping with the active synthetic state of the cell, it is euchromatic; that is, the nuclear chromatin is generally dispersed when seen with the electron microscope and the nucleus usually has a vesicular appearance when viewed with the light microscope (Fig. 8–10). The nuclear envelope, with its nuclear pores, is typical of that of all eukaryotic cells (Fig. 8–13). One, and sometimes two or even three prominent nucleoli are present within the nucleus; their fine structure is also typical of that in other protein-synthesizing cells. Associated with the nucleoli may be one or more "satellites," of which the female sex chromatin (corresponding to the heterochromatic X chromosome) is the best known (Fig. 8–14); this satellite was first described in neurons by Barr. These so-called Barr bodies may be attached to the nucleolus, to the inner face of the

---

[1]At one time it was thought that the nuclei of many large neurons (for example, those of the pyramidal cells of the hippocampus and the Purkinje cells of the cerebellum) were tetraploid, but this appears to have been due to a technical error in measuring the cells' DNA content.

nuclear membrane, or to both. Other nucleolar satellites and crystalline or filamentous intranuclear particles are occasionally seen, but they are uncommon and of uncertain significance.

The Perikaryon. Perhaps the most striking feature of the perikarya of neurons is the large amount of ribosomal material that they contain, a material that indicates the high rate of protein synthesis in these cells. As seen in the electron microscope, the ribosomal material is mainly in the form of multiple stacks of rough endoplasmic reticulum, but a great many free ribosomes and polyribosomal rosettes are also present. These clustered masses of free and attached ribosomes are strongly basophilic, and when nervous tissue is stained with basic dyes and viewed in the light microscope, many neurons are seen to contain irregularly shaped clumps of intensely stained cytoplasmic inclusions. These inclusions are customarily called *Nissl bodies* after the German neurologist F. Nissl, who first used aniline dyes to study the nervous system. Although the cytoplasm of all neurons is basophilic because of their rich content of RNA, not all neurons have distinct Nissl bodies. Such bodies can be seen particularly well in the large motoneurons of the spinal cord (Figs. 8–10 and 8–13) and in large dorsal root ganglion cells; the cytoplasm of smaller neurons merely shows a diffuse, dustlike basophilia.

The *Golgi complex* is also prominent in all neurons; at the electron-microscopic level, it is commonly seen as several groups of flattened and dilated smooth-walled sacs and vesicles of variable size, usually near the nucleus but sometimes extending into the bases of the larger dendrites (Figs. 8–13 and 8–15). The reason for this well-developed Golgi complex is incompletely understood; but by analogy with its appearance in other secretory cells it probably is engaged in both the glycosylation of proteins and the packaging of secretory products within membrane-bound vesicles. The most common vesicles found in neurons are the *synaptic vesicles*, which are present in large numbers in axon terminals and appear to contain the neurochemical transmitter agents that mediate synaptic function (see p. 309). We do not know to what extent these vesicles are produced in the perikaryon or in axon terminals. However, the cell bodies of some types of neuron contain variable numbers of membrane-bound dense vesicles that represent their main neurosecretory product or en-

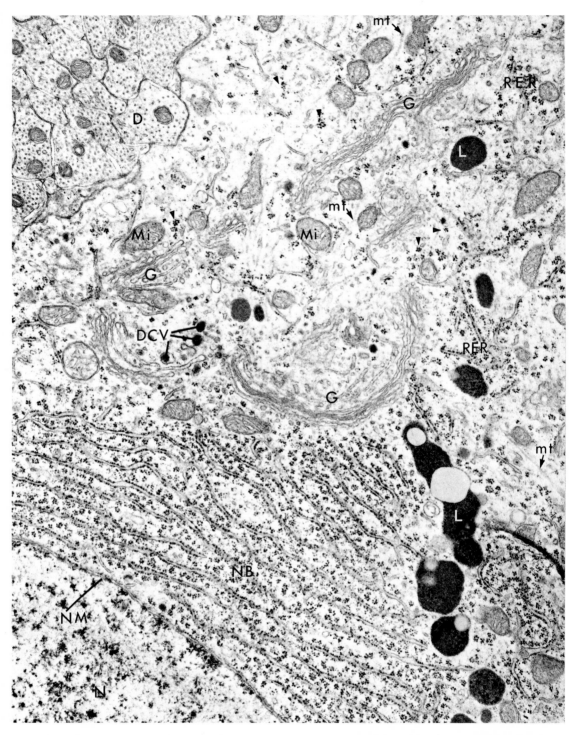

8–13 An electron micrograph of a pyramidal cell from the cerebral cortex showing the nucleus (**N**) with its surrounding envelope (**NM**), a prominent Nissl body (**NB**), several lysosomes (**L**), mitochondria (**Mi**), dense-core vesicles (**DCV**), and microtubules (**mt**). The cell has an extensive Golgi complex (**G**), a good deal of rough endoplasmic reticulum (**RER**), and free ribosomes (**arrowheads**) outside the obvious Nissl body. In the upper left corner there are several transversely sectioned dendrites (**D**) containing microtubules cut in transverse section. × 25,000.

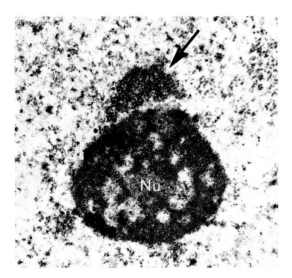

8–14 Nucleolus **(Nu)** and nucleolar satellite **(arrow)** from cortical neuron of a female rat. × 29,000.

zymes involved in its synthesis. In certain small neurons of the autonomic nervous system, for example, many dense-core vesicles about 600 to 800 Å in diameter are present in the perikaryon as well as in the axons and their terminals. These vesicles contain catecholamines which, when condensed with formaldehyde, cause the neurons to be intensely fluorescent under ultraviolet light (Fig. 8–16).

Neurosecretory products that do not act as chemical transmitter agents at synapses but are released into the general circulation are such polypeptide hormones as oxytocin and vasopressin, and the various hypothalamic-releasing hormones. These hormones are produced by the neurons in the hypothalamus and are transported in membrane-bound vesicles down their axons for release near the blood vessels of the neurohypophysis or the median eminence. The neurosecretory material is synthesized in the endoplasmic reticulum, packaged in the Golgi complex, and transported in large (approximately 2,000 Å) membrane-bound, dense-core vesicles. Aggregations of these vesicles in the axons and their terminals may be selectively stained by means of the Gomori technique, and in the light microscope they appear as large granular masses called *Herring bodies*.

As might be expected in metabolically active cells, *mitochondria* are also present in very large numbers in neuronal perikarya (Fig. 8–13). They vary a great deal in size, density, and general configuration, but probably not more so in these than in other cells.

Some of the most ubiquitous elements in neuronal perikarya are the large numbers of *microtubules* and *neurofilaments*. Aside from the fact that they are found in all parts of the perikaryon, the microtubules (which have a diameter of about 250 Å) appear to be identical to those in

8–15 An osmic-acid-stained preparation of a spinal ganglion to show the reticular appearance of the Golgi apparatus. × 500.

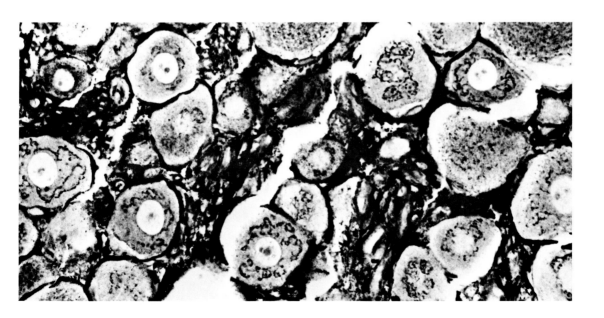

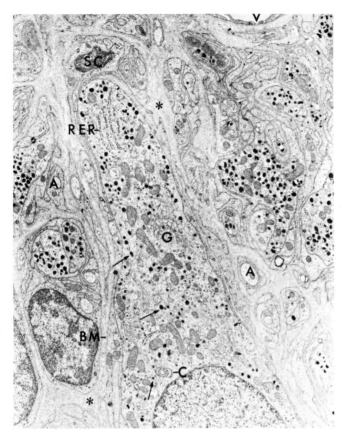

8–16 Electron micrograph of a catecholamine-synthesizing neuron from the nodose ganglion of a cat. Note the dense-core vesicles in the cytoplasm **(arrows). RER,** rough endoplasmic reticulum; **G,** Golgi region; **C,** cilium; **V,** blood vessel. × 13,500. (From Grillo, M. A., Jacobs, L., and Comroe, J. H., Jr. 1974. J. Comp. Neurol. 153:1; courtesy of M. A. Grillo.)
◁

8–17 Lipofuscin granules **(arrows)** in the cytoplasm of neurons in the human superior cervical ganglion. **C,** satellite Schwann cells. × 300.   ▽

other cells (Figs. 8–13 and 8–19). At present it is not known if neurofilaments (which have a diameter of about 100 Å) are identical to the intermediate filaments (Fig. 8–19B) seen in other cells, and until their substructure and chemical composition have been adequately characterized, this will remain unsolved. Of course, both microtubules and neurofilaments are visible only at the electron-microscopic level. However, when neurons are stained with certain heavy metals (especially silver salts), thick, intertwined fibrillar strings up to 2 or 3 μm in diameter can be seen; they are known as *neurofibrils* (Fig. 8–24). It is thought that they represent metallic silver deposited on bundles of neurofilaments; but in some cases, at least, the silver deposits may be around microtubules as well. As in the case of Nissl bodies, neurofibrils appear most distinctly in large neurons; in smaller cells the neurofibrillar methods give a more diffuse staining of the cytoplasm, although the staining is probably still associated with neurofilaments.

Lysosomes of various kinds are also found in neurons. They appear as dense, or multivesicu-

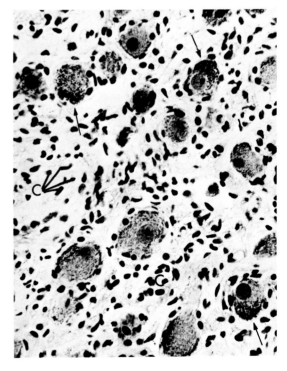

lar, bodies exhibiting positive acid phosphatase activity. Their number varies from neuron to neuron and seems to increase with the age of the individual. The yellowish pigment *lipofuscin,* which accumulates in neurons with advancing age, probably represents insoluble residues remaining from lysosomal activity. In the human brain, the yellowish lipofuscin pigment may build up with age to the extent that it may occupy more than half the cross-sectional area of the somata of certain cells (Fig. 8–17). Its ultrastructural counterpart is a heterogeneous membrane-bound body composed of dense particles and lipid-filled vacuoles (Fig. 8–13). Other pigments occur naturally in certain groups of neurons. Perhaps the best known is the melanin of the nerve cells in the substantia nigra of the midbrain. The pigment seems to be absent in human infants, but by puberty it has reached its maximal development. This pigment is also enclosed in membrane-bound structures resembling lysosomes.

Neurons also frequently contain one or two typical centrioles, usually associated with a cilium that may protrude for some distance from the cell surface. Their significance is quite obscure; possibly they simply reflect the epithelial origin of the nerve cells.

The Structure of Dendrites

In some respects, dendrites can be regarded as extensions of the cell soma. For example, at both the light- and electron-microscopic levels it is difficult to define the point at which the soma ends and a dendrite begins. The dendrites appear as though they were "drawn out" from the soma, and most of the organelles typical of the perikaryon extend for considerable distances into the dendrites. The main-stem dendrites of larger neurons can usually be seen in material stained with routine neurohistological stains, because they often contain Nissl bodies or dispersed Nissl substance as distinct as that found in the soma (Figs. 8–10 and 8–22A). By electron microscopy, considerable amounts of rough-surfaced endoplasmic reticulum, free ribosomes, and components of the Golgi complex are often seen in the proximal portions of dendrites (Fig. 8–18).

As they extend away from the soma, the dendrites taper and the successive generations of branches to which they give rise are always of smaller diameter than the parent trunk. In some

neurons the dendrites appear to be beaded with irregular dilatations and constrictions. In some instances, this appearance may be artifactual; but in others, the beading clearly reflects the natural state of the dendrites.

As the dendrites extend away from the soma, the rough endoplasmic reticulum and other organelles become progressively diminished; and in the more peripheral dendrites, rough endoplasmic reticulum and free ribosomes are sparse or lacking entirely. The presence of ribosomal material is important, however, because at the electron-microscopic level it serves to distinguish dendrites from axons. But the most striking feature of dendrites is the presence of many microtubules and neurofilaments (Figs. 8–18 and 8–19). In general, they are much more conspicuous than in the soma and are more regularly aligned along the axis of the dendrite. The number of filaments and tubules seems to vary with the diameter of the dendrite and the distance from the soma. Some microtubules and neurofilaments may extend from the soma almost to the tips of the dendrites; as the dendrites branch, bundles of filaments and tubules diverge into the branches. The microtubules are thought to be involved in the transport of various materials, including proteins and such organelles as mitochondria, from the perikaryon to the distal portions of the dendrites. By tracing the movement of labeled proteins after injecting radioactive precursors into the soma, it has been possible to demonstrate "dendritic transport" with a rate of about 3mm/h, a rate comparable to that at which certain materials move down the axon. This transport is inhibited by drugs, such as colchicine and vinblastine, which cause a breakdown of microtubules. The role of the neurofilaments is unknown.

One of the most distinctive features of dendrites is the presence on their surfaces of synaptic contacts made by the axon terminals of other neurons. The structure and general distribution of synapses will be discussed elsewhere. Here we need only note that all dendrites receive synaptic contacts at various points along their length. In addition, the dendrites of many (but by no means all) classes of neurons have multiple small protrusions (dendritic spines) that are specialized to receive synaptic contacts.

As seen in Golgi preparations, a typical dendritic spine is a pedunculated structure with an expanded tip measuring 0.5 to 2 μm in diameter, and a narrow stalk 0.5 to 1 μm long (Fig. 8–20).

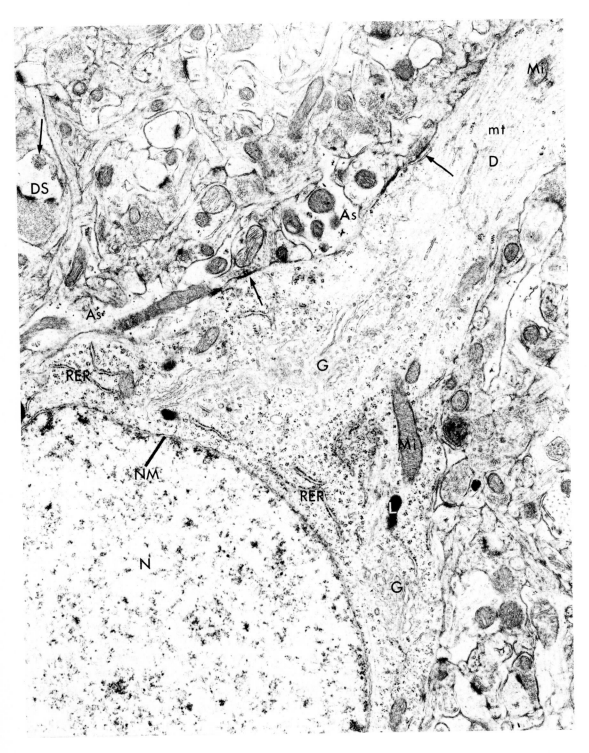

8–18 An electron micrograph of the apical portion of a pyramidal neuron from the cerebral cortex, with its apical dendrite extending toward the upper right corner. **N,** nucleus; **NM,** nuclear envelope; **RER,** rough endoplasmic reticulum; **G,** Golgi complex; **L,** lysosome; **Mi,** mitochondrion; **mt,** microtubules; **D,** dendrite; **As,** astrocytic processes; **DS,** dendritic spine with spine apparatus **(arrow).** The **arrows** in the cell soma mark the sites of two synapses on the surface of the neuron. × 15,000.

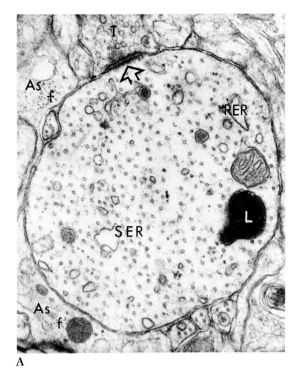

A

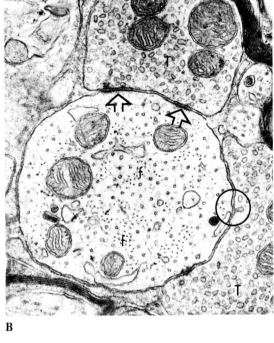

B

By electron microscopy the stalk can often be seen to contain one or more microtubules; but the expanded tip usually appears as an amorphous matrix (Fig. 8–21), except at the point of synaptic contact where a considerable amount of electron-dense material is attached to the postsynaptic membrane. In many spines, one or more smooth-walled vesicular or saclike structures are seen, often alternating with bands of electrondense material; they constitute a special organelle of unknown function called the spine apparatus.

On any given neuron, the spines may vary considerably in shape and size. Generally, those situated most distally are the longest and may even be bifid, and those near the soma are the smallest and are often simple, sessile protrusions of the dendritic surface, usually without a spine apparatus. There is also a fairly consistent relationship between the number of dendritic spines and the distance from the soma. Generally, there are few or no spines on the proximal portions of the stem dendrites but their amount quickly increases to a maximum, maintained over the middle portion of the dendritic system, and then declines again toward the distal portions of the dendrites (Fig. 8–37). Although the significance of this characteristic spine distribution is difficult to assess, it is clear that, when present, the

8–19 Electron micrographs of two transversely sectioned dendrites that contain saccules of smooth endoplasmic reticulum (**SER**), many microtubules, and neurofilaments (**f**). The dendrites are contacted by axon terminals (**T**), which form distinct synapses at the points marked by the large **open arrows**. The dendrites are surrounded by astrocytic processes (**As**), which also contain filaments (**f**). **L**, lysosome. The circled area in **B** shows an endocytotic vesicle thought to indicate retrieval of synaptic vesicle membrane from membrane of terminal. **A**, ×38,500; **B**, ×29,000 (From Rockel, A. J., and Jones, E. G., 1973. J. Comp. Neurol., 147:61.)

spines represent the principal synaptic surface on the dendrites. The dendritic spines may also be labile structures in the sense that they may disappear after deafferentation or sensory deprivation and possibly with increasing age.

Structure and Function of Axons

Unlike dendrites, the axon usually appears as a unique and sharply defined process. It usually arises from the soma as a conspicuous conical elevation called the axon hillock (Figs. 8–22 to 8–24), but it may also arise from the basal portion of a stem dendrite. The *initial segment* of the axon is commonly the narrowest portion of

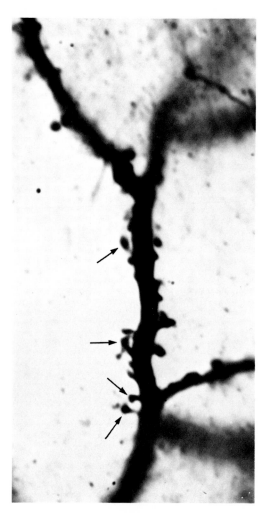

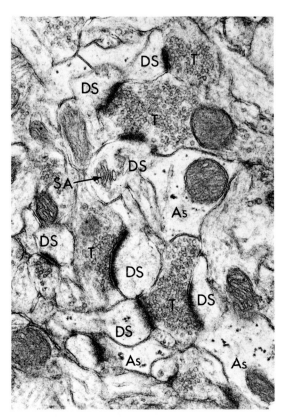

8–21 Electron micrograph of a series of dendritic spines **(DS)**, each contacted by an axon terminal **(T)**. One spine contains a spine apparatus **(SA)**. **As,** astrocytic cytoplasm. Cerebral cortex of rat. × 28,000.

8–20 A high-power light micrograph of a portion of a dendrite of a cell in the inferior colliculus of a cat, stained by the Golgi method, to show the appearance of the dendritic spines **(arrows)**. × 1,800. (From Rockel, A. J., and Jones, E. G. 1973. J. Comp. Neurol. 147:11.)

the process, and, like the axon hillock, has a number of distinctive morphological features. The most obvious feature of the axon hillock is the relative absence of free ribosomes and rough-surfaced endoplasmic reticulum, so that in Nissl-stained preparations it appears as a palely stained, triangular or fan-shaped area free of Nissl granules. In electron micrographs, the most obvious ultrastructural feature of the axon hillock is the presence of many microtubules and neurofilaments streaming from the perikaryon into the initial segment. The extent of the initial

segment is easiest to define in cells whose axons subsequently acquire a *myelin sheath;* in them the segment reaches from the apex of the axon hillock to the beginning of the myelin sheath. It is characterized by the absence of ribosomes and rough-surfaced endoplasmic reticulum and by two special features (Fig. 8–22B). The first feature is the presence of an electron-dense "undercoating" beneath the plasma membrane (or *axolemma*). The undercoat measures about 200 Å in thickness and is deficient only beneath the regions of synaptic contact that are sometimes made by the terminals of other axons on the initial segment. The membrane of the initial segment generally has the lowest threshold of excitability, and is therefore commonly the site of initiation of the nervous impulse. To what extent the dense membrane undercoat facilitates this is not known, but it is noteworthy that a similar

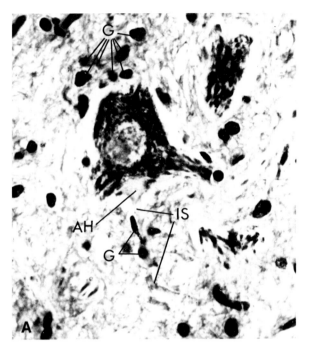

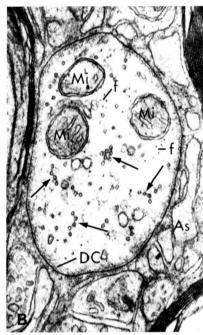

dense undercoat is found at the nodes of Ranvier in myelinated axons (see below).

The second distinguishing feature of the initial segment is the fact that the microtubules passing through it are collected into small bundles. In these bundles the individual microtubules are linked at intervals to one or more of their neighbors by multiple small cross-bridges best seen in cross sections of the initial segment (Fig. 8–22B). When seen in longitudinal sections, the electron-dense cross-bridges resemble the rungs on a ladder, which in myelinated axons can be followed to the point where the myelin sheath is acquired. In axons that do not acquire a myelin sheath, the fasciculation of the microtubules and the dense membrane undercoat cease at a comparable distance from the soma. These two features of the initial segment seem to be peculiar to the central nervous system; they have not been found in neurons of the dorsal root ganglia or autonomic nervous system.

In addition to the microtubules, the axon contains a variable number of neurofilaments of unknown function (Fig. 8–53). They are commonly regarded as semirigid structures that provide a skeletal framework for the axon, but this has not been proved; other suggestions—for example, that they guide the axon toward its destination during development—are dubious. We do know,

8–22 In a Nissl-stained preparation the axon hillock **(AH)** and initial axonal segment **(IS)** appear essentially unstained. An electron micrograph of a transversely sectioned initial segment shows a characteristic electron-dense undercoating beneath the axolemma **(DC)**, and fasciculated clusters of microtubules **(arrows)**. **Mi,** mitochondria; **f,** neurofilaments; **G,** glial cells; **As,** astrocytic cytoplasm. **A,** motoneuron of cat, thionin stain, × 650. **B,** electron micrograph from cat inferior colliculus, × 40,000.

however, that in cold-blooded animals the number of neurofilaments increases during cold adaptation, and in all animals their number increases after injury to the axon.

The Terminations of Axons

Axons end by forming functional contacts with other nerve cells, muscle fibers, or gland cells. In the central nervous system the axon of a neuron terminates on other nerve cells in the specialized junctions already referred to as synapses. As an axon approaches the region of the nervous system in which it terminates, it generally branches repeatedly; if it has a myelin sheath, the initial branches are myelinated, but as they approach the neurons with which they are destined to

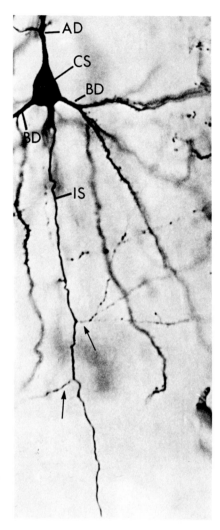

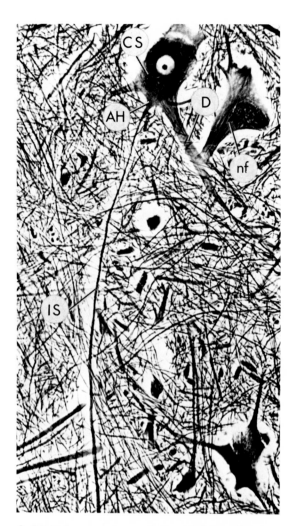

8–23 Pyramidal cell from the cerebral cortex of a
monkey showing collateral branches **(arrows)**
arising from initial segment of axon **(IS)**. **BD**, basal
dendrites; **CS**, cell soma; **AD**, apical dendrite. Golgi
stain. × 700.

8–24 Motoneuron from spinal cord of a cat showing
axon hillock **(AH)** and initial segment **(IS)**.
Dendrites **(D)** and cell soma **(CS)** contain neurofibrils
(nf) best seen in part of second cell to right. Bodian
stain. × 850.

make synaptic contact, they usually branch again
(Figs. 8–25 and 8–26), and the final branches are
unmyelinated.[2]

The appearance of the endings in silver-
stained preparations is variable, but because they

are usually in the form of tiny swellings on the
axon branches, they are customarily called synaptic *boutons* (or buttons) (Figs. 8–26 to 8–28).
A synapse is formed where a synaptic bouton becomes closely associated with a portion of the
membrane of another nerve cell (commonly its
soma or dendrites) and where, by means of a series of morphological specializations to be described below, the release of a neurochemical
transmitter agent from the axon terminal can influence the conductance of the recipient (or *postsynaptic*) cell. Synaptic boutons may occur as
swellings at the very ends of the terminal
branches of an axon, in which case they are

[2]The individual branches making up the terminal spray en-
gendered by a long axon are commonly called *telodendria* (sin-
gular, *telodendron*). This term, which means "branches at a
distance," is often inappropriate if applied to the branches of
a short, unmyelinated axon belonging to a Golgi type II neuron,
for in the highly branched axonal plexus commonly engen-
dered by such a cell, it is not possible to distinguish a major
parent trunk much beyond the initial segment.

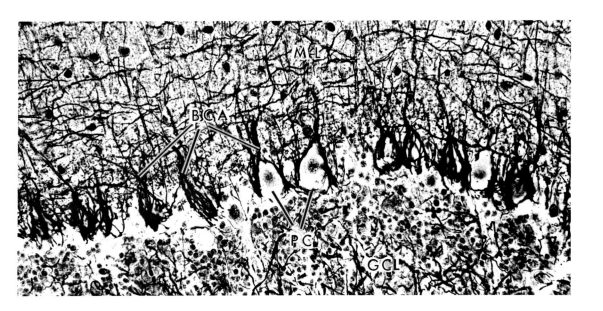

8–25 Basket cell axons **(BCA)** traversing molecular
layer **(ML)** of cat cerebellum and descending to
form terminal baskets over somata of Purkinje cells
(PC). **GCL,** granule cell layer. Reduced silver stain.
× 500.

8–26 Terminal axon **(open arrow)** branching **(arrow)**
and terminating as a series of terminal boutons
(arrow heads) on soma **(CS)** and axon initial segment
(IS) of a pyramidal cell in the cerebral cortex of a
monkey. **AD,** apical dendrite; **DS,** dendritic spines.
Golgi stain. × 500. (From Jones, E. G. 1975. J. Comp.
Neurol. 160:205.)

called *boutons terminaux*. Some axon terminals
are exceedingly large and may cover a great deal
of the surface of the postsynaptic cell, in which
case they may be called *calyces,* or *baskets*
(Figs. 8–9 and 8–25). Other synaptic contacts
may occur at intervals along a terminal segment
of an axon or, in the case of a short axon, along
most of its length. In this situation, they are usually called *boutons en passant* (or *boutons de
passage*) (Figs. 8–26 and 8–27). The term synapse was introduced by Sherrington in 1897, and
even at that time there was good physiological
evidence (based on the direction of transmission
of nervous impulses from cell to cell and the differential sensitivity of the junctional region to
pharmacological agents such as nicotine) that
this was a functionally specialized part of the
nervous system. Morphological evidence about
the nature of the synapse rested solely on the
knowledge that axonal boutons terminaux could
be seen making contact with the somata and dendrites of nerve cells. Only since electron microscopy has been used to study the nervous system
have the structural correlates of synaptic activity
become fully understood.

A typical synapse in the central nervous system consists of a presynaptic element and a post-

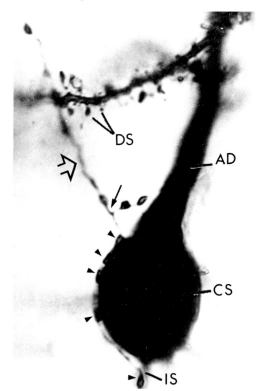

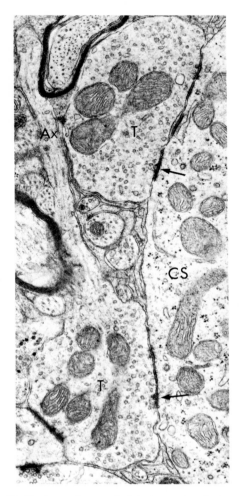

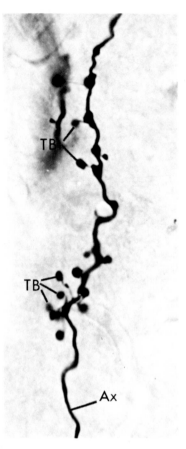

8–28 Terminal portion of an axon **(Ax)** in inferior colliculus of cat showing terminal boutons **(TB)**. Golgi stain. × 1350. (From Rockel, A. J., and Jones, E. G. 1973. J. Comp. Neurol. 147:11.)

8–27 Electron micrograph showing preterminal axon **(AX)** and two terminal boutons **(T)** making synaptic contact **(arrows)** on cell soma **(CS)** of a neuron in inferior colliculus of a cat. × 18,000. (From Rockel, A. J. and Jones, E. G. 1973. J. Comp. Neurol. 147:61.)

synaptic element in close association with one another at a region of membrane specialization and separated only by a narrow extracellular cleft (Figs. 8–27 and 8–29). The commonest form of synapse in the central nervous system is one in which the presynaptic element is a synaptic bouton and the postsynaptic element a dendrite. This type of synapse will be used to illustrate the general form (Fig. 8–30). The membranes of the pre- and postsynaptic elements are aligned to one another with a gap of only 200 to 300 Å between them and without any intervening tissue elements. The region of apposition between the axon terminal and the dendrite is usually some-

what more extensive than the region of membrane specializations that seems to constitute the active zone of the synapse. At the apparently active zone, the gap between the pre- and postsynaptic profiles, usually called the *synaptic cleft*, often becomes slightly wider than the 150- to 200-Å gap that separates other contiguous profiles in the nervous system, and it may contain fine filaments or dense material derived from the outer leaflets of the opposed pre- and postsynaptic membranes, which are much more electron-dense than elsewhere. In addition to being denser, the membrane specializations appear thicker than the rest of the dendritic or axonal membrane, because attached to them is electron-dense material that extends for a variable distance into the pre- and postsynaptic cytoplasm (Figs. 8–30 and 8–31). On the presynaptic side

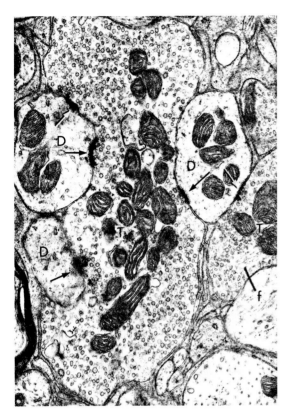

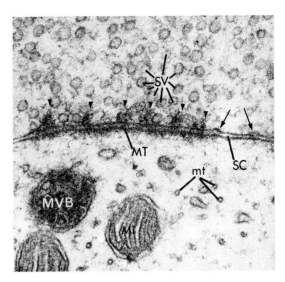

8–30 Electron micrograph of a synapse, showing synaptic vesicles **(SV)**, presynaptic dense projections **(arrowheads)**, and possible sites **(arrows)** of incorporation of synaptic vesicle membrane into membrane of terminal. **MT,** membrane thickening; **SC,** synaptic cleft. Postsynaptic dendrite contains mitochondria **(Mi)**, a multivesicular body **(MVB)**, and microtubules **(mt)**. × 57,000. (From Rockel, A. J., and Jones, E. G. 1973. J. Comp. Neurol. 147:61.)

8–29 Electron micrograph from inferior colliculus showing two terminal boutons **(T)** of the type illustrated in Fig. 8–28. They make synaptic contacts **(arrows)** with small dendrites **(D)**. One terminal contains a small cluster of neurofilaments **(f)**. × 27,000 (From Rockel, A. J., and Jones E. G. 1973. J. Comp. Neurol. 147:61.)

the material appears as a series of conical protrusions from the membrane. On the postsynaptic side, there is often a greater amount of dense material attached to the inner surface of the postsynaptic membrane; it is more homogeneous than on the presynaptic side and can extend for a considerable distance into the dendritic cytoplasm. The membrane thus appears "thicker" than that on the presynaptic side. In other words, the synaptic membrane specializations are asymmetrical. The pre- and postsynaptic membranes and their associated dense material most probably have a different protein composition from the rest of the nerve cell membrane. One clear manifestation of this is the fact that they may be selectively stained in electron-microscopic preparations with phosphotungstic acid.

The second distinguishing feature of a synapse is the presence in the presynaptic element of large numbers of clear-centered vesicles (*synaptic vesicles*) with diameters ranging from 400 to 600 Å. These vesicles contain neurotransmitter substances that are the basis of chemical synaptic action. The concentration of the vesicles is usually greatest near the presynaptic membrane specialization, and many lie between the presynaptic dense projections of the membrane. As an action potential invades the axon terminal, synaptic vesicles fuse with special "release sites" in the presynaptic membrane between the dense projections and there discharge their content of transmitter into the synaptic cleft. The transmitter then diffuses to the postsynaptic membrane where it interacts with special receptor molecules in the postsynaptic membrane; this leads to a change in the membrane conductance of the postsynaptic neuron.

The only other consistent components of every synapse are mitochondria in the presynaptic process, their number varying with the size of the terminal (Figs. 8–27 and 8–29). In addition, a few sacs or tubules of agranular endoplasmic reticulum may be present and in some

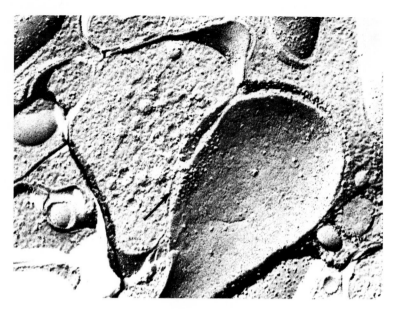

8–31 Freeze-etch preparation of a synaptic contact in cerebellum. **Arrow** indicates synaptic cleft. Note synaptic vesicles in terminal **(left)** and particles in postsynaptic membrane of Purkinje cell dendritic spine **(right)**. × 79,000. (From Landis, D. M., and Reese, T. S. 1974. J. Comp. Neurol. 155:93; courtesy of Dr. T. S. Reese.)

cases microtubules and neurofilaments also extend into the axon terminal. The neurofilaments, if found in the presynaptic process, are either diffusely scattered or occasionally aggregated in a single bundle that forms a loop or ring around a central cluster of mitochondria. In the latter case, neurofibrillar stains often show the axon terminals as ringlike boutons (Fig. 8–75B).

From electrophysiological studies, we know that synapses may be either *excitatory* or *inhibitory* depending on whether their activation drives the membrane potential of the postsynaptic neuron toward or away from its threshold level for firing nerve impulses. In chemical synapses these effects are usually mediated by different neurotransmitter agents because, as a general rule, an individual nerve cell releases only one kind of transmitter agent from its axon terminals. Certain transmitters that have differing actions at different postsynaptic sites presumably do so because of differences in the postsynaptic receptors or in the properties of the postsynaptic membranes.

In parts of the vertebrate central nervous system, inhibition has often been found to involve Golgi type II neurons. Such neurons are, therefore, often termed *inhibitory interneurons*. Examples of such inhibitory interneurons are the basket cells of the cerebellum and the Renshaw cells of the spinal cord. However, not all inhibitory neurons are of the Golgi type II variety; the Purkinje cells of the cerebellum have relatively long axons, but we now know that they act to inhibit the cells of the deep cerebellar nuclei. Conversely, not all neurons with short axons are inhibitory; some (for example, the granule cells of the cerebellum) are clearly excitatory.

Synapses in the central nervous system vary in their morphology. The earliest indication of this came from the work of E. G. Gray, who noted in 1959 that synapses could be divided into two categories on the basis of differences in the width of the synaptic cleft and in the extent of the postsynaptic membrane thickenings. The typical axodendritic synapse described on page 306 is an example of what Gray referred to as a *type I synapse* (Fig. 8–32). The two characteristics of this type of synapse are a widening of the intercellular gap at the synaptic cleft to approximately 300 Å and a pronounced accumulation of dense material beneath the postsynaptic membrane. The most striking feature of these synapses is the asymmetry in the pre- and postsynaptic membrane specializations; thus they are now referred to as *asymmetrical synapses*. In Gray's second type of synapse (type II synapses, Fig. 8–33) the synaptic cleft is only slightly wider than the normal intercellular gap (approximately 200 Å) and the postsynaptic membrane specialization is less marked. Little or no dense material is seen attached to the deep surface of the postsynaptic membrane, and because the two apposed membranes appear equally "thick," such synapses are now usually called *symmetrical synapses*.

Although the pre- and postsynaptic mem-

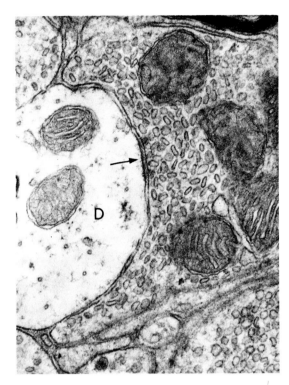

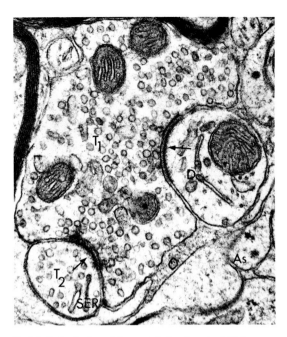

8–33 Spherical vesicle-containing terminal **(T₁)** making asymmetrical synaptic contacts **(arrows)** with a dendrite **(D)** and another axon terminal **(T₂).** Thalamus of cat. **SER,** smooth endoplasmic reticulum; **As,** astrocytic processes. × 35,000.

8–32 Flattened vesicle-containing axon terminal making symmetrical synaptic contact **(arrow)** with a dendrite **(D)** in inferior colliculus of cat. × 36,000. (From Rockel, A. J., and Jones, E. G. 1973. J. Comp. Neurol. 147:61.)

brane specializations appear in single electron micrographs as linear structures, they are, in fact, fairly extensive plaquelike structures that may measure as much as 1×1 μm. The postsynaptic plaques of asymmetrical synapses are frequently perforated in one or more places, so that in a section passing perpendicularly through the plaque, the axon terminal appears to be associated with two or more postsynaptic "thickenings" (Fig. 8–29). Perforation of the postsynaptic plaques seems to be uncommon in symmetrical synapses.

Although to some extent the asymmetrical and the symmetrical synapses represent the extremes of a continuum, most synapses encountered can be placed readily in one or the other class. The significance of this is emphasized by the observation that the synaptic vesicles in the presynaptic processes associated with the two classes may also differ. If nervous tissue is fixed in aldehyde-containing solutions with buffers of relatively high osmolality, the synaptic vesicles in some axon terminals become "flattened,"

ovoid, or disc-shaped (Fig. 8–32), whereas those of other terminals retain the spherical form commonly seen after osmium tetroxide fixation alone (Fig. 8–33). Uchizono first noted that in the cerebellar cortex, where the functions of most synaptic contacts are known, this flattening of the synaptic vesicles occurs only in the terminals of known inhibitory neurons. Furthermore, because the synaptic vesicles in the terminals of the granule cell axons (which are known to be excitatory) remain spherical (S vesicles) under the same conditions of fixation, it was suggested that the presence of flattened (or F) vesicles in aldehyde-fixed material might serve as an identifying marker for inhibitory synapses and that spherical vesicles might always be associated with excitatory synapses. The subsequent association of flattenable synaptic vesicles with symmetrical membrane specializations and spherical vesicles with asymmetrical membrane thickenings, made first by Colonnier for synapses in the cerebral cortex, strengthened the idea that there was a close relationship between vesicle morphology and functional synaptic type. The flattening of the synaptic vesicles is clearly an artifact in-

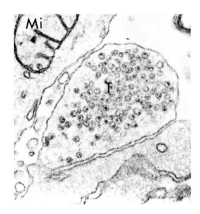

8–34 Noradrenergic terminal **(T)** from tissue culture
of rat superior cervical ganglion. Note large
proportion of dense-core vesicles demonstrated by
soaking tissue $10^{-5}M$ norepinephrine before fixation.
Mi, mitochondrion. × 40,000. (Courtesy of Dr. M. I.
Johnson.)

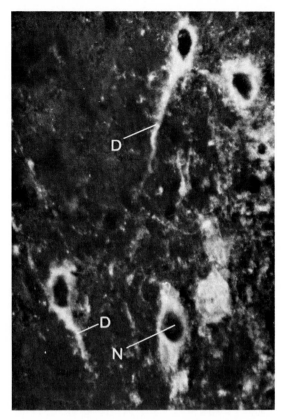

8–35 Noradrenergic neurons in locus coeruleus of a
rat demonstrated by binding of a fluorescent-
labeled antibody to enzyme dopamine-β-hydroxylase.
D, dendrites; **N,** nucleus × 950. (Courtesy of B. K.
Hartman and L. W. Swanson.)

duced by the high osmolality of the aldehyde fixative solutions, but in many parts of the brain
and spinal cord, the flattening is sufficiently consistent to provide a useful basis for classifying
synapses. However, it has become clear that the
association of flattened synaptic vesicles and the
presence of an inhibitory synaptic transmitter is
not universal. Several instances are now known
in which the presynaptic process exerts an inhibitory influence but contains spherical vesicles. The mechanism responsible for the flattening of certain synaptic vesicles is not clear, but it
presumably reflects some basic differences either
in the vesicle membrane or possibly in its content of synaptic transmitter. In some situations
the vesicles that become flattened in aldehyde-
fixed material are clearly of the same size as
those that remain spherical, but others that become irregular in shape (or pleomorphic) are distinctly smaller in diameter.

A third distinct class of synaptic vesicle has
been recognized in axons that are known to release catecholamines or indoleamines. This will
be considered in greater detail in the section on
the autonomic nervous system, but we shall note
here that the terminals of certain classes of ami-
nergic neurons in the central nervous system
contain small, spherical vesicles with electron-
dense "cores" identical to those found in sympathetic nerve terminals (Fig. 8–34). These vesicles have diameters of 400 to 600 Å, with dense
cores approximately 250 Å in diameter. In rou-
tinely fixed material the granular vesicles of

these "G synapses" are not particularly prominent, because the material in the dense cores is
not well retained. However, if the tissue is fixed
in potassium permanganate or presoaked in the
appropriate biogenic amine, the cores are seen to
be present in most of the vesicles.

Such small dense-core vesicles are to be distinguished from a larger type that is found in
small numbers in virtually every type of axon
terminal in the nervous system. The larger vesicle has a diameter of approximately 1,000 Å and
a core diameter of approximately 500 Å. One or
more of them may be found in terminals containing small dense-core vesicles or clear vesicles,
either spherical or flattened, and occasionally
they are even found in the neuron soma. Their
significance is unknown.

Other, even larger dense-core vesicles (up to
2,000 Å in diameter) are associated with the
transport and release of various hormones by the

neurosecretory neurons of the hypothalamus (*see* p. 131 and Chap. 29).

The site of formation of the clear and smaller dense-core vesicles is not certain. Some evidence suggests that they may be formed in the Golgi complex of the neuronal soma and that they are transported down to the terminals as part of the general "axoplasmic flow." This view is based partly on the known functions of the Golgi complex and partly on the fact that the neuronal soma usually contains considerable amounts of the appropriate neurotransmitter substance and of the enzymes involved in its synthesis. For example, the somata of neurons that release norepinephrine at their axon terminals contain norepinephrine and the enzyme dopamine-β-hydroxylase (which produces norepinephrine from dopamine—the amine of dihydroxyphenylalalanine) (Fig. 8–35). On the other hand, smooth-walled, clear-centered vesicles are rarely seen in axons or in the somata of neurons, and since it is known that substantial amounts of most neurotransmitters can be synthesized in axon terminals, it is evident that many vesicles must be formed locally within nerve endings, possibly from the smooth endoplasmic reticulum. Direct evidence for this comes from studies on the uptake of exogenous proteins by axon terminals (Fig. 8–36). If a histochemically identifiable marker such as the enzyme horseradish peroxidase is present in the extracellular space surrounding the terminals of an axon, it is rapidly taken up by the terminals in coated vesicles. At a slightly later stage, peroxidase-laden coated vesicles can be seen to fuse with the cisternae of smooth endoplasmic reticulum in the terminal and to lose their coats or shells, which appear to remain free in the terminal. Synaptic vesicles, containing horseradish peroxidase, then bud off from the cisternae and are free to pass toward the presynaptic membrane, to fuse with it, and in the process to release the enzyme (and whatever transmitter may have been incorporated into the vesicles) into the synaptic cleft. If the terminal is subjected to repetitive stimulation, it can also be shown that as it becomes depleted of synaptic vesicles, its circumference is progressively enlarged. These experimental observations suggest a continuous recycling of the synaptic vesicle membrane, with the vesicular membrane first becoming incorporated into the presynaptic membrane, then moving to one side of the presynaptic specialization, and finally being returned to the interior of the axon terminal in the form of a coated vesicle.

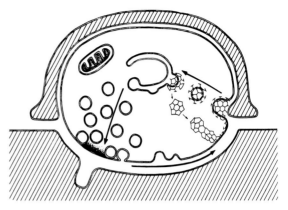

8–36 Postulated mechanism for recycling of synaptic vesicle membrane at neuromuscular junction. Vesicles discharge contents by exocytosis and membranes are incorporated into membrane of terminal; moving away from synaptic region, incorporated membrane is taken up as coated vesicle by endocytosis; joining smooth endoplasmic reticulum, it loses dense coat and is pinched off as new synaptic vesicle. (From Heuser, J. S., and Reese, T. S. 1973. Evidence for recycling of synaptic vesicle membrane during transmitter release at the frog neuromuscular junction. J. Cell Biol. 57:315; courtesy of T. S. Reese.)

The Distribution of Synapses. Axon terminals may make synaptic contacts with any portion of the surface of another neuron (Fig. 8–37). Although the majority occur on dendrites and perikarya, the axon terminals of one neuron may also contact the axon of another; the only parts of nerve cells that have never been seen to receive a synapse are those segments of an axon covered by a myelin sheath.

Synapses on dendritic spines are usually termed *axospinous synapses*. They are usually found on the expanded tips of spines, and each spine receives at least one. Because not all neurons have spines on their dendrites, axospinous synapses are not always present; however, when they are present, they tend to be of the asymmetrical type, and the weight of evidence points to their being excitatory in function. Synapses on the shafts of dendrites are called *axodendritic synapses*. They may be either symmetrical or asymmetrical, and their relative distribution and density depends on the type of neuron. The dendrites of some cells are covered with both types of synapse, whereas others have relatively few of one or the other type, and some have few of either type. Generally, the symmetrical synapses predominate on the larger dendritic trunks near

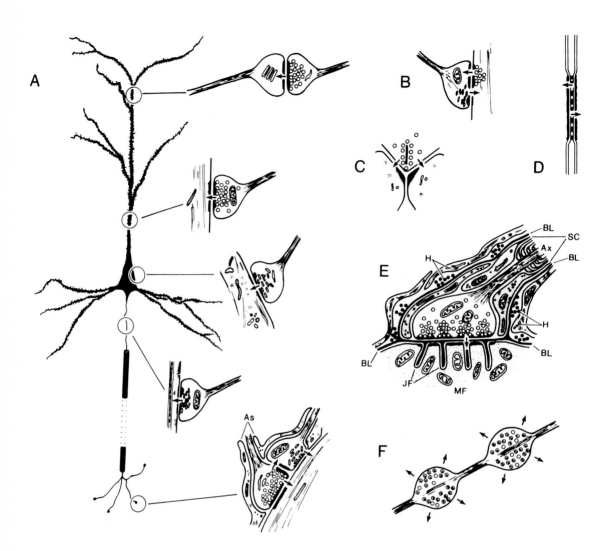

8–37 Types of synapse; **arrows** indicate direction of transmission. **A.** Types of synaptic contact received or made by pyramidal cell of cerebral cortex. From above, down: axospinous; axodendritic, axosomatic; initial segment synapse; axoaxonic, and serial synapse. **As,** astroglial covering. **B.** Reciprocal synapse of olfactory bulb. **C.** Ribbon synapse of retina. **D.** Electrical (gap junction) synapse. **E.** Motor end plate. **Ax,** myelinated axon; **BL,** basal lamina; **H,** fibroblast processes and collagen bundles forming sheath of Henle; **JF,** junctional folds; **MF,** muscle fiber; **SC,** Schwann cell processes; **T,** axon terminal. **F.** Adrenergic terminal in sympathetic nervous system.

the soma. Synapses on the perikaryon are known as *axosomatic synapses*. Again, their numbers and type vary from cell to cell; cells that receive few axosomatic synapses tend to have only symmetrical synapses on the soma; those that receive

many tend to have both types. Where a synapse is found on the initial segment of the axon or adjacent axon hillock of a neuron, it may be referred to as an *initial-segment synapse*. Because of the critical role of the initial segment in impulse initiation, synapses located on or near it are in a unique position to influence the discharge of the cell. It is significant therefore that wherever such synapses have been observed, they have invariably been of the symmetrical type, and it is generally assumed that they exert an inhibitory effect on the postsynaptic cell. In some instances a terminal from one axon may form a synapse on a terminal of another: this arrangement is called an *axoaxonic synapse*. Axoaxonic synapses seem to be involved in the phenomenon of *presynaptic inhibition*, because their action tends to reduce the amount of transmitter released by the postsynaptic axon terminal. Occasionally axoaxonic synapses of this type are serially arranged so that one process is postsynaptic at one synapse and presynaptic (on another process) at a second synapse. Such arrangements are *serial synapses*.

The remaining classes of synapses are all rather unusual and have been demonstrated in only a few sites in the nervous system. In some cases dendrites have been found to contain clusters of synaptic vesicles and membrane specializations indistinguishable from those seen in axon terminals. Such processes are termed *presynaptic dendrites*, and because they usually contact other dendrites, the synapses they form are *dendrodendritic synapses*. Such dendrodendritic synapses have now been described in several sites such as the thalamus where they are of the symmetrical type and the presynaptic dendrite usually contains flattened vesicles. A special type of dendrodendritic synapse has been found in the olfactory bulb between the dendrites of the mitral cells and the processes of granule cells. In this case the mitral cell dendrites form asymmetrical synapses (associated with spherical synaptic vesicles) on the granule cell processes; usually within a few microns of such a contact, the same granule cell process forms a *reciprocal synapse* on the mitral cell dendrite. The granule cell processes usually contain flattenable synaptic vesicles and form symmetrical synapses (which are known to be inhibitory) on the mitral cells. *Somatodendritic* and *somatosomatic* synapses have also been described in certain amphibia and in the sympathetic ganglia of mammals. As the names suggest, the presynaptic element in both cases is the cell body of a neuron.

Another form of synapse is the so-called *ribbon synapse*, the best known examples of which are found in the retina. In these cases the axonal process of one type of cell makes synaptic contact with the juxtaposed processes of two other cell types (see Chap. 33). These "triad" synapses are characterized by the presence in the presynaptic element of an electron-dense synaptic ribbon. The synaptic ribbon is invariably aligned perpendicular to the presynaptic membrane and the synaptic vesicles are gathered about it instead of aggregated at the presynaptic membrane.

All the synapses described so far are chemical synapses because they act through the intermediary of a chemical synaptic transmitter. A final synaptic type (relatively infrequent in mammals but very common in other vertebrates and in invertebrates) is the so-called *electrical synapse*. In these synapses the pre- and postsynaptic elements are joined through low-resistance gap junctions so that the electrical activity set up in one cell readily spreads to the next cell without a significant delay. The gap junctions found between neuronal processes are identical to those found in other tissues in which electrical coupling occurs (*see* Chap. 3). In certain cases, an axon terminal may make both a conventional (chemical) and an electrical synapse with a postsynaptic element. The best-known example of such a mixed chemical and electrical synapse is in the ciliary ganglion of birds, but similar contacts have been found in the lateral vestibular nucleus and in the mesencephalic nucleus of the trigeminal nerve of mammals.

Neuroglia and Other Supporting Cells

Although neurons tend to dominate any microscopic section of nervous tissue, they form only a relatively small percentage of the total population of cells present in the section. In most regions they are far outnumbered by the generally smaller nonneuronal or supporting cells, which in the central nervous system are collectively referred to as *neuroglial cells*. Such cells may account for more than one-half the total weight of the brain, and they may outnumber the neurons by as much as 10:1 to 50:1.

The supporting cells are characterized by their generally small size, their ubiquity, and their large numbers. Because of their small size, only their nuclei are seen in routine preparations (Figs. 8–10, 8–22A, and 8–38). The nuclei vary in diameter from 3 to 10 μm, which is about the same size as the very smallest neurons. They are found between neuronal somata and within fiber tracts. Unlike neurons, probably all supporting cells retain the capacity to proliferate under appropriate circumstances.

The Supporting Cells of the Central Nervous System

Two main classes of supporting cell are recognized in the brain and spinal cord (Fig. 8–39). The first consists of *astrocytes* and *oligodendrocytes*, sometimes known collectively as the macroglia. The second class is a heterogeneous group of cells, including the *ependymal cells*, which form the epithelial linings of the choroid plexuses, of the ventricular system of the brain, and of the central canal of the spinal cord; a va-

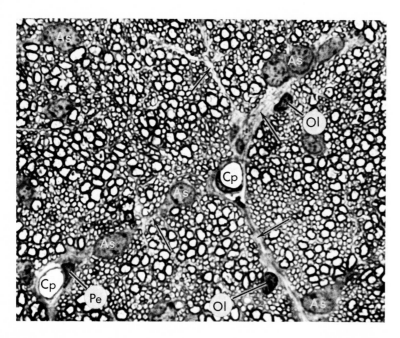

8–38 Cross section of monkey optic nerve showing myelinated axons, astrocytes **(As)**, and oligodendrocytes **(Ol)**. Septa **(arrows)** formed by astrocytic cytoplasm contain capillaries **(Cp)**, one of which is associated with a pericyte **(Pe)**. Toluidine-blue stained plastic section. × 1,600.

riety of vascular and perivascular cells; and cells commonly called *microglial cells*, once thought to be mesodermal rather than neurectodermal in origin but now regarded as immature, or resting, glioblasts.

Astrocytes. As the name implies, astrocytes are star-shaped when demonstrated by heavy metal preparations that impregnate the whole cell (Fig. 8–40A and B). A small, irregularly shaped cell soma gives rise to a number of pro-

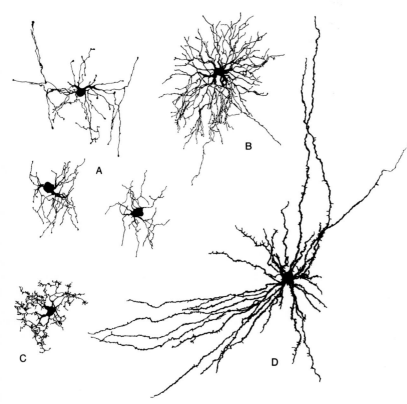

8–39 Camera lucida drawings at same magnification (× 1,000) showing oligodendrocytes **(A)**, protoplasmic astrocyte **(B)**, microglial cell **(C)** and fibrous astrocyte **(D)**. Golgi stain, cerebral cortex of monkey.

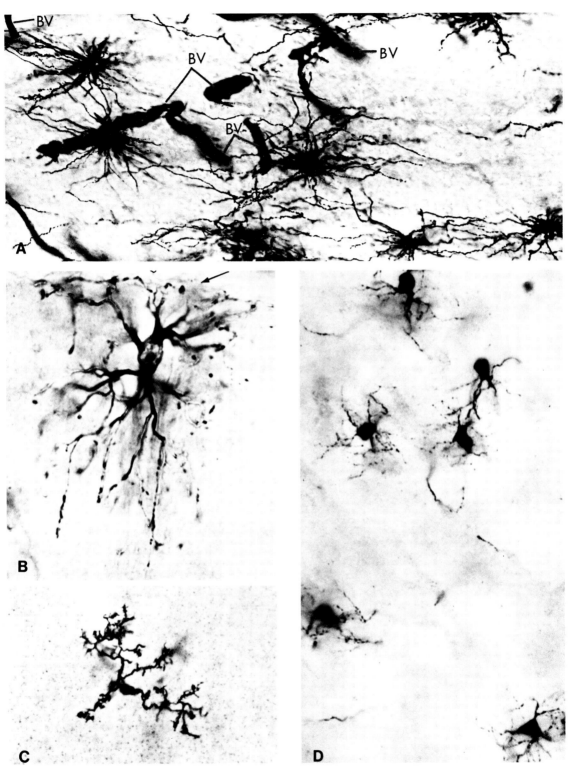

8–40 Photomicrographs of neuroglial cells from cerebral cortex of monkey, Golgi stain.
A. Fibrous astrocytes. **BV,** blood vessels. × 1,000.

B. Protoplasmic astrocyte. **Arrow,** brain surface.
× 1,900. **C.** Microglial cell. × 1,700.
D. Oligodendrocytes. × 1,900.

cesses of variable thickness, length, and branching pattern, which ramify between the perikarya and processes of nerve cells. Astrocytes near the surface of the brain or spinal cord usually have one or more processes extending to the pial surface where they expand to form "end feet;" others have similar end feet on the walls of blood vessels. Two types of astrocyte have traditionally been recognized: *fibrous astrocytes* and *protoplasmic astrocytes*. Fibrous astrocytes (Figs. 8–39, 8–40A, 8–42, and 8–43), found predominantly in white matter, have long, slender, generally unbranched processes containing many delicate fibrils when stained with the usual metallic methods. Protoplasmic astrocytes are found predominantly in gray matter and have shorter, stouter, much more highly branched processes that give to the cells a "fluffy" appearance (Figs. 8–40B, 8–41A, 8–42, and 8–43). These two types of astrocyte are, in fact, modulations in the form of a single cell type, and the appearance of the cells apparently depends on their location and possibly on their metabolic state.

Although the full extent of individual astrocytes can be demonstrated only by using special metallic stains, it is more common to see them in routine neurohistological preparations. In such preparations generally only the nuclei of the cells are seen, because the amount of perikaryal cytoplasm they contain is small and their cytoplasmic processes are thin. The nuclei are usually oval in shape, vesicular, and somewhat larger than the nuclei of oligodendrocytes (see below).

In electron micrographs, astrocytes are distinguished by their relatively organelle-free cytoplasm and their euchromatic nuclei (Figs. 8–44 and 8–45). Ordinarily the nucleus is oval and indented, and distinct nucleoli are not seen. Only a small amount of cytoplasm is usually seen around the nucleus in single sections; however, these sections give a very incomplete picture of the extent of the cytoplasm, for several irregularly shaped cytoplasmic processes emanate from the perikaryon and often extend for considerable distances. As they do so, they give rise to branches and protrusions that align themselves along blood vessels or along the pial surface and insinuate themselves between the somata and processes of nerve cells and other glial cells. Some of these processes are stout and lengthy, but others are thin and sheetlike.

The cytoplasm contains few free ribosomes and little rough-surfaced endoplasmic reticulum. A Golgi complex is always present, and lyso-

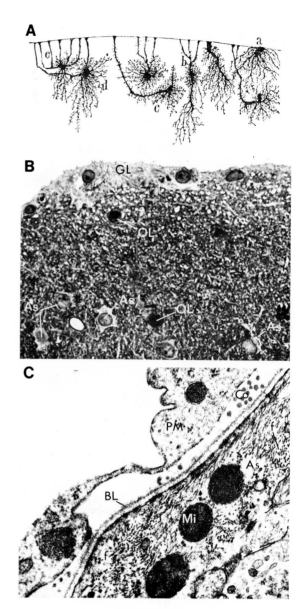

8–41 A. Protoplasmic astrocytes at surface of cerebral cortex in a Golgi preparation. **B.** Protoplasmic astrocytes forming the glia limitans **(GL)** at surface of cerebral cortex of a monkey. Other astrocytes **(AS)** and oligodendrocytes **(OL)** are more deeply situated. Toluidine-blue-stained plastic section. × 800. **C.** Electron micrograph showing cell process **(PM)** and collagen bundles **(Co)** of pia mater lying loosely on basal lamina **(BL)** of monkey cerebral cortex. Beneath the basal lamina lie astrocytic processes **(As)** containing mitochondria **(Mi)** and many microfilaments **(f).** × 30,000. (Part A from Cajal, S. Ramón y. 1909. Histologie de Système Nerveux de l'Homme et des vertébrés, vol. 1. Republished 1952. Madrid: Consejo Superior de Investigaciones Cientificas.)

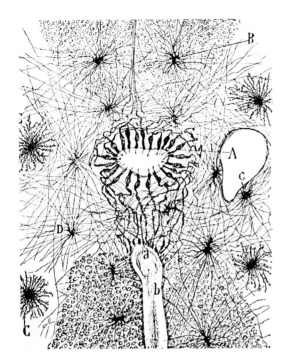

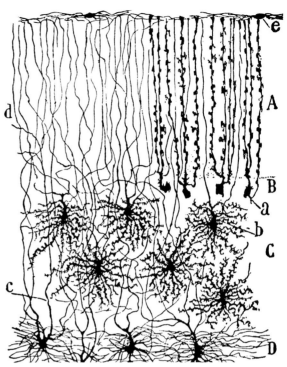

8–42 Astrocytes and ependymal cells in human spinal cord, Golgi stain. Ependymal cell foot processes reach surface at **a**. (From Cajal, S. Ramón y. 1909. Histologie de Système Nerveux de l'Homme et des Vertébrés, vol. 1. Republished 1952. Madrid: Consejo Superior de Investigaciones Cientificas.)

8–43 Astrocytes in human cerebellar cortex, Golgi stain. **a,** Bergmann glial cells; **b,** protoplasmic astrocytes; **c,** fibrous astrocytes. (From Cajal, S. Ramón y. 1911. Histologie de Système Nerveux de l'Homme et des Vertébrés, vol. 2. Republished 1952. Madrid: Consejo Superior de Investigaciones Cientificas.)

somes and glycogen granules are common. The most distinctive astrocytic organelles are the glial filaments, which are similar in appearance to the neurofilaments of nerve cells (Figs. 8–41C and 8–44). Variably sized bundles of these filaments are found in the perikaryal cytoplasm and in most of the processes of all astrocytes. Such bundles of filaments clearly form the basis of the fibrils that are seen with the light microscope.

Two special types of modified astrocyte are known. One is the *Müller cell* of the retina, which is an elongated columnar cell extending across the thickness of the neural retina (*see* Chap. 34). Müller cells have expanded foot processes that form the inner and outer limiting membranes of the retina. The second type is the *Bergmann glial cell* of the cerebellum (Fig. 8–43). The somata of Bergmann glial cells lie at the Purkinje cell layer, and each glial cell has several processes with short side branches that ascend and envelop the Purkinje cell dendrites.

The functions of astrocytes in the normal central nervous system are unknown, but some features about their distribution are suggestive.

Many of their processes are aligned at interfaces between the nervous system and other tissues. Such interfaces occur at the surface of the brain and spinal cord where neural tissue abuts the meninges and along the walls of blood vessels within the central nervous system (Figs. 8–41A to C, 8–46, and 8–47). The largest concentration of astrocytic processes is found beneath the pial surface where many astrocytic foot processes form the *glia limitans.* The outer surface of this zone of astrocytic processes is in contact with the *basal lamina,* which surrounds the brain and spinal cord and derives from the original basal lamina of the embryonic neuroepithelium (Fig. 8–41C). Similarly, as the larger blood vessels enter or exit from the central nervous system, they are invariably separated from the neural tissues proper by the basal lamina and by a *perivascular space* that is continuous with the subarachnoid space surrounding the brain and spinal cord (Fig. 8–46). Again, the basal lamina

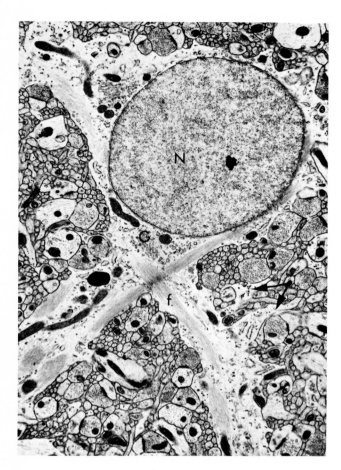

8–44 Electron micrograph of an astrocyte from cerebral cortex of a cat. **N,** nucleus; **f,** filaments; **G,** Golgi complex; **arrows,** cell processes. × 8,000.

is underlain by stacked astrocytic processes. As the vessels penetrate farther into the brain or spinal cord, they progressively lose their muscle coats and the perivascular space becomes obliterated (Fig. 8–47). Finally the capillaries, deep within the substance of the brain or cord, are invested by a continuous basal lamina, which remains ensheathed by astrocytic end feet.

The presence of astrocytic processes at these interfaces suggested to earlier workers that they might serve as diffusional barriers and, in particular, that they might represent the morphological basis of the well-known blood–brain barrier. However, we now know that the intercellular spaces within the brain and spinal cord freely communicate with the subarachnoid space through channels between the astrocytic foot processes; and even though there are occasional gap junctions between adjoining processes, they do not prevent passage of even large molecules between the cerebrospinal fluid and the neural parenchyma. The structural basis of the

blood–brain barrier clearly consists of occluding tight junctions between the capillary endothelial cells.

Astrocytes and their processes also divide the brain and spinal cord into sectors of varying distinctiveness, in some places, such as the spinal cord and optic nerve (Fig. 8–38), actually forming septa. It has been suggested, therefore, that their major role is to provide a form of scaffolding, or structural support, on which the neurons and their processes are assembled. It is doubtful that this could be their sole, or even principal, purpose, although in some parts of the nervous system they may serve to isolate groups of neurons or, more often, groups of synapses from their neighbors. Interestingly, the initial segments of most axons and the "bare" segments at nodes of Ranvier are usually ensheathed in astrocytic processes; in many situations, groups of axon terminals ending on a particular neuron, or part of a neuron, are separated from other cells and their processes by an almost complete enve-

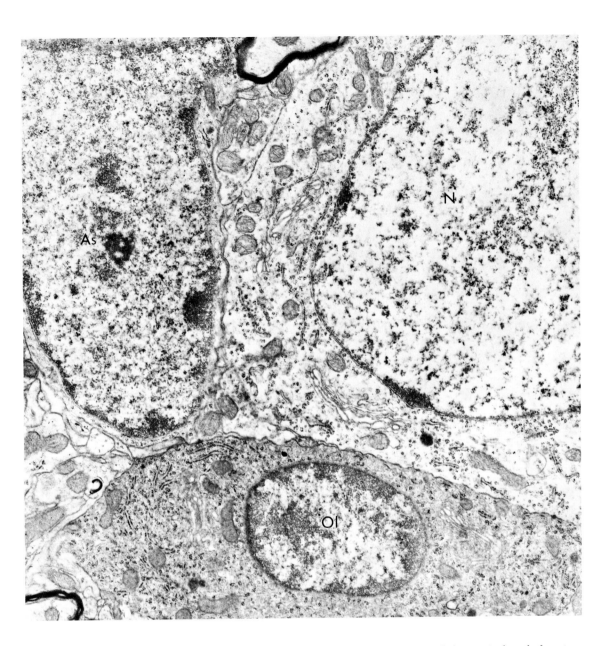

lope of astrocytic processes. Such glial-en-
sheathed synaptic aggregations are sometimes
called *glomeruli* (Fig. 8–37).

Some astrocytes undergo a slow depolarization when neighboring nerve cells are repeatedly
activated. This depolarization appears to be due
to the uptake by astrocytes of excess potassium
from the extracellular space, which accumulates
during prolonged neuronal activity. The ability
to serve as a "potassium sink" is extremely important, although we should point out that at
least some invertebrate neurons can be stripped

8–45 Electron micrograph from spinal cord of a rat
showing distinguishing features of neuron **(N)**,
astrocyte **(As)**, and oligodendrocyte **(Ol)**. Label is on
nucleus in each case. × 15,000.

of their glial ensheathment and yet continue to
function for considerable periods of time.

Finally, under various pathological conditions
astrocytes play a key role in removing neuronal
debris and in sealing off damaged brain tissue
(see p. 327).

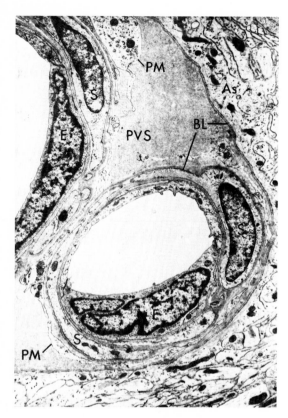

8–46 Electron micrograph of two blood vessels lying in a perivascular space **(PVS)** as they enter cerebral cortex of a cat. **E,** endothelial cells; **S,** smooth muscle cells; **BL,** basal lamina; **PM,** pia mater; **As,** astrocytic processes. × 7,500. (From Jones, E. G. 1970. J. Anat. [Lond.] 106:507.)

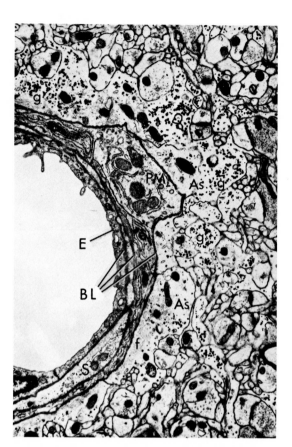

8–47 Electron micrograph showing a small blood vessel with a cell process of the pia mater **(PM)** caught between it and basal lamina of brain. **As,** astrocyte foot processes containing filaments **(f)** and glycogen **(g)**; **BL,** basal lamina; **E,** endothelial cell. Cat cerebral cortex. × 17,500. (From Jones, E. G., and Powell, T. P. S. 1970. Philos. Trans. R. Soc. Lond. [Biol. Sci.] 257:1.)

Oligodendrocytes. Oligodendrocytes are small neuroglial cells with relatively few processes. In light-microscopic preparations (Fig. 8–38) their nuclei are smaller, more irregular, and more deeply staining than those of astrocytes. There are two main types of oligodendrocytes, *interfascicular oligodendrocytes* and *perineuronal satellite* cells (Figs. 8–39 and 8–40D). As the names suggest, interfascicular oligodendrocytes are found among the bundles of axons constituting the white matter of the brain and spinal cord. Perineuronal satellite cells, on the other hand, are found in close association with the perikarya of neurons in areas of gray matter. Although the interfascicular form tends to be more elongated than the perineuronal satellite form, the two types are essentially similar.

In electron micrographs, the oligodendrocyte is generally a much denser cell than the astrocyte (Figs. 8–45 and 8–48). The nucleus is heterochromatic and the cytoplasm is filled with organelles, especially large numbers of free and attached ribosomes, the latter associated with numerous short cisternae of endoplasmic reticulum. The Golgi apparatus is also extensive, and many mitochondria are present. Perhaps the most striking cytoplasmic feature is the large number of microtubules that permeate the perikaryal cytoplasm and extend into the processes of the cell.

The close association of perineuronal satellite oligodendrocytes with neurons has suggested to some workers that these oligodendrocytes may be in some way involved in maintaining the metabolic state of the neurons with which they are

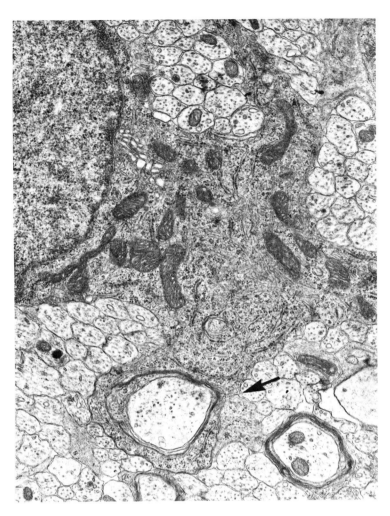

8–48 Electron micrograph of a myelin-forming oligodendrocyte in the developing optic nerve of a rat. **Arrow** indicates mesaxon. × 12,500. (From Vaughn, J. E. 1969. Z. Zellforsch. Mikrosk. Anat. 94:293; courtesy of J. E. Vaughn.)

associated. However, this has never been satisfactorily demonstrated. Only one function can be attributed with confidence to the oligodendrocytes. Both interfascicular and perineuronal oligodendrocytes are the *myelin-forming* cells of the central nervous system (Fig. 8–49).

In a myelinated axon, the sheath begins at the end of the initial segment, usually a few microns from the axon hillock, and ends near the region of termination of the axon (Figs. 8–50 and 8–51). With the light microscope the myelin sheath appears as an elongated tube that is interrupted at regular intervals along its length at the *nodes of Ranvier*. The segments of myelin between consecutive nodes of Ranvier are termed *internodal segments*, or *internodes*. The thickness of the myelin sheath and the length of the internodal segments are fairly constant for a given axon and have been found to be proportional to the diameter (or more strictly, the circumference) of the contained axon.

In the central nervous system, each internodal segment of myelin is formed by a cytoplasmic process of an oligodendrocyte wrapping itself around the axon in a spiral fashion (Figs. 8–48 and 8–49). The process becomes extremely attenuated as it approaches the axon, and this portion of the process is known as the *external tongue* (Fig. 8–50). As the process spirals around the axon, the cytoplasmic faces of its plasma membrane fuse to form what appears in section as a dense line (about 25 to 30 Å thick), called the *major dense line*. A myelin internode is made up of repeated wrappings or lamellae of the oligodendrocytic process and therefore appears as a regularly arranged, repeating series of major dense lines. They are separated from one another by an electron-lucent zone approximately 90 Å

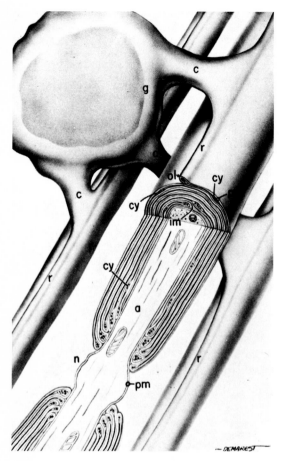

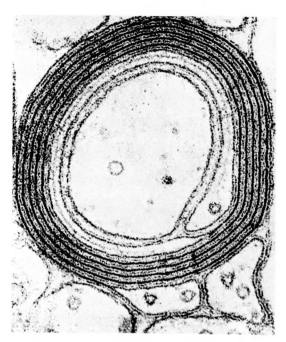

8–50 Electron micrograph of a small myelinated axon in the central nervous system showing inner and outer tongues of oligodendrocytic cytoplasm and major and minor dense lines of myelin sheath. × 161,000. (From Hirano, A., and Dembitzer. H. M. 1967. J. Cell Biol. 34:555; courtesy of A. Hirano.)

8–49 Schematic drawing of an oligodendrocyte forming internodes on three adjacent axons. **r,** outer tongue; **n,** node of Ranvier. (From Bunge, M. B., Bunge, R. P., and Ris, H. 1961. J. Biophys. Biochem. Cytol. 10:67; courtesy of M. B. Bunge and R. P. Bunge.)

wide—referred to as the *intraperiod line*—that contains a faint line somewhat thinner than the major dense line. The intraperiod line is formed by the fused outer faces of the plasma membranes of adjoining wrappings of the oligodendrocytic process.

The outermost major dense line of a myelin internodal segment is directly continuous with the external tongue of the oligodendrocytic process. The innermost major dense line splits apart as it approaches its end to form a similar tongue of cytoplasm known as the *internal tongue*. The intraperiod line disappears as the inner and outer tongues emerge. The internal tongue is the leading edge, as it were, of the oligodendrocytic process. The thickness of a myelin sheath is de-

termined by the number of wrappings of oligodendrocytic cytoplasm and in axons of increasing diameter, the number of major dense lines and intraperiod lines becomes progressively greater. In myelinated axons, one lamella is added for approximately every 0.2-μm increase in axonal diameter. The great concentration of plasma membranes in the myelin sheath accounts for the high concentration of lipids and lipoproteins that gives it a high affinity for fat stains (Fig. 8–51) and also accounts for its intense staining in electron-microscopic preparations.

Oligodendrocytes have several processes and, therefore, unlike Schwann cells in the peripheral nervous system (see pp. 329–330), can each form several internodal segments. In the optic nerve of the rat, a single oligodendrocyte may give rise to as many as 40 or 50 internodal segments. If the portions of an oligodendrocyte that form myelin internodes could be unwrapped, they would appear as extensive flattened sheets roughly trapezoidal in shape. The extent of the cell is there-

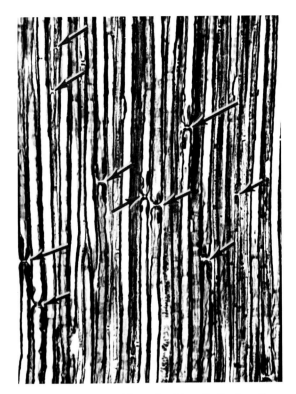

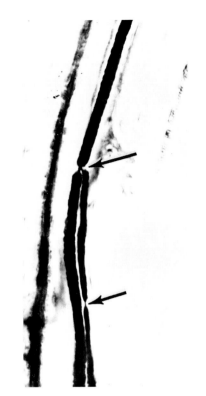

8–51 Osmium-tetroxide–stained longitudinal section of peripheral nerve of cat showing myelin sheaths and nodes of Ranvier **(arrows).** × 300.

8–52 Gold-chloride–stained, teased preparation of myelinated nerve fiber branching at a node **(upper arrow).** Thinner branch has shorter internodal distance (to **lower arrow**). Muscle nerve of a marsupial. × 500.

fore actually much greater than is shown in even the best specimens impregnated with metallic salts, for here the tenuous connections between the parent oligodendrocytic processes and the myelin internodal segments are not visualized. Even in electron micrographs, clear demonstrations of the continuity are limited to occasional fortuitous examples.

The "naked" portions of the axon at the nodes of Ranvier (Figs. 8–52 and 8–53) are highly specialized regions of high capacitance and low electrical resistance, responsible for the self-regenerative capacity of the conducted action potential. During the passage of an action potential, significant changes in membrane conductance occur almost exclusively at the nodes; thus, the wave of depolarization leaps from node to node, a form of conduction known as "saltatory." The structure of the axonal membrane is modified at the node by the addition of a dense membrane undercoat similar to that seen at the initial segment. The outer surface of the membrane is free of any oligodendrocytic covering and is usually

separated from astrocytic processes by the 200-Å wide extracellular cleft seen between all processes in the central nervous system. The remainder of the axon is unchanged at the node, although occasionally a typical axon terminal may bulge from its side, and when myelinated axons branch, the branching always occurs at a node (Fig. 8–52). In such cases, three or more internodal segments come together.

At the nodes of Ranvier the edges of the spirally wrapped myelin lamellae separate at each major dense line and form a series of tonguelike processes. These processes, of course, contain oligodendrocytic cytoplasm; microtubules and other organelles are usually seen in each tongue. The tongues of cytoplasm are best visualized in longitudinal sections where they collectively form the *paranodal region* of the myelinated fiber (Figs. 8–49 and 8–53). In the paranodal region, each tongue is in contact with the axolemma; thus the tongue arising from the most

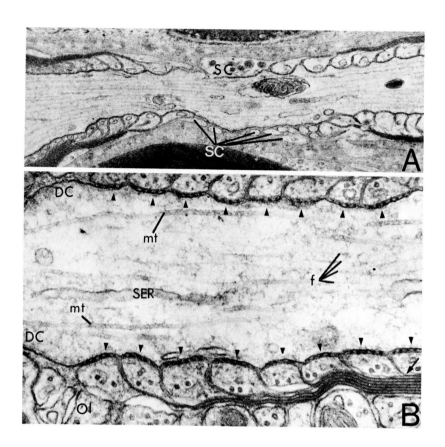

8–53 **A.** Electron micrograph of node of Ranvier in trigeminal nerve of rat. **SC,** Schwann cell processes. × 25,000. **B.** Electron micrograph of paranodal region of myelinated axon in inferior colliculus of cat. **Arrowheads** indicate dense bars joining tongues of oligodendrocytic cytoplasm to axon. **Arrow** indicates formation of major dense line. **DC,** dense undercoating of naked part of axonal membrane; **f,** neurofilaments; **mt,** microtubules; **Ol,** oligodendrocytic processes; **SER,** smooth endoplasmic reticulum. × 54,000.

superficial major dense line adjoins the naked part of the axon at the node, whereas the tongue arising from the innermost major dense line is the deepest and lies farthest from the node. Because of the spiral nature of the myelin wrapping, the tongues are continuous with one another; and if they could be displayed three-dimensionally they would appear as a helix spiraling around the paranodal segment of the axon.

The tongues of oligodendrocytic cytoplasm at the paranodal region are much more intimately associated with the axolemma than is the innermost myelin wrapping of the rest of the inter-

node. At the paranodal region the gap between the tongues and the axolemma is reduced at intervals to a form of close junction in which the adjoining plasma membranes are separated by a gap no more than 20 to 30 Å wide. Within this gap, a series of regularly spaced, short, dense bands are seen extending from the axolemma to the oligodendrocytic tongues (Fig. 8–53B). These dense bands appear to form a continuous spiral around the paranodal region, with about 3 to 5 bands associated with each tongue. Despite the close proximity of the membranes of the oligodendrocyte tongues and the spiral bands, there seems to be fairly free diffusion of ions and even larger particles between the axon and the innermost lamella of the myelin sheath, for electron-dense markers such as lanthanum can readily penetrate between them.

When first formed, all nerve fibers are unmyelinated. In the human embryo, myelination begins at about the fourteenth week of intrauterine life and accelerates in the last trimester of pregnancy. However, a considerable amount of myelination occurs postnatally; and in some animals, such as the rat, which is born in a relatively immature state, the brain may be largely devoid of myelin at birth. In fiber pathways that normally myelinate after birth, the process of myelination is in general related to the functional maturation of the system to which the pathway belongs. For example, in the human infant the myelination of the major descending pathways that control voluntary movements starts at birth, and essentially all of the fibers have acquired a myelin sheath by the time of walking. Thereafter, no new internodal segments are added, but existing internodes increase in length as the brain and spinal cord grow and the nerve fibers elongate.

Other Neuroglial Cells and Pathology of Neuroglia

When the central nervous system is injured or diseased, glial cells proliferate, become phagocytic, and may form a scar. The extent to which astrocytes and oligodendrocytes are involved in these three processes is still much debated, and the role of blood-borne and other macrophages is also uncertain. For some time it was believed that a specific class of cells, the so-called microglia, was the major source of phagocytes in the central nervous system. In light-microscopic preparations, this cell is usually described as being the smallest of the glial elements, with a deeply staining, angular nucleus. When impregnated with heavy metal salts, it resembles a small oligodendrocyte, but with rather more spikelike projections from its slender processes (Fig. 8–40C). Microglia are said to be present in small numbers in the normal central nervous system. The neuropathologist del Rio Hortega believed that they were mesodermal rather than neurectodermal in origin, and that they invaded the brain and spinal cord with the capillary network during the period of vascularization. In areas of neural damage, or during inflammatory disease processes, the microglial cells have been thought to proliferate and become actively phagocytic. As they ingest more and more debris, such as degenerating myelin, they enlarge and become globular in shape and filled with large vacuoles, lipid droplets, and other inclusions; they are then termed *compound granular corpuscles*, or *Gitterzellen*.

At the electron-microscopic level, it has been extremely difficult to identify microglia. Many workers, finding that virtually all glial cells can be fairly readily classified as either astrocytes or oligodendrocytes, would prefer to regard the resting microglial cell of convential light microscopy as simply a variety of oligodendrocyte. If this is the case, unless the vasculature of the nervous system is damaged, all the phagocytes in an area of neuronal death will be derived from astrocytes and oligodendroyctes. If the integrity of the vascular system is damaged, extraneous cells may invade the damaged or diseased central nervous system. Many of these cells are blood-borne phagocytes, but some appear to be vascular pericytes associated with the walls of blood vessels. In experiments in which the brain was subjected to heavy-particle irradiation, it was found that the pericytes (Fig. 8–38), which are normally surrounded by the basal lamina of the capillaries, can break through the basal lamina, invade the brain, and become phagocytic. The pericytes are thus regarded by some as being the source of microglial cells. Another possible source is the meninges, for the presence of infective agents or other foreign material in the subarachnoid space may cause many of the cells of the pia and arachnoid to detach themselves and to invade the brain, particularly by way of the perivascular spaces.

Several recent studies have led to the suggestion that there may be a third class of glial cell normally resident in the central nervous system that, under the appropriate stimulus, may proliferate and become the major source of phagocytic cells in pathological states. These cells are more or less intermediate in fine structure between oligodendrocytes and astrocytes. The developing optic nerve may contain a considerable proportion of such cells, but their numbers decline as astrocytes and oligodendrocytes become more prominent. It has been claimed that they are a form of glial precursor cell derived from the neurectoderm, or the subventricular zone, which persists in small numbers into adulthood and retains the capacity to produce both oligodendrocytes and astrocytes. In regions of axonal degeneration, these precursor cells may become phagocytic and for this reason are regarded by some researchers as the source of the phagocytic microglia.

The Ependyma and the Choroid Plexus

The central canal system of the brain and spinal cord is lined by a layer of closely packed cuboidal or columnar epithelial cells known collectively as the *ependyma* (Fig. 8–42). These cells are the remnants of the embryonic neuroepithelium and retain their original position after the neuroblasts and glioblasts have migrated into the mantle layer. The ependymal cells have many microvilli at their luminal surfaces and commonly have one or more cilia, although the distribution of cilia is patchy and large areas of the lining of the central canal system may be devoid of them. The ependyma is only one cell thick, but its thickness varies because the constituent cells are of variable height in different regions. In parts of the third ventricle overlying the median eminence of the hypothalamus and over certain specializations of the ventricular walls (such as the subcommissural organ and the area postrema) the cells may be very attenuated and even absent. Elsewhere, they are tall and columnar. The ependymal cells are bound to their neighbors near their luminal surfaces by the usual junctional complexes, including close junctions and zonulae adhaerentes. There are, however, no occluding junctions (except in the modified ependymal lining of the choroid plexus): solutes, and even moderately large protein molecules seem to be able to reach the brain parenchyma by passing between the ependymal cells. In this way the cerebrospinal fluid of the ventricular system can communicate freely with the intercellular spaces of the central nervous system.

Ependymal cells usually have a pronounced apical accumulation of mitochondria, but in most other respects their fine structure resembles that of astrocytes. Rough endoplasmic reticulum is not prominent and the cells contain bundles of filaments 60 to 80 Å in diameter. Many ependymal cells have lengthy processes extending from their basal aspects. In the embryo, these processes often reach the surface of the developing brain and spinal cord; but in the mature nervous system, this arrangement is rare except in certain sites such as the anterior median fissure of the spinal cord, where the central canal is relatively close to the surface (Fig. 8–42).

In the four ventricles of the brain, the ependyma is modified to form the special secretory epithelium of the *choroid plexuses* (Figs. 8–54 and 8–55). The choroid plexuses are formed at regions where the *roof plate* of the developing neural tube becomes extremely attenuated so that the ependyma and the overlying pia mater come into direct contact with one another over an area known as a *choroidal tela*. The portion of the pia mater entering into the formation of the choroidal tela becomes richly vascularized,

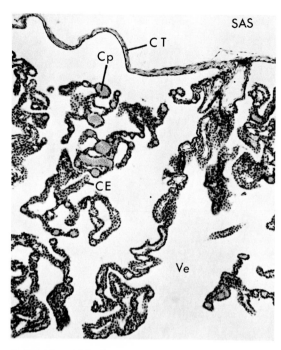

8–54 Choroidal tela **(CT)** and choroid plexus from fourth ventricle **(Ve)** of a cat. **Cp**, capillary; **CE**, choroidal epithelium; **SAS**, subarachnoid space. Hematoxylin and eosin stain. × 32.

and this highly vascular tissue becomes invaginated into the ventricle as a mass of villous-like processes collectively known as the choroid plexus. The line of invagination of the choroidal tela is the *choroid fissure*.

Electron micrographs of the choroid plexus reveal an essentially trilayered structure (Fig. 8–55): (1) At the ventricular surface there is a row of closely packed, columnar ependymal cells with many microvilli but no cilia. The sides and bases of the cells are thrown into numerous interdigitating cytoplasmic processes, and near their luminal surfaces the cells are joined by zonulae adhaerentes and true tight junctions (zonulae occludentes) that encircle the cells so as to occlude the intercellular cleft. (2) The basal surfaces of these modified ependymal cells rest on a basal lamina continuous with that covering the rest of the brain. (3) Deep to this is a thin connective tissue space containing free-lying pia-arachnoid cells, small irregular bundles of collagen fibers, and many small blood vessels. The endothelial cells lining the choroidal capillaries are highly fenestrated and the constituents of blood plasma, including proteins, can pass freely

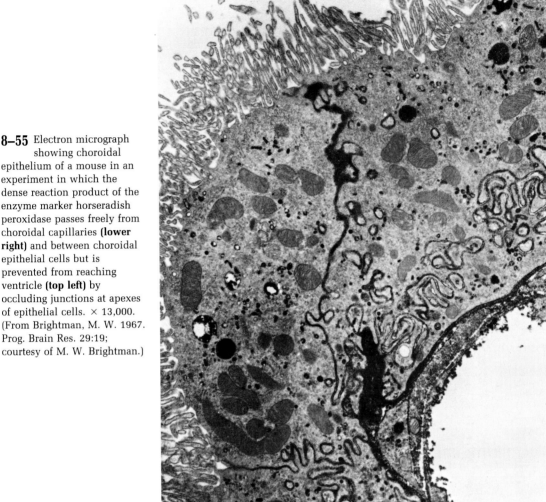

8–55 Electron micrograph showing choroidal epithelium of a mouse in an experiment in which the dense reaction product of the enzyme marker horseradish peroxidase passes freely from choroidal capillaries **(lower right)** and between choroidal epithelial cells but is prevented from reaching ventricle **(top left)** by occluding junctions at apexes of epithelial cells. × 13,000. (From Brightman, M. W. 1967. Prog. Brain Res. 29:19; courtesy of M. W. Brightman.)

into the connective tissue spaces. However, these materials are prevented from reaching the ventricles by the apical tight junctions surrounding the epithelial cells. Thus, despite the permeability of the choroidal capillaries to plasma proteins, the cerebrospinal fluid under normal conditions contains little or no protein.

The secretion of cerebrospinal fluid is an active process requiring energy and can be readily inhibited by carbonic anhydrase inhibitors and by ouabain, which blocks sodium transport. Moreover, it can continue despite an adverse pressure gradient, as in the case of an obstruction to its outflow (thus resulting in hydrocephalus).

Cerebrospinal fluid is produced in humans at the rate of approximately 0.5 liter/day. The fluid flows out into the subarachnoid space through the median and lateral apertures of the fourth ventricle and is absorbed primarily into the cranial venous sinuses through tufts of pia-arachnoid cells (arachnoid villi), which protrude through the walls of the sinuses into the lumen.

Supporting Cells in the Peripheral Nervous System

The supporting cells of the peripheral nervous system are the *Schwann cells*, associated with all peripheral nerve fibers and forming the capsular or satellite cells of the dorsal root and au-

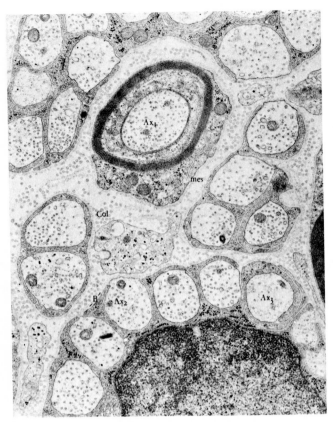

8–56 Electron micrograph of cross section of sciatic nerve of rat showing relationship of Schwann cells and their processes to myelinated and unmyelinated axons. **B,** basal lamina; **Col,** collagen; **mes,** mesaxon. × 21,000. (From Peters, A., Palay S. L., and Webster, H. deF. 1976. The Fine Structure of the Nervous System. Philadelphia: W. B. Saunders; courtesy of A. Peters.)

tonomic ganglia. They are derived from the neural crest. Like their counterparts in the central nervous system, all the peripheral supporting cells are small cells, and cytologically they are unexceptional. The outer surfaces of their plasma membranes are always associated with a basal lamina.

Schwann Cells in Peripheral Nerve Trunks.
The Schwann cells of peripheral nerve trunks are sometimes known as neurilemmal or sheath cells because of the manner in which they enfold the constituent axons (Fig. 8–56). Every axon in the peripheral nervous system, from the dorsal and ventral roots to the most distal branches of the sensory or motor fibers, is surrounded over most of its length by a series of Schwann cells; in the case of axons with a diameter greater than about 1 μm each of these Schwann cells forms a single myelin internodal segment (Fig. 8–57). In two respects the association of Schwann cells with peripheral axons differs from that between the supporting cells of the central nervous system and central axons: (1) unmyelinated axons in the central nervous system lack any form of ensheathment; and (2) whereas each Schwann cell forms only a single internodal segment, each oligodendrocyte may form 50 or more internodal segments and be associated with a comparable number of axons.

Peripheral nerves have several coverings, of which the Schwann cell constituent is most intimately related to the axons. Aside from the Schwann cells, there are three connective tissue coats (Figs. 8–58 and 8–59): an epineurium, perineurium, and endoneurium. An *epineurium* made up of dense fibrous connective tissue encloses the entire nerve as in a sleeve. This covering is sufficiently thick to be sutured in operations involving nerve repair. Within the epineurium the axons of the nerve are formed into longitudinally running bundles, or *fasciculi*, of variable size. These fasciculi are also enclosed in a sleeve of moderately dense fibrous connective tissue called the *perineurium*. This sheath is not completely limiting, however, since axons may leave one fasciculus to join another. Within the perineurium the axons and their as-

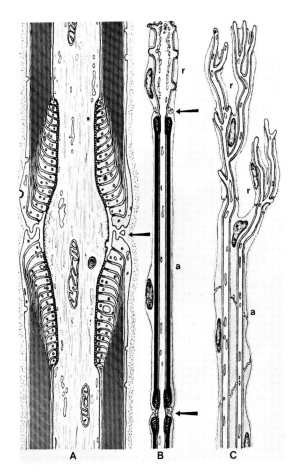

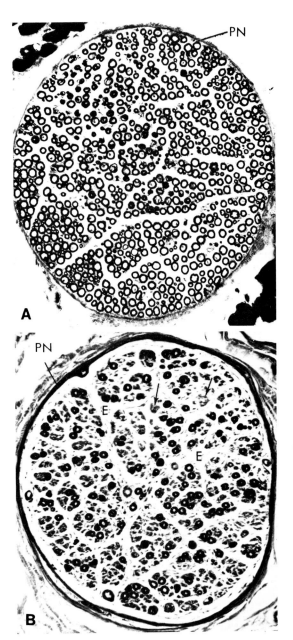

8–57 Schematic drawings of a node of Ranvier in peripheral nervous system **(A)**, terminal portion of a myelinated sensory nerve fiber **(B)**, and terminal portions of two unmyelinated sensory nerve fibers **(C)**, showing relationship of axon to investing Schwann cells. (From Andres, K. H., and von Düring, M. 1973. Handbook of Sensory Physiology, vol. 2. New York: Springer-Verlag, New York, Inc.; courtesy of K. H. Andres.)

sociated Schwann cells are surrounded by a small amount of delicate, loose connective tissue known as the *endoneurium*. Generally, a small number of blood vessels, the *vasa nervorum*, are also present; they penetrate the epineurial and perineurial sheaths and break up into a loose capillary plexus in the endoneurium.

Although Schwann cells are found along the length of peripheral nerve fibers, any short segment of the fiber is associated with only a single Schwann cell. To a greater or lesser degree, all fibers are invaginated into the Schwann cells.

8–58 **A.** Cross section of part of a spinal ventral root of a cat showing bimodal myelinated fiber spectrum. **PN**, perineurium. Osmium tetroxide stain. × 125. **B.** Cross section of a fascicle of a small cutaneous sensory nerve showing unmyelinated **(arrows)** as well as large and small myelinated fibers. **E**, endoneurium. Osmium tetroxide stain. × 165.

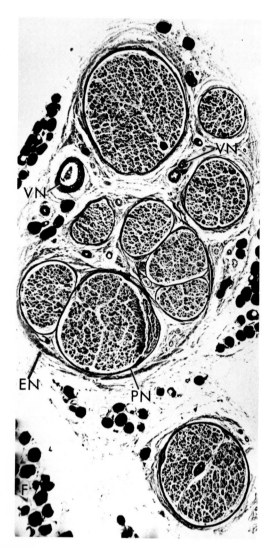

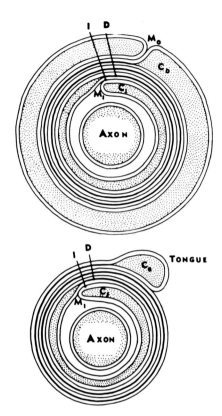

8–60 Schematic figure showing mode of formation of myelin in peripheral nervous system **(top)** and central nervous system **(bottom). C_i, C_o,** inner and outer cytoplasmic leaflets; **D,** major dense line; **I,** intraperiod line; **M_i, M_o,** inner and outer mesaxon. (From Peters, A. 1960. J. Biophys. Biochem. Cytol., 7:121; courtesy of A. Peters.)

8–59 Cross section of small peripheral nerve consisting of several fascicles surrounded by epineurium **(EN)** and perineurium **(PN). F,** fat cells; **VN,** vasa nervorum. Osmium tetroxide stain. × 50.

The line of the invagination, which usually forms a narrow cleft leading from the endoneurium to the enclosed axon, is known as the *mesaxon* (Fig. 8–56), by analogy with the mesenteries of the alimentary canal. *Schwann cells* associated with unmyelinated fibers may invest as many as 20 such fibers, and surrounding the whole cell and the associated fibers is the basal lamina. Where one Schwann cell comes to an end, it is overlapped by the next cell in the chain of Schwann cells (Fig. 8–57), and there is no gap comparable to the nodes of Ranvier of myeli-

nated fibers. In the case of myelinated fibers, each Schwann cell is associated with only a single fiber.

Although the general form of myelin in the peripheral nervous system is similar to that found in the central nervous system, its mode of formation is rather different. In the peripheral nervous system the axon to be myelinated first becomes invaginated into the Schwann cell. Then one of the lips of cytoplasm adjoining the mesaxon appears to insinuate itself between the adjoining lip and the axon; and by the continued elongation of the lips of the mesaxon, a spiral wrapping made up of many lamellae is formed (Fig. 8–60). By the alternate fusion of the inner leaflets of the plasma membranes (belonging to the same lamella) and of the outer leaflets of the plasma membranes (belonging to adjoining lamellae), the major dense and intraperiod lines are respectively established. The exact manner in which the spiral wrapping occurs is uncertain, but there is some evidence from observations in tissue culture that at least in the initial phase the whole Schwann cell may rotate around the axon.

The innermost major dense line expands to form an inner tongue of Schwann cell cytoplasm, and the cleft formed by the associated separation of the innermost intraperiod line is usually called the *inner mesaxon*. This cleft is originally continuous with the initial line of invagination of the fiber, which constitutes the *outer mesaxon*. At the outer mesaxon, the outermost major dense line splits and becomes continuous with what is usually a substantial amount of Schwann cell cytoplasm—far greater than the small outer tongue of oligodendrocytic cytoplasm seen in the central nervous system. If the myelin sheath is seen in a longitudinal section or in a cross section near the middle of an internode, the nucleus of the Schwann cell will also be present; and, as in the case of unmyelinated fibers, the cell is surrounded by a basal lamina.

Nodes of Ranvier are present in myelinated peripheral nerve fibers, as in the central nervous system (Fig. 8–53). The nodal portion of the axon has a dense membrane undercoat, and the Schwann cells of the two adjoining internodes form comparable tongues of cytoplasm in the paranodal regions. The spiral bands between the tongues and the outer leaflet of the axolemma are usually less distinct than in the central nervous system. However, the major difference between nodal regions in the central and peripheral nervous systems is that at peripheral nodes the nerve fiber is not completely bare. Although devoid of a myelin sheath, the nodal segment is covered by large overlapping processes of Schwann cell cytoplasm derived from the cells that give rise to the two adjoining internodes, and the whole region is surrounded by a basal lamina.

Myelin internodes in the peripheral nervous system often show a series of small clefts or splittings running obliquely for some distance across the thickness of the myelin sheath. They are called *Schmidt-Lanterman incisures*, or *clefts*, and they represent regions in which the major dense lines are separated over a short distance so that a small amount of Schwann cytoplasm is inserted into the myelin wrapping. Where the cleavage affects all lamellae, the cleft will form a helical wrapping around the sheath,

but sometimes only a few adjacent major dense lines are affected.

Supporting Cells in the Peripheral Ganglia. Schwann cells, often called *satellite cells*, are found in large numbers in both dorsal root ganglia and autonomic ganglia. In the dorsal root ganglia (Fig. 8–61A) and in the sensory ganglia of certain of the cranial nerves, they tend to surround the pseudounipolar neurons and are, therefore, sometimes called *capsular cells* (Fig. 8–61B). In autonomic ganglia, the investment of individual neurons is rarely so complete (Fig. 8–62), and most neurons are associated with a relatively small number of satellite cells.

The capsular cells are distinguished by their small size relative to the neurons and, in light micrographs, by their paucity of cytoplasm. In electron micrographs they usually appear to be embedded in depressions in the ganglion cell cytoplasm, and the neurons may invaginate finger-like extensions into the capsular cell. The cytoplasmic processes of adjacent capsular cells overlap to a variable extent, and the thickness of the capsular layer is usually proportional to the size of the ganglion cell. Because the cells are Schwann cells, it is not surprising that the entire "capsule" is invested by a basal lamina. No synapses are present in dorsal root ganglia, but in autonomic ganglia the capsule is deficient at several points to allow for the passage of the terminal portions of the preganglionic axons that form synapses on the cells. In some cases, capsular cells form myelin around the enclosed neurons. In mammals, this unusual situation is mainly confined to the ganglia of the vestibulocochlear nerve in which the somata of the bipolar cells commonly have a thin covering of loose myelin.

The capsular cells continue without interruption onto the initial segment of the axon, and portions of the same capsular cell may line both the perikaryon and the axon. In many animals, and particularly in humans, the initial stem processes of the dorsal root ganglion cells, before bifurcating into central and peripheral branches, are highly coiled, forming what is usually referred to as a *glomerular segment* (Fig. 8–62C). The enveloping cells follow the contours of this convoluted structure and normally give rise to one or more myelin internodes just before the point of branching. The branching occurs, as always, at a node.

The Schwann cells continue along the central processes of the sensory ganglion cells to the

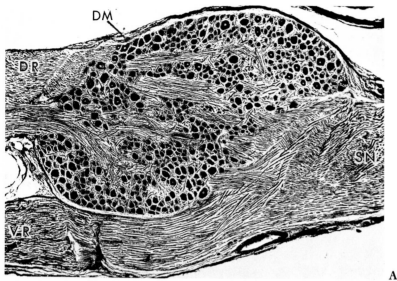

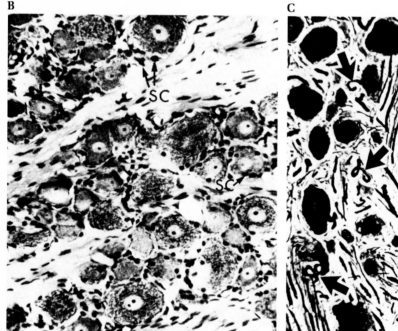

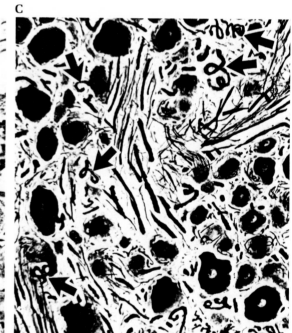

8–61 **A.** Bodian-stained preparation of dorsal root ganglion of a cat showing covering of dura mater **(DM)**, ventral root **(VR)**, dorsal root **(DR)**, and spinal nerve **(SN)**. × 90. **B.** Thionin-stained section showing dorsal root ganglion cells of varying size and enveloping Schwann (capsular) cells **(SC)**. × 480. **C.** Higher-powered view of a part of **A**, showing coiled initial axon segments of ganglion cells **(arrows)**. × 480.

spinal cord or brainstem. The point at which these cells disappear and the oligodendrocytes assume the responsibility for forming the myelin sheath of the central process has not been studied intensively. The changeover seems to occur not at a sharp boundary line but over a long region of transition.

Schwann Cells in Degeneration and Repair of Peripheral Nerves. Degeneration of a peripheral nerve after a transection or some injury at a more proximal level is always accompanied by reactive changes in the Schwann cells. The axons that are severed from their trophic center, the cell body, degenerate distal to a transection. This degenerative process is known as *Wallerian degeneration* after the neurologist A. V. Waller, who first described it in 1850. It includes the whole distal portion of an axon and its terminal ramifications. Although the earliest stages of de-

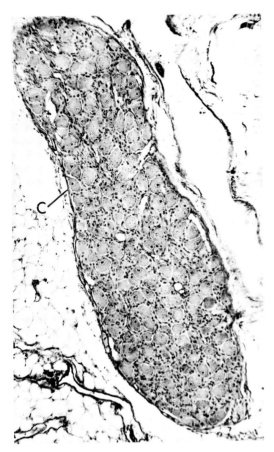

8–62 Longitudinal section of otic ganglion of a dog showing sympathetic neurons and intervening small nuclei of satellite Schwann cells. **C**, capsule. Hematoxylin and eosin stain. × 250.

generation may be seen close to the severed end, the changes affect the whole distal portion more or less simultaneously. The first changes are seen at the nodes of Ranvier, where the axon swells and the mitochondria are disrupted. Within a few hours the paranodal portions of the myelin sheath start to fragment and clefts resembling Schmidt-Lantermann incisures appear in large numbers in the internodes. This is followed by fragmentation of the whole myelin sheath, which appears in myelin-stained preparations as a chain of ovoid or vesicular masses. These masses become denser and further fragmented, and they and the fragments of degenerating axoplasm are phagocytosed by the Schwann cells and by macrophages that invade the degenerating portion of the nerve from the blood stream. These cells become filled with large heterogeneous dense bod-

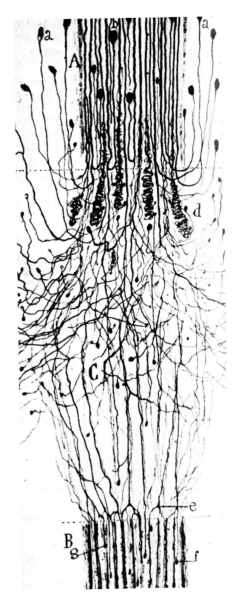

8–63 Some of the earliest degenerative and regenerative changes seen at the site of interruption of a nerve bundle. The proximal stump **(A)** in the upper part of the figure shows numerous retraction bulbs, convoluted spiral structures, and newly formed axon sprouts, some of which have grown toward the Schwann tubes of the distal stump **(B)**. (From Cajal, S. Ramón y. 1928. Degeneration and Regeneration of the Nervous System. Republished 1958. New York: Hafner Pub. Co.)

ies and vacuoles containing lipids derived from the further degradation of the myelin fragments.

The Schwann cells hypertrophy and markedly increase in number. The proliferation may continue for as long as 3 weeks and the number of cells may increase to more than 10 times the original population. Clearly, large portions of the plasma membrane of the Schwann cell are disrupted in the course of fragmentation of the myelin sheath, but few cells actually appear to die. The proliferating Schwann cells seem to free themselves from their surrounding basal laminae, which remain as a series of longitudinally oriented tubes. Along these tubes, the Schwann cells form a complexly interdigitated mass of cytoplasmic processes that, together with the tubes of basal lamina, appear to guide the regenerating axonal sprouts into the degenerated distal segment and toward their peripheral target (Fig. 8–63). The extracellular compartments formed by the interdigitating Schwann cell processes and the basal laminae are often referred to as *Schwann tubes.*

As regeneration of the axons proceeds, the Schwann cells become more orderly in their arrangement and gradually form linear arrays within the persisting tubes of basal laminae. The regenerated axons become invaginated within the Schwann cells and those larger than 1 μm become remyelinated. The new myelin internodes are generally shorter and thinner than those in the normal nerve. The shortness is perhaps to be expected, in view of the marked proliferation of Schwann cells, but it is uncertain what proportion of the newly produced Schwann cells survive to form internodes or to ensheath unmyelinated fibers.

The Peripheral Terminations of Nerve Fibers

In the peripheral nervous system, the processes of neurons either synapse with other nerve cells, as in the case of autonomic preganglionic neurons, or enter into a functional relationship with the cellular components of other tissues, as in the case of the dorsal root ganglion cells, the motoneurons of the spinal cord or the autonomic postganglionic neurons. The structure of autonomic ganglia is described below. Here we shall be concerned primarily with the peripheral terminations of dorsal root ganglion cells, of spinal motoneurons, and of autonomic postganglionic neurons.

The peripheral processes of dorsal root ganglion cells and of the cells in the sensory cranial ganglia terminate in association with specialized connective, epithelial or muscular tissues that in many cases facilitate the sensory transduction process leading to the discharge of action potentials in the nerve fiber and to their propagation toward the central nervous system. The pseudounipolar ganglion cells are, therefore, *receptor* neurons and their peripheral terminals are specialized sensory receptors. Motoneurons in the spinal cord and brainstem and the autonomic postganglionic neurons are *effector* neurons, and their axons terminate respectively on skeletal muscle cells and on smooth muscle or gland cells. In these cases, the peripheral terminal is an effector or "motor" ending, comparable in its general structure and function to a central synapse, although the effect on the target organ is, of course, to induce muscular contraction or glandular secretion.

The Structure and Function of Peripheral Sensory Receptors

The peripheral sensory receptors are concerned with the transduction of various forms of energy into neural activity, which, if of sufficient intensity, results in the discharge of nerve impulses whose frequency and pattern constitute the neural code that is interpreted centrally as a sensory experience. Before describing individual receptors three general points may be made. (1) For the most part, the type or *modality* of sensation mediated by a particular axon is specific for each axon, and its specificity resides within the axon itself. As a rule, each axon is concerned with only one sensory modality. (2) The sensory transduction process occurs within the axon itself rather than in the specialized end formations that may be associated with it. (3) Not all activity in sensory receptors is consciously perceived; much of it is concerned with various reflexes and other adjustments to changes in the external or internal environment, of which the subject is often wholly unconscious. The use of the term *sensory* is synonymous with *afferent* and does not necessarily imply conscious *sensation.*

Sensory receptors may be classified in several ways. Among the oldest is that of Sherrington, who spoke of (1) *exteroceptors,* specialized for the reception of stimuli on or beyond the surface of the body; (2) *interoceptors,* concerned with the reception of stimuli arising within the body itself; and (3) *proprioceptors,* which are a special group of interoceptors specialized for the re-

ception of information about the position of the
body, or its parts, in space; this group includes
the receptors in the vestibular apparatus and
those in muscles and joints. More recent physiological classifications tend to emphasize the
nature of the stimulus that the receptors are
equipped to deal with. Hence we may speak of
*mechanoreceptors, thermoreceptors, nocicep-
tors* (for pain), *chemoreceptors, photoreceptors*
(in the retina), and so on.

A useful anatomical classification rests on the
fact that in most parts of the body, the terminal
portions of the peripheral processes of cranial or
spinal ganglion cells fall into one of three
groups: (1) *Free nerve endings,* which in this
case, are the terminal branches of the processes
that lose all their coverings (including their
Schwann cell investment) and end without specialization among the epithelial, connective tissue, or other cells of the innervated region (Fig.
8–57). (2) *Expanded tip endings,* which are
found more especially in the skin. Here the terminal branches end in a series of bulbous expansions that make contact with the bases of dome-
like aggregations of specialized epithelial cells.
(3) *Encapsulated endings,* in which the terminal
axon ends inside a distinct connective tissue
capsule in relation to either groups of connective
tissue or muscle cells; such endings are apparently specialized for determining the direction or
type of displacing force that acts on the contained sensory nerve terminal. We shall follow
this classification but, for convenience, describe
the sensory nerve terminals in relation to three
main groups of tissues: skin and subcutaneous
tissue, muscles and joints, and blood vessels and
viscera.

Sensory Receptors in the Skin and Subcutaneous Tissues

As the peripheral branches of a cutaneous nerve
penetrate the subcutaneous tissues and approach
the skin, they form an intricate plexus of interconnected bundles just beneath the dermis (Fig.
8–64). Several branches of a single nerve, and
branches of different nerves, usually contribute
to this *subcutaneous plexus.* From the subcutaneous plexus, branches pass to deep receptors,
and many fine bundles of axons ascend to form
a second *dermal plexus* beneath the epidermal
ridges. From this plexus, terminal branches pass
into the dermal papillae and into the epidermis.
Unless otherwise specified, what follows refers
to both hairy and nonhairy (*glabrous*) skin, but it

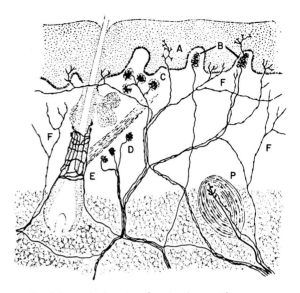

8–64 Schematic drawing showing innervation
pattern of hairy skin. **A,** intraepithelial
endings; **B,** Meissner corpuscles; **C,** Krause's end
bulbs; **D,** Ruffini endings; **E,** endings associated with
hairs; **F,** free endings; **P,** Pacinian corpuscle. (From
LeGros Clark, W. E. 1965. The Tissues of the Body.
Fairlawn, N. J.: Oxford University Press.)

should be noted that in addition to the sensory
fibers, each plexus also contains sympathetic
postganglionic fibers that supply the blood vessels, sweat glands, and arrector pili muscles of
the skin.

Free Nerve Terminals. Free nerve terminals
form the majority of the sensory receptors in the
skin. All are derived from unmyelinated axons of
small diameter (approximately 1 μm or less) and
a single fiber often branches profusely over a
wide area. On approaching the deepest layer of
the epidermis, the basal lamina of the Schwann
cells fuses with that beneath the epidermis, and
the naked nerve fibers pass into the epidermis
within deep invaginations in the epidermal cells.
In this way they may penetrate the epidermis almost as far superficially as the stratum corneum.
They display no obvious structural specialization, but evidence suggests that different fibers
are functionally specialized to respond to painful
stimuli, to warmth or cold, and to mechanical
displacement of the skin. Such receptors are connected to unmyelinated (Fig. 8–57) or finely
myelinated axons in the peripheral nerve trunks.

**Sensory Nerve Endings in Relation to
Hairs.** Hairs are associated with such a rich in-

nervation that they should probably be considered as one of the more elaborate forms of sensory receptor. At least 80% of the finely myelinated fibers in a cutaneous nerve terminate in relation to hairs. Different categories of hair may be identified, and each type is associated with sensory nerve fibers that signal different types of information to the central nervous system. In what follows, we shall be concerned only with the generalities of this system and shall not consider the details of the different types.

Every hair follicle receives several fine unmyelinated axons, most of which are ultimately derived from thinly myelinated parent axons 1 to 5 μm in diameter in the peripheral nerve trunk. Others appear to be branches of thicker myelinated fibers with diameters up to 12 μm.[3] A single parent fiber may branch many times and innervate several hundred follicles, so the *peripheral receptive field* from which the parent nerve fiber or its dorsal root ganglion cell can be activated may be very large. The various fibers innervating a single hair follicle form an encircling meshwork containing both longitudinally and circumferentially running branches that surround the greater part of the hair follicle as it traverses the dermis. Most of the terminal portions of the axons are enclosed in Schwann cells, but the ultimate portion is naked and embedded in the glassy membrane that forms the outermost covering of the follicle. The nerve endings are thus in a position to be activated when the hair is deflected.

Nerve Terminals with Expanded Tips. Two kinds of sensory receptor with expanded nerve terminals are found in glabrous and hairy skin. The most distinctive of these is the *Merkel's touch corpuscle* (Fig. 8–65). As a cutaneous nerve approaches one of these epithelial specializations, it gives rise to a number of unmyelinated branches that lose their Schwann cell covering and penetrate the basal lamina of the epidermis. Each terminal expands to form a flattened disc or plate that is closely applied to a modified epidermal cell (Merkel cell). These cells are attached to the neighboring cells by desmosomes, and they have many flattened cytoplasmic protrusions that enclose the terminal discs of the nerve fiber. Where it is in close contact with the nerve ending, the Merkel cell con-

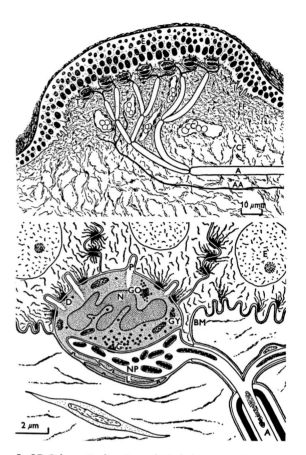

8–65 Schematic drawings of Merkel-type touch corpuscles from footpad of a cat. Merkel cell (indicated by shading in lower figure) contains granular vesicles **(G)** and is contacted by platelike axon terminal **(NP)**. (From Iggo, A., and Muir, A. R. 1969. J. Physiol. [Lond.], 200:763; courtesy of A. Iggo.)

tains many large, dense-core vesicles approximately 1,000 Å in diameter. The nerve terminal itself does not contain vesicles. The myelinated nerves whose terminals end in Merkel's corpuscles are of large diameter (7 to 12 μm) and are usually excited by pressure applied directly to the touch corpuscles.

A simpler form of epithelial cell–nerve terminal complex, in which expanded terminals of an axon end in relation to normal basal epidermal cells, has been identified as a cold receptor. In these cases, the parent axons are myelinated and are about 1 to 6 μm in diameter; they are specifically activated by localized cooling of the epidermis over their terminals. No specialized receptors have yet been identified for the reception of warm stimuli.

---

[3]Fiber diameters indicated here refer to primates. Diameters of the largest fibers in some experimental animals (e.g., cats) may be up to 15–16 μm.

Encapsulated Nerve Terminals. Although numerically in the minority, encapsulated receptors have tended to dominate descriptions of the innervation of the skin and subcutaneous tissues because of their large size and distinctive appearance. Three main types are usually recognized: *Pacinian corpuscles, Ruffini endings,* and *Meissner's corpuscles.* Other types, less distinct and not recognized by all authorities, are *Krause's end bulbs* and *Golgi-Mazzoni corpuscles.* All these encapsulated endings are distinguished by the presence of a lamellated connective tissue sheath surrounding the nerve terminals. The form of the connective tissue ensheathment and of the nerve terminal is extremely variable but sufficiently characteristic for each type of receptor to be readily recognized. Each is innervated by a single myelinated axon, 6 to 12 μm in diameter, which is usually derived from a parent trunk that supplies many lamellated endings of the same type.

The Pacinian Corpuscle. This is one of the largest sensory receptors, often with a diameter of 1 mm. They are found in subcutaneous tissues below both hairy and glabrous skin and are especially numerous just beneath the dermis of the digits; they are also present in large numbers in the deep musculoskeletal tissues, especially in the periosteum, and in the mesenteries of the peritoneal cavity. The capsule is ellipsoidal and made up of 30 or more concentric rings of flattened fibroblast-like cells that are continuous with the endoneural sheath of the nerve terminating in the capsule (Fig. 8–66). The lamellae of the capsule are formed by the overlapping processes of several cells and each lamella is separated from its neighbor by a fluid-filled space. The nerve fiber enters one pole of the capsule and its last one or two myelin internodes are usually contained within the capsule. However, the greater part of the axon within the sheath is unmyelinated. This part is straight and terminates near the other pole of the corpuscle as a small spray of knoblike branches (Fig. 8–67). Like all other sensory nerve terminals, the axon endings display no unique structure at the electron-microscope level. The unmyelinated part of the axon is surrounded by multiple lamellae of flattened Schwann cells that are closely packed and form an *inner core* within the encircling fibrous connective tissue lamellae (the *outer core*). Pacinian corpuscles are exquisitely sensitive to mechanical displacement: the corpuscle can respond to vibratory stimuli up to about 700 per

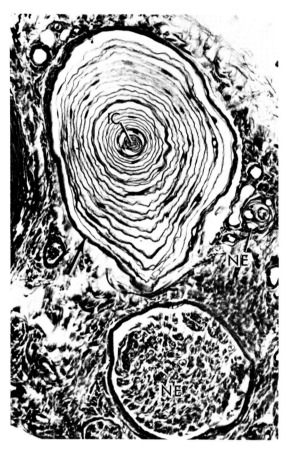

8–66 Pacinian corpuscle with numerous concentric lamellae and inner core **(IC)** containing the terminal part of the innervating axon that is usually derived from a nearby nerve bundle **(Ne)**. **Arrow** indicates capsule of Pacinian corpuscle. Hematoxylin and eosin stain. × 200.

second. The capsule is not essential for the responsiveness of the terminal (since all the outer core and much of the inner can be removed without affecting the response of the nerve terminal to directly applied mechanical stimuli). However, it seems to serve as a mechanical filter, and its elastic components ensure that the nerve responds in a rapidly adapting manner both when the stimulus is applied and when it is removed.

Meissner's Corpuscles. These receptors are found in the dermal papillae of glabrous skin (Fig. 8–68). They are particularly common near the tips of the fingers and toes. The corpuscle is smaller (approximately 150 μm long) and more cylindrical than the Pacinian corpuscle. The flat-

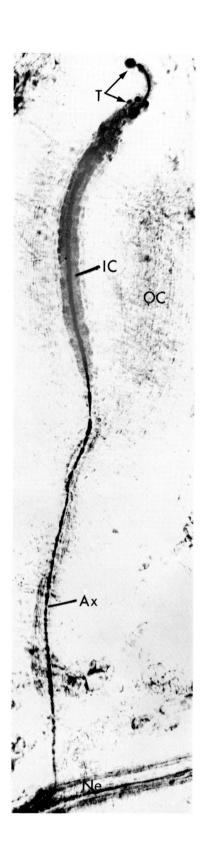

8–67 A myelinated nerve fiber **(Ax)** leaving a nerve bundle **(Ne)** to innervate a Pacinian corpuscle. The inner core of the corpuscle **(IC)** is clearly shown, as are the naked terminal expansions of the nerve fiber **(T).** The outer capsular lamellae **(OC)** are lightly stained. Gold chloride stain. × 1,000.

tened cells form the greater part of its mass and are arranged in multiple-stacked lamellae within a thin, fibrous connective tissue outer coat. Most of the lamellar cells appear to be modified Schwann cells, and the unmyelinated terminal part of the axon threads its way among the lamellae to the superficial pole of the corpuscle. Commonly, more than one axon may enter a sin-

8–68 Schematic drawing of a Meissner corpuscle showing linkage by tonofibrils to overlying epidermis. **ax,** axons; **cp,** blood vessel; **pn,** perineurial sheath; **ra,** receptor part of axons; **SC,** Schwann cells. (From Andres, K. H., and von Düring, M. 1973. Handbook of Sensory Physiology, vol. 2. New York: Springer-Verlag, New York, Inc.; courtesy of K. H. Andres.)

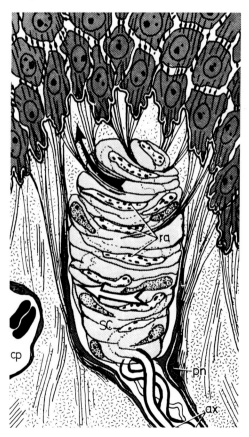

gle Meissner's corpuscle, but it is not clear whether they are branches of the same or of different parent axons. Meissner's corpuscles seem to be sensitive tactile receptors usually activated by moving the epidermal ridges of the glabrous skin over a surface. Although they too are rapidly adapting, they seem to respond best to low-frequency stimuli (approximately 30–40 per second).

Ruffini Endings. Although once considered artifacts of metallic impregnation, these endings are now regarded as one of the commonest forms of slowly adapting mechanoreceptor (Fig. 8–69). They are elongated fusiform structures, up to 1 to 2 mm in length, and are found in the dermis of both hairy and glabrous skin, in subcutaneous tissues, and in joint capsules. They are the least highly lamellated of the encapsulated receptors and consist of a thin connective tissue capsule enclosing a fluid-filled space. This space is traversed by bundles of collagen fibers that often pass through the capsule and are joined to other collagen fibers in the dermis and adjacent tissues. A single myelinated axon, 5 to 12 μm in diameter, enters the capsular space, loses its myelin sheath, and breaks up into a large number of unmyelinated branches that intertwine with the collagen bundles. The receptors are activated by displacement of the surrounding con-

8–69 Camera lucida drawing of nerve terminal from a gold-chloride-impregnated Ruffini ending in knee-joint capsule of a cat. Capsule of ending and other connective tissue elements are not shown. (From Skoglund, S. 1956. Acta Physiol. Scand. 36 (Suppl.) 124:1)

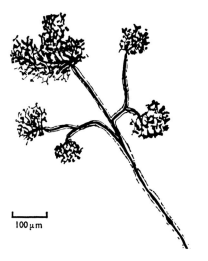

100 μm

nective tissues and they usually respond with a regular, sustained discharge to a maintained mechanical stimulus.

Sensory Receptors in Muscles and Joints

Sensory Receptors in Muscle. Skeletal muscles contain some of the most highly organized encapsulated sensory receptors, together with many free nerve endings (Fig. 8–70). The encapsulated endings are the *muscle spindles* and the *Golgi tendon organs*, both of which are *proprioceptors*.

Muscle Spindles. *Muscle spindles* are found in all human striated muscles but are occasionally absent from some muscles, such as the tongue and the extraocular muscles, in other animals. Their numbers vary from muscle to muscle: in general, muscles that are capable of delicate movements and are subject to the highest degree of central nervous control contain the highest numbers of muscle spindles. For example, the intrinsic muscles of the hand, and the neck muscles at the base of the skull that are responsible for the delicate postural adjustments of the head on the spinal column contain a greater relative number of spindles than do such large muscles as the gluteus maximus and latissimus dorsi.

Each muscle spindle consists of an ovoid connective tissue capsule, about 1.5 mm long and 0.5 mm wide, enclosing a fluid-filled space (Figs. 8–71 and 8–72). This space is traversed from pole to pole by a bundle of special striated muscle fibers that are associated with specialized sensory and motor nerves. The capsule is composed of several circumferential lamellae of flattened fibroblasts (Fig. 8–72), joined to one another at intervals by desmosomes. At the poles of the spindle the lamellae are closely applied to the contained muscle fibers, but elsewhere they enclose a dilated *capsular space* containing tissue fluid, a little delicate endomysial connective tissue, and the neuromuscular apparatus of the spindle. The muscle fibers within the spindle are termed *intrafusal fibers* to distinguish them from the main contractile elements of the muscle, which are termed *extrafusal fibers*. The intrafusal fibers are much smaller, both in diameter and length, than extrafusal fibers, but their orientation is the same, so that the muscle spindles are said to be *in parallel* with the extrafusal fibers.

Each small bundle of intrafusal fibers contains

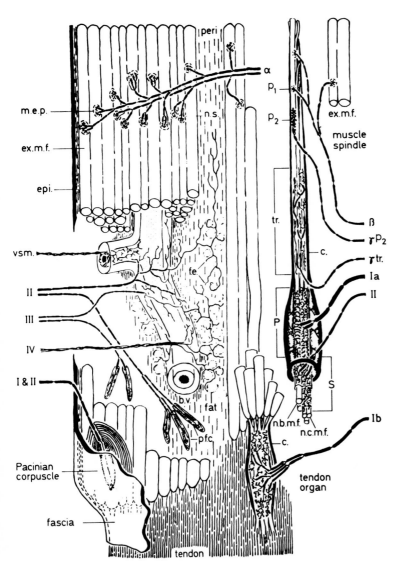

8–70 Schematic drawing showing pattern of innervation of skeletal muscle. Nerve fiber groupings indicated to left and right innervate structures shown. **bv**, blood vessel; **fe**, free endings; **pfc**, "Paciniform" corpuscles; **vsm**, vasomotor (sympathetic) endings. (From Barker, D. 1974. Handbook of Sensory Physiology, vol. 3, part 2. New York: Springer-Verlag, New York, Inc., Courtesy of D. Barker.)

from two to 20 or more intrafusal fibers. In most mammals they are of two main types: a longer, somewhat thicker form that extends well beyond the poles of the spindle capsule, its ends being inserted into endo- or perimysial connective tissue; and a shorter, thinner form whose ends do not extend much beyond the poles of the capsule. Every spindle contains one or two of the thicker type and many more of the smaller type. Both types are striated over much of their length and have dark-staining, peripherally placed nuclei. As they approach the widest part of the capsular space (the "equator" of the spindle) they usually lose their striations. In the larger form of intrafusal fiber, there is a large central aggrega-

tion of nuclei in the equatorial region; for this reason these fibers are known as *nuclear bag fibers* (Fig. 8–72). On each side of this central aggregation, the nuclei form a single row (the "myotube" region); beyond this, they are progressively replaced by myofibrils and peripheral nuclei. Some nuclear bag fibers may enter a second spindle capsule at some distance from the first and give rise to a nuclear bag in the second as well. This arrangement constitutes a *tandem spindle*.

The shorter and more numerous form of intrafusal fiber has only a single row of vesicular nuclei in its central nonstriated portion. It is thus known as a *nuclear chain fiber* (Fig. 8–72). Nu-

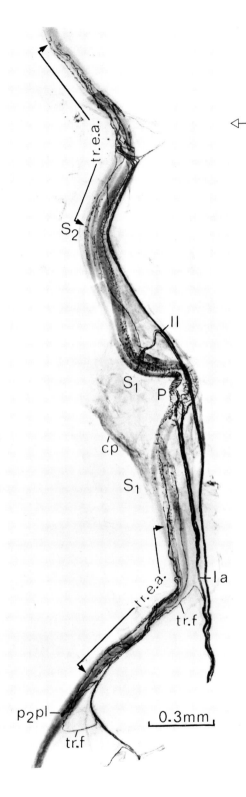

8–71 Silver-stained, teased, whole preparation of a muscle spindle from muscle of a cat. **cp,** capsule; **P** primary ending; **p₂pl,** plate ending; **S₁, S₂,** secondary endings; **tr.e.a., tr. f.,** trail endings and trail fiber. (From Barker, D., Stacey, M. J., and Adal, M. N. 1970. Philos. Trans. R. Soc. Lond. [Biol. Sci.] 258: 315; courtesy of D. Barker.)

clear chain fibers and some nuclear bag fibers have been found to be more rapidly contracting than other nuclear bag fibers and they usually have a less-regular pattern of myofilaments with much intervening sarcoplasm and well-developed M lines. The other nuclear bag fibers have a more orderly array of myofilaments, less intervening sarcoplasm, and no M lines. These nuclear bag fibers seem to contract in a tonic fashion, and their activation is not associated with a propagated action potential. They therefore resemble the "slow" muscles of lower vertebrates. The contraction of nuclear chain fibers is more twitchlike and is associated with propagated action potentials. Note that because of the lack of myofilaments in the equatorial regions, the cen-

8–72 A muscle spindle in cross section showing the appearance of the connective tissue capsule **(C),** the capsular space **(CS),** two large nuclear bag intrafusal fibers **(NB),** and several smaller nuclear chain fibers **(NC).** The spindle as a whole is in parallel with the extrafusal muscle fibers **(MF).** Van Gieson stain. × 350.

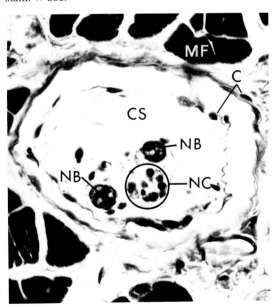

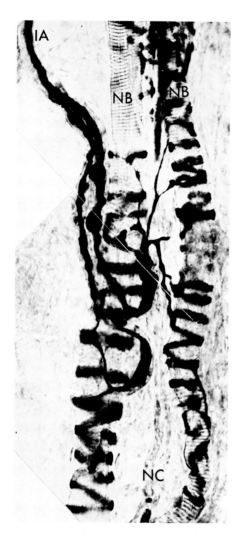

8–73 A group **IA** fiber terminating as spiral primary endings on two nuclear bag fibers **(NB)** in muscle spindle of a marsupial. Nuclear chain fibers **(NC)** do not appear to receive a primary ending in this methylene-blue-stained, teased preparation. × 400. (From Jones, E. G., 1967. J. Anat. [Lond.] 100:733.)

tral parts of the intrafusal fibers are essentially noncontractile.

The sensory nerves to a muscle spindle enter through the capsule and terminate near the equatorial region of the intrafusal muscle fibers (Figs. 8–71 and 8–73). Every spindle receives a single, large, myelinated afferent fiber about 12 to 20 μm in diameter. This fiber loses its myelin sheath close to the intrafusal bundle and gives rise to several branches that end in a series of ribbon-like spirals that partially or completely encircle the central portion of each nuclear bag and nu-

clear chain fiber (Fig. 8–73). Electron microscopy shows that the terminal spirals and rings may be deeply invaginated into folds in the sarcolemma of the intrafusal fibers without any intervening basal lamina. The whole terminal complex is known as the *primary sensory ending* of the spindle, and its parent fiber (which may supply primary endings to more than one spindle capsule) is usually called a *group Ia* afferent fiber.

Many spindles, although not all, also receive one or more smaller (group II) afferent fibers, about 6 to 8 μm in diameter. These fibers lose their myelin sheath as they branch within the spindle capsule and form terminal spirals, rings, and sprays similar to those of the primary ending but predominantly on the nuclear chain fibers. This complex constitutes the *secondary sensory ending* of the spindle. Both the primary and secondary endings of a spindle are activated by any stretching force acting on the muscle as a whole, which would tend to lengthen the intrafusal bundle. The primary ending responds most vigorously during the dynamic phase of the stretch; secondary endings are more responsive to maintained stretch. That is, the primary endings exhibit *dynamic sensitivity*, the secondary endings *static sensitivity*.

The spindles are also innervated by a number of small motor nerve fibers that end on the striated portions of the intrafusal fibers near both poles of the capsule (Fig. 8–71). The parent nerve fibers are small, myelinated axons 2 to 8 μm in diameter arising from a specific group of small motoneurons in the ventral horn of the spinal cord. These fibers innervate only intrafusal muscle fibers and are known as γ *motoneurons*, or *fusimotor neurons*; the axons that provide the motor innervation to the spindle are, thus, termed γ *efferents*, or *fusimotor fibers*. Less commonly, some of the large α motor fibers that supply the extrafusal musculature (see p. 346) also provide a branch to one or more intrafusal fibers in a neighboring spindle. Two types of motor nerve terminal are seen on the intrafusal fibers. Some are localized and closely resemble the motor end plates on extrafusal muscle fibers. Others are long, diffuse endings that ramify widely over the surface of the intrafusal fiber and make multiple *en passant* terminal contacts. The "plate" type of ending is found mainly on nuclear bag fibers, and the diffuse "trail" type, mainly on nuclear chain fibers; but both types can at times be found on the same fiber. Activity in the fusimotor fibers causes the intrafusal fibers to contract and thus effectively

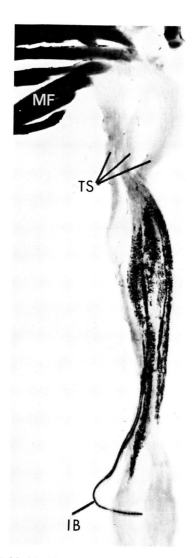

8–74 Gold-chloride-stained, teased preparation of a Golgi tendon organ from myotendinous junction of a marsupial. Group **IB** fiber branches widely among tendinous slips **(TS)** attached to several skeletal muscle fibers **(MF)**. × 80.

stretch the nonstriated part of the fiber that carries the sensory endings. This leads to a state of increased sensitivity of the sensory endings so that they discharge more readily and at increased rates when the muscle in which they lie is stretched.

Golgi Tendon Organs. These receptors, found primarily at musculotendinous junctions, consist of a thin, fibroblastic capsule that is filled with a number of large, collagenous fiber bundles continuous with those of the tendon in which the

organ lies (Fig. 8–74). The whole complex may be about 1 mm long, and since a variable number (3 to 25) of extrafusal muscle fibers are inserted into the collagenous tendon slips that make up the greater part of the tendon organ, these receptors are said to be *in series* with the extrafusal fibers. This arrangement permits the sensory nerve fibers to be activated during both contraction and stretching of the relevant muscle.

Each tendon organ receives a single, large, myelinated sensory nerve fiber having a diameter of 12 to 15 μm; afferent fibers of this type fall within the group Ib class of muscle afferents (see below). The terminal branches of the fiber lose their myelin sheaths after entering the capsule of the tendon organ and give rise to a number of longitudinally running unmyelinated branches that terminate in small sprays of naked terminals wrapped around, and insinuated between, the bundles of collagen fibers.

Sensory Receptors in Joints. The capsules and periarticular tissues of joints are richly endowed with proprioceptors, which, along with muscle receptors, are believed to contribute to the conscious awareness of movement and position (*kinesthesis*). The majority of receptors found in joints have already been described. There are many free nerve endings derived from both unmyelinated and finely myelinated parent fibers, some of which penetrate as far as the synovial membrane. The major type of encapsulated ending found in joint capsules is the Ruffini ending, but some Pacinian corpuscles are also present. In the ligaments associated with the joint capsule, Golgi tendon organs are common. The function of these different receptors in kinesthesis is not clear; recent evidence suggests that the stretch receptors of the muscles acting on a joint may signal small variations in joint angle. The Ruffini endings seem to discharge in response to movement in one direction, and some show a substantial response when the joint is held in a fixed position. The small Pacinian corpuscles seem to respond only to movements. The role of the free nerve terminals is uncertain, but many are thought to be nociceptive.

Sensory Nerve Endings in Blood Vessels and Viscera

The walls of the larger blood vessels, and all the thoracic and abdominal viscera, contain a fairly rich complement of mechanoreceptors. In many regions nociceptors are also present and individual organs may have other special kinds of receptors that reflect their particular functions. Collectively, these receptors are termed *interoceptors*.

Most interoceptors are free, or relatively poorly organized, nerve endings that ramify beneath and between epithelial cells and in the submucosal, muscular, and serosal coats of hollow viscera. The parent nerves are usually of small diameter (unmyelinated or thinly myelinated) and are distributed with the autonomic nerves. In some sites, such as the mesenteries, encapsulated endings (and especially Pacinian corpuscles) are also seen.

The best-defined interoceptors are those associated with the aortic arch and with the carotid body and sinus. They monitor circulating blood gas levels and blood pressure and mediate a variety of cardiovascular and respiratory reflexes. The receptors that are sensitive to changes in oxygen and carbon dioxide tension and blood pH are called *chemoreceptors* and are found in the carotid body and in similar bodies on the arch of the aorta. Those sensitive to changes in blood pressure are called *baroreceptors* and are found in the walls of the carotid sinus and aortic arch. Each has a rather similar structure consisting of glomerular aggregations of large globular cells (which are thought to be the actual receptors) on which the highly branched afferent nerve fibers terminate. In the case of the chemoreceptors, the large cells are filled with dense-core vesicles 1,000 to 2,000 Å in diameter and contain rich stores of catecholamines. Many arteriovenous anastomoses are also present and apparently serve to regulate blood flow through the carotid and aortic bodies. Free nerve endings are also found in the subendocardial layers of the heart, particularly near the valves and in the atrial walls close to the point of entry of the great veins.

In the hollow viscera of the alimentary and genitourinary tracts the free nerve endings seem to be excited mainly by distension of the viscus or by peristaltic or other muscular activity. In certain regions, groups of free receptor terminals in the epithelium are thought to be specifically excited by changes in intraluminal pH, by changes in glucose concentration, or by the presence of certain amino acids and polypeptides.

In the respiratory tract, free nerve endings in and beneath the epithelium of the larynx, trachea, and bronchi are sensitive to irritant particles and gases, and when stimulated evoke a coughing reflex. In the lungs themselves, the pulmonary stretch receptors are mainly free nerve endings associated with the smooth muscle of the bronchi. Their afferent fibers are myelinated and are among the fastest conducting interoceptive afferents. Other free endings in the interstitial tissue around the alveoli are thought to be sensitive to changes in the interstitial fluid, particularly those brought about by vascular congestion and irritant vapors.

The Peripheral Terminations of Efferent Nerve Fibers

Motor Nerve Fibers to Skeletal Muscle. Striated muscles are innervated by the axons of motor nerve cells (motoneurons) situated in the ventral horn of the spinal cord or in the motor nuclei of certain of the cranial nerves. Two classes of myelinated fiber are involved: (1) large fibers with diameters of 12 to 20 μm, commonly termed α *motor fibers*, which innervate the extrafusal muscle fibers; (2) thinner fibers, 2 to 8 μm in diameter, termed γ *efferents*, or *fusimotor fibers*, which innervate the intrafusal fibers of the muscle spindles. Because the latter have already been described, the following account will be concerned solely with the α fibers.

The α motor axons, which are among the largest in the peripheral nervous system, seldom branch before entering the muscle they innervate. However, they branch profusely in the muscle so that a single parent axon may innervate anything from 1 or 2 muscle fibers to 500 or more. On the other hand, each muscle fiber is usually innervated by only one axon. A single motor axon and all the extrafusal fibers it supplies are referred to as a *motor unit*.

As the branches of an axon approach the muscle fibers they are to innervate, they lose their myelin sheaths; covered only by their Schwann cell investment, they form specialized terminal formations known as *motor end plates* (Figs. 8–37, 8–75A, 8–76, and 8–77). Typically a motor end plate is made up of the expanded terminal portion of an α motor axon and its sheath, a junctional cleft, and a specialized portion of the underlying extrafusal muscle fiber. On the surface of the muscle fiber, the axon forms a number of interconnected terminal bulbs of varying size within a fairly circumscribed round or oval zone (Fig. 8–77). In the light microscope this zone appears slightly elevated because the terminal bulbs are overlain by Schwann cells and by the

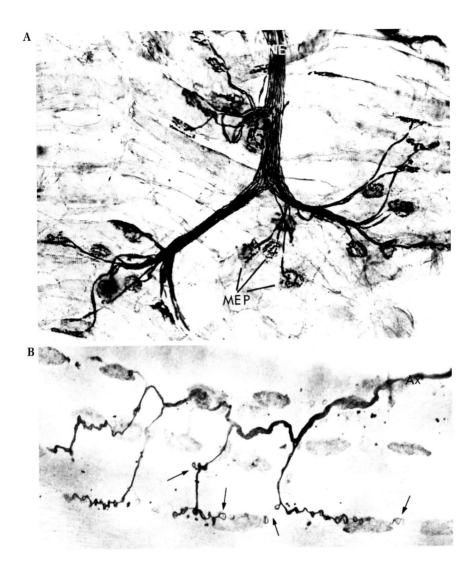

8–75 **A** Gold-chloride-stained, teased preparation of human intercostal muscle showing intramuscular nerve **(NE)** branching to supply motor end plates **(MEP)** on skeletal muscle fibers. × 70. **B.** Silver-stained, teased preparation showing motor axon **(Ax)** branching to supply diffuse multiterminal endings in slow muscle of a tortoise. **Arrows** indicate neurofibrillar rings. × 650.

cells of the endoneurium, which become continuous with the endomysium. This connective tissue layer, external to the Schwann cells, is termed the *sheath of Henle* (Fig. 8–37).

In electron micrographs the terminals resemble synaptic boutons, being filled with large numbers of clear vesicles (approximately 400 Å in diameter) and many mitochondria. Fingers of Schwann cell cytoplasm cover the individual terminal bulbs and may penetrate between them and the muscle fiber (Fig. 8–76). The plasma membranes of the axon terminal and the underlying muscle fiber are separated by an extracellular cleft approximately 500 Å in width, which is filled with the basal lamina of the muscle fiber. The presynaptic membrane shows no dis-

tinctive specialization; but over the whole length of its approximation to the sarcolemma, the latter is thrown into a large number of folds that deeply invaginate the underlying sarcoplasm. Like the cleft, these infoldings are filled with basal lamina (Figs. 8–37 and 8–76).

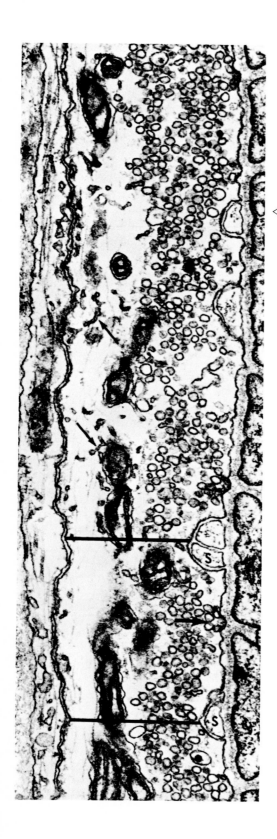

8–76 Electron micrograph of a frog neuromuscular junction. Terminal is separated by basal lamina from junctional folds of muscle fiber (to right). Schwann cell process covers it to far left and some Schwann cell processes **(S)** intervene between terminal and basal lamina. **Large arrow** indicates one of several aggregations of synaptic vesicles about a presynaptic density, site of active synaptic vesicle release. **Small arrows** indicate smooth endoplasmic reticulum. × 40,000 (From Heuser, J. E., and Reese, T. S. 1973. J. Cell Biol. 57:315; courtesy of T. S. Reese.)

The plasma membrane of the muscle fiber usually has a small amount of dense material attached to it along the crests between each infolding. This region thus resembles the postsynaptic specialization seen at central synapses and is thought to represent the "active site" of the neuromuscular junction. In the portion of the axon terminal immediately opposite each of the junctional folds, there is usually a ridge and a small accumulation of synaptic vesicles (Figs. 8–37, 8–76, and 8–78). During prolonged stimulation of a motor nerve, synaptic vesicles move toward these sites. The sarcoplasm beneath the nerve terminal is often called the *sole plate* and is usually devoid of myofilaments but rich in free ribosomes, rough endoplasmic reticulum, and mitochondria. There is also an accumulation of nuclei in this region that are somewhat larger

8–77 Gold-chloride-stained preparation of two motor end plates from a human intercostal muscle. Dark bulbs are terminal contacts. × 1,100.

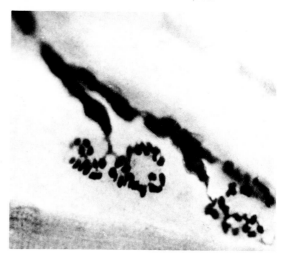

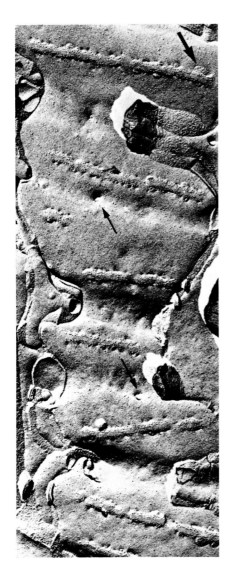

8–78 Freeze-fracture preparation showing surface of nerve terminal at a frog neuromuscular junction. Transverse ridges with membrane particles correspond to presynaptic regions indicated by large arrow in Fig. 8–76. Grooves between ridges correspond to regions occupied by Schwann cell processes. **Arrows** indicate presumed re-formation of synaptic vesicles by endocytosis. × 30,000. (From Heuser, J. E., Reese, T. S., and Landis, D. M. D. 1974. J. Neurocytol. 3:109; courtesy of T. S. Reese.)

and more vesicular than other muscle nuclei; they are the *sole plate nuclei.*

Motor end plates vary in structure, depending on the type of muscle in which they lie. In mammals, the motor end plates of *fast-twitch muscles* have many long and often branched sarcolemmal infoldings. In *slow-twitch muscles* the sarcolemmal infoldings are fewer and shallower; the axon terminals also contain fewer synaptic vesicles than do those ending on fast-twitch muscles. True *slow muscles,* which do not show propagated action potentials and which are capable of sustained, graded contractions, are uncommon in mammals. When present (for example, in the extraocular muscles) they are characterized by diffuse, multiterminal (or *en grappes*) motor endings; the terminal motor axon spreads diffusely over much of the surface of the muscle fiber and gives off terminal bulbs at intervals (Fig. 8–75B). Individual bulbs may be separated from one another by several hundred microns. Each of these bulbs contains synaptic vesicles and makes a contact in every way similar to a motor end plate, but there are no associated sarcolemmal infoldings.

The Peripheral Terminations of Autonomic Nerve Fibers

The axons of the neurons in sympathetic and parasympathetic ganglia are extremely fine (approximately 1 μm) and in most cases unmyelinated. The postganglionic fibers of the sympathetic division of the autonomic nervous system are distributed in peripheral nerves (which they join via the gray rami communicantes), or in plexuses associated with the larger blood vessels (Fig. 8–79A), or in the splanchnic nerves. In the autonomic plexuses of the abdominopelvic cavity, sympathetic preganglionic fibers are distributed with the postganglionic fibers, since not all preganglionic fibers synapse in the sympathetic chain. Parasympathetic preganglionic fibers derived from the vagus are also found in the visceral autonomic plexuses.

Although the sympathetic nervous system is in general a diffusely distributed system, the density and diffuseness of the innervation varies from organ to organ. For example, the postganglionic axons supplying the sphincter pupillae muscle branch little before entering the iris and give rise to a relatively sparse terminal plexus within it, whereas those innervating the gut branch profusely and give rise to a widespread plexus in the gut wall. The terminal ramifications of sympathetic postganglionic fibers in an organ are called the *sympathetic ground plexus.* This consists of a large number of fine, often interconnected, axons that ramify over the surfaces

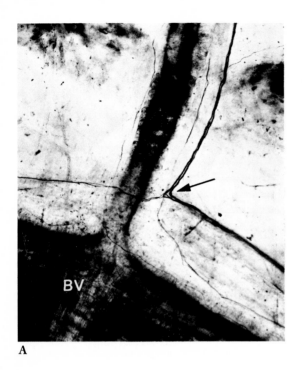

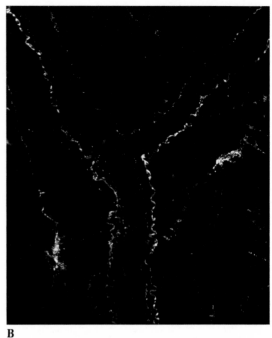

A

B

8–79 A. Silver-stained, teased preparation showing several unmyelinated axons accompanying a large blood vessel **(BV). Arrow** indicates point of bifurcation of certain fibers. × 500. **B.** Fluorescence photomicrograph showing a small branching blood vessel in the mucous membrane of the alimentary tract outlined by thin axons. The axons contain the peptide transmitter, substance P, and have been labeled immunocytochemically with a monoclonal antibody to this peptide. × 250. (Courtesy of A. C. Cuello and M. A. Matthews.)

of smooth muscle and gland cells. At regular intervals each terminal branch has a series of bulb-like expansions that are regions of transmitter release (Fig. 8–37).

At the electron microscopic level, these bulb-like expansions appear rather like synaptic boutons, because they contain large aggregations of synaptic vesicles and mitochondria. However, they are usually not in intimate contact with the underlying smooth muscle or gland cells, and the characteristic pre- or postsynaptic membrane densities seen at central synapses are rarely present. In some places such as the vas deferens and the sphincter pupillae, the terminal bulbs may approach to within 150 to 200 Å of the smooth muscle fibers and no Schwann cell processes intervene: in these sites it is possible that all or most muscle cells are contacted by at least one terminal bulb. In other sites, such as the gut, most terminal varicosities lie at some distance (1,000 Å) from the target cells and are thought to exert their effects by releasing their transmitters into the general intercellular space. Because smooth muscle cells are electrotonically coupled by means of gap junctions, the excitation of one cell rapidly spreads from cell to cell throughout the tissue.

The terminals of most sympathetic postganglionic axons release *norepinephrine (noradrenaline)*, but some release *acetylcholine*. In the case of noradrenergic endings, most of the synaptic vesicles present are small (about 500 Å) and contain dense cores (Fig. 8–34). These dense cores are especially obvious if the tissue has been "loaded" with the transmitter or with an analog, such as 6-hydroxydopamine, or if it has been fixed in potassium permanganate. A few larger, dense-core vesicles (approximately 1,000 Å) are also found in adrenergic terminals. Both types probably contain norepinephrine and the final enzyme involved in its synthesis, *dopamine-β-hydroxylase*.

Cholinergic nerve terminals in the sympathetic system generally resemble the adrenergic terminals with the notable exception that the vesicles they contain are clear, comparable to those seen in motor nerve terminals in skeletal muscle. Although much less work has been done on the peripheral terminations of parasympathetic postganglionic fibers, they too appear to be of this type. Parasympathetic preganglionic fibers end in such sites as the sinoatrial and atrioventricular nodes and on the postganglionic neurons by means of terminals containing clear vesicles and with definite (asymmetric) pre- and postsynaptic membrane thickenings.

The walls of the alimentary tract possess extensive plexuses of nerve fibers that derive partly from pre- and postganglionic sympathetic and parasympathetic fibers and partly from neurons that are intrinsic to the gut wall (see Chap. 19). These plexuses are concerned with maintaining the rhythmic peristaltic activity of the alimentary canal, although the intrinsic neuronal system is itself capable of maintaining this activity when the sympathetic and parasympathetic nerves are destroyed.

The two major plexuses of the gut wall are the *myenteric* (or Auerbach's) *plexus*, which lies between the longitudinal and circumferential muscle coats, and the *submucosal* (or Meissner's) *plexus*, which lies in the submucosa. Each of these contains localized aggregations of moderately large, multipolar neurons resembling those of the sympathetic and parasympathetic ganglia. The adrenergic nerve terminals in these plexuses may be derived from sympathetic neurons situated in the sympathetic chain or in the ganglionated plexuses. They take the form of chains of bulbous terminals containing large numbers of small, dense-core vesicles. Such terminals form axodendritic and axosomatic synapses on the intrinsic neurons. Unlike adrenergic terminals elsewhere, definite membrane specializations are present. Other nerve terminals within the plexuses contain small, clear vesicles and also end axosomatically and axodendritically. These may be the terminals of both sympathetic and parasympathetic fibers. The intrinsic neurons themselves appear to have short axons that end as varicose, clear-vesicle-containing terminals among the smooth muscle cells adjacent to the plexus; they appear to utilize a variety of neurotransmitters.

A third smaller plexus of fine nerve fibers is found in the gut wall at the level of the muscularis mucosae. It contains relatively few nerve cells and seems to be composed predominantly of sensory fibers whose finer branches ramify beneath the epithelium, sending naked terminal processes between adjoining epithelial cells. The sensory nerve fibers supplying the mucous membrane have their cell bodies in the dorsal root ganglia, but they are distributed with the autonomic nerves and thus pass through the myenteric and submucosal plexuses en route to the mucosa.

The Fiber Spectra of Peripheral Nerves

In the foregoing accounts of sensory, motor, and autonomic nerves and their terminations, we have frequently pointed out that different types of nerve endings are customarily supplied by axons whose diameter and degree of myelination are fairly constant for a particular category of ending. Because the diameter of an axon is closely related to its conduction velocity, fibers in a particular diameter range will also fall within a fairly constant range of conduction velocities. The range of fiber diameters in a nerve is known as the *fiber spectrum* of that nerve (Fig. 8–58A and B), and because of the relationship between diameter and conduction velocity, such a fiber spectrum also effectively indicates the range of conduction velocities in the fibers of that nerve.

On the basis of their diameters, conduction velocities, and certain other properties that need not concern us here, peripheral nerve fibers have been grouped into several classes. A summary of the two main classifications in current use is given in Table 8–1. The alphabetic classification into groups A, B, and C was made in the 1930s by Erlanger and Gasser and is based on the conduction velocities of mixed peripheral nerve fibers as revealed by the peaks of the compound action potentials recorded after electrical stimulation of the various peripheral nerves. Group A contains fibers with the fastest conduction velocities, and within it two subgroups are now identified. These subgroups (in order of decreasing diameter) are the $A\alpha$ and $A\delta$ fibers. The B group is formed principally by autonomic preganglionic fibers, and the C group is composed of unmyelinated fibers (including both afferent fibers entering the spinal cord in the dorsal roots and autonomic postganglionic fibers).

A second widely used classification was originally introduced by Lloyd to describe the afferent fibers in muscle nerves. Four groups of fibers were recognized on the basis of their diameters: groups I, II, III, and IV. This is perhaps the more

Table 8–1 Classification of Peripheral Nerve Fibers

Fiber type	Aα			Aδ	C
	Group I		Group II	Group III	Group IV (unmyelinated)
Diameter (includes myelin sheath, where present)	12–20 μm	5–20 μm	5–12 μm	2–5 μm	0.1–1.5 μm
Conduction velocity	70–120 m/s	30–120 m/s	30–70 m/s	5–30 m/s	0.5–2 m/s
Receptor types	Primary endings in muscle spindles (Ia) Golgi tendon organs (Ib)		Secondary endings in muscle spindles Most other encapsulated endings Larger diameter mechanoreceptors and interoreceptors	Thermoceptors Nociceptors Smaller diameter mechanoreceptors and interoreceptors	
Other fiber types	α motor fibers, 12–20 μm		γ motor fibers, 2–8 μm	Autonomic preganglionic fibers 1.5–4 μm (B fibers)	Autonomic postganglionic fibers; olfactory nerve fibers, 0.1–1 μm

useful classification (since it also takes into account the peripheral terminations of sensory fibers). However, it is not usually applied to non-sensory nerves even though they can be made to fit into the scheme (Table 8–1).

Some Aspects of Neuronal Organization

Up to this point we have considered neurons more or less as isolated units. After their migration from the neuroepithelium or the neural crest, however, most neurons normally aggregate with other similar nerve cells to form characteristic neuronal populations. Here we shall consider some general principles of neuronal organization and indicate how the more common neural aggregates are constructed. The three most common types of neural aggregate are (1) the ganglia of the peripheral nervous system, including the sensory ganglia associated with the cranial and spinal nerves, and the ganglia of the autonomic nervous system; (2) various cellular groups in the central nervous system, usually re-

ferred to as *nuclei*; and (3) cortical formations, also found in the central nervous system.

Sensory Ganglia

The cells of all the spinal ganglia (Fig. 8–61A) and most of those in the sensory ganglia associated with the cranial nerves are derived from the neural crest. The cells of certain cranial nerve ganglia are derived from the associated placodal epithelia. The factors leading to the segregation of the neural crest cells that give rise to the sensory ganglia from those that give rise to other crest derivatives are not known. After migrating to their definitive location, they aggregate to form the presumptive ganglion. The key morphogenetic event—the coming together of cells of like kind—represents the first step in the formation of any neuronal population.

Subsequently, a high percentage of the neurons that were initially generated die, usually about the time that the cells in the population as a whole make their synaptic or peripheral sensory connections. This *histogenetic cell death* appears to be a general feature of the formation of most neuronal populations in both the peripheral and central nervous systems: in all populations that have been analyzed quantitatively, only about 30 to 60% of the cells survive to maturity. The factors responsible for the death of so many neurons are not known, but it is generally thought that the cells that die are unable to establish either the appropriate number or the appropriate type of synaptic or sensory connections.

At present the most complete accounts of the development of the sensory ganglia derive from the study of these structures in chick embryos. In these ganglia, two distinct neuronal populations appear: initially a large-celled ventrolateral group of neurons (thought to be proprioceptive) arises; and somewhat later in development a smaller-celled dorsomedially located population is generated. Although at a later stage the topographic segregation of the two populations is obscured, they are clearly different. For example, after the early removal of a developing limb, the larger cells degenerate extremely rapidly, whereas the small-celled population usually persists for a much longer period. Conversely, the developing small-celled population appears to be particularly sensitive to the action of the neurotrophic protein, nerve growth factor (NGF). The precursors of this population and the postganglionic sympathetic neurons are said to be the only cells that proliferate under the influence of NGF. A process of *functional specification* of the ganglion cells must then occur. This process determines not only the peripheral and central connections of the cells but also the sensory modality to which they will respond. The nature of this specification is poorly understood: we do not yet know whether it is an intrinsic property of the developing neurons or if it is imposed on them by the peripheral tissues they innervate. In the adult animal a number of different functional classes of ganglionic cell are present, corresponding to each of the various modalities of somatic sensibility, but except for variations in size (Fig. 8–61B) and in the relative amounts of Nissl material and other organelles that the cells contain, no distinct morphological differences exist within the population of ganglion cells. However, cells innervating closely adjacent peripheral receptive fields and projecting their central processes into the same dorsal root filament tend to lie together. This tendency for neurons that innervate a particular region to be closely related to each other topographically is one of the fundemental prinicples of neuronal organization and is found at virtually all levels of the nervous system. Throughout the somatosensory system, the arrangement is commonly called the *somatotopic organization*, reflecting the systematic central nervous mapping of the body surface; but comparable patterns of organization are found in the other sensory systems where the organizing feature is either topographic (for example, the retinotopic organization of the visual system) or functional (for example, the tonotopic organization of the auditory system).

Interestingly, both the large and small neurons in the sensory ganglia undergo chromatolysis when their peripheral processes are interrupted but not when their central processes are cut. This may be related to the observation that substantially more of the materials synthesized in the perikaryon are transported into the peripheral than into the central processes. Because impulse transmission in these sensory neurons seems to proceed directly from the peripheral to the central process (either without invading the soma or by invading it only after some delay), and inasmuch as there are no synapses on the perikaryon, it appears that the principal role of the ganglion cell soma is trophic, in the sense that the soma serves primarily to maintain the integrity of the processes.

The Ganglia of the Autonomic Nervous System

The second major class of peripheral nerve cell aggregation comprises the ganglia associated with the sympathetic and parasympathetic divisions of the autonomic nervous system (Fig. 8–62). The structure of the para- and prevertebral sympathetic ganglia and the principal cranial and sacral parasympathetic ganglia is essentially the same. Certain of the ganglionic arrangements in the viscera (for example, the gut plexuses) are different and have already been briefly outlined.

Like the sensory ganglia, the ganglia of the autonomic nervous system are invested by a fairly dense fibrous connective tissue capsule that is continuous with the epineurium of the related pre- and postganglionic nerve trunks. Within the ganglia the nerve cells are surrounded by satellite cells, which, like the neurons, are of neural crest origin. However, these ganglia differ from the sensory ganglia in two important respects. First, the neurons are all *multipolar*, usually with several dendrites of varying length and with a single, usually unmyelinated, axon that passes out into the appropriate postganglionic trunk. Second, all the so-called principal ganglion cells (and these constitute most of the neurons in each ganglion) receive synapses from the preganglionic fibers. These synapses are all cholinergic in type. The great majority of them are distributed to the dendrites rather than to the cell soma. As a rule, each ganglion cell receives an input from several preganglionic fibers, and conversely each preganglionic fiber forms synapses with several neurons. There are exceptions to this pattern (for example, in the ciliary portion of the avian ciliary ganglion there is a one-to-one relationship between preganglionic fibers and postsynaptic cells), but such exceptions are rare in the mammalian autonomic nervous system.

The ganglion cells themselves are not uniform in type. In most ganglia there is a class of principal cells that are relatively large, with ovoid or spherical nuclei and an abundance of rough endoplasmic reticulum. Those cells that are adrenergic (as are most principal ganglion cells) contain large numbers of small, dense-core vesicles both in their somata and throughout their processes, but especially at the sites of presumed transmitter release from their axons. As we have seen, these dense-core vesicles contain the neurotransmitter norepinephrine (noradrenaline) and the last enzyme involved in its synthesis, dopamine-β-hydroxylase. The presence of these two substances provides the basis for two common methods for displaying postganglionic sympathetic fibers: namely, the Falck-Hillarp method in which the norepinephrine is condensed by formaldehyde vapor to form a highly fluorescent compound; and an immunohistochemical method, using a peroxidase or fluorescently labeled antibody to dopamine-β-hydroxylase (Fig. 8–35).

In many sympathetic ganglia a second, smaller cell type is found that is intensely fluorescent when treated with formaldelyde vapor. These so-called SIF (small, intensely fluorescent) cells appear to be a class of *dopaminergic* interneurons, but their functional role remains to be determined. At their most numerous they constitute only a small percentage of the total number of ganglion cells. Their nuclei are smaller, often ellipsoidal or convoluted, and more heterochromatic than those of the principal cells. They contain many large dense-core vesicles and are

presynaptic to the principal cells, but they may also release their contents directly into the blood stream (Fig. 8–16).

The Organization of Neuronal Aggregates in the Central Nervous System

Compared with the relatively simple organization of peripheral neural aggregates, the central nervous system presents a bewildering display of different neuronal patterns. No two regions of the central nervous system are identical in their organization, although from animal to animal within any species, and even between different species and different classes, homologous structures usually show a surprisingly consistent neural architecture. Only two of the more common patterns will be considered here. These are the so-called central *nuclei* and certain laminated or *cortical* structures. Each of these different types of neuronal aggregate can be readily recognized at a fairly gross level in preparations stained either by the Nissl method or by one of the common methods for myelinated fibers; the analyses of neural organization at this level are called *cytoarchitectonic* or *myeloarchitectonic* studies, respectively, and constitute an essential preliminary to any serious study of the central nervous system.

Central Cell Masses or "Nuclear Groups." Collections of neurons of similar type in the central nervous system are usually termed nuclei (a term that should not be confused with the nuclei of individual neurons) (Figs. 8–80 and 8–81). The neurons in such nuclei are usually generated over a restricted period of time in a well-defined region of the neuroepithelium. From this region the postmitotic, but still immature, neurons migrate to their definitive location where they aggregate with other neurons of the same type. The mechanisms responsible for this selective cell aggregation are generally thought to involve the presence on the surfaces of the cells of certain cell-type-specific macromolecules (probably glycoproteins) that serve to "recognize" other cells of similar type. This does not imply that all the cells in a given nucleus are absolutely identical in structure or function. In fact, in nearly every center that has been carefully studied in adult animals, two or more distinct cell types have been found. One type, which we may again refer to as the principal cell, usually gives rise to the efferent axons that connect the cell mass to other

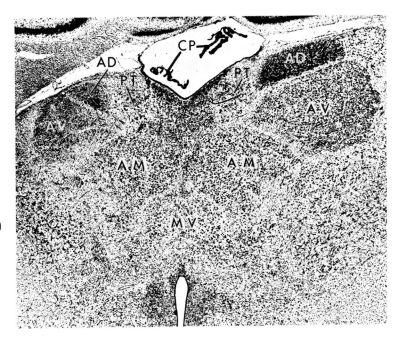

8–80 Frontal section of diencephalon of a rabbit brain from which cingulate region of cerebral cortex was removed several weeks previously. Anterodorsal **(AD)** and anteroventral **(AV)** nuclei of left thalamus have undergone profound retrograde degeneration characterized by cell death and gliosis. Other nuclei **(AM, PT, MV)** remain normal. **CP,** choroid plexus. Thionin stain. × 70.

parts of the central nervous system. These cells have relatively long axons and are usually the largest cells in the nucleus. Often, but not always, the afferent input to the nucleus ends on the dendrites or somata of the principal cells. There is usually a second population of cells, usually smaller than the principal cells. These cells are thought to serve as interneurons, being interposed either between the major source of af-

ferents to the cell mass and the principal cells or between axon collaterals of some principal cells and other, adjacent principal cells. In the first case, they are usually excitatory in nature; in the second, inhibitory. Such small cells are generally Golgi type II neurons with short, locally ramifying axons; but, evidently many of them may be axonless and act through "presynaptic dendrites."

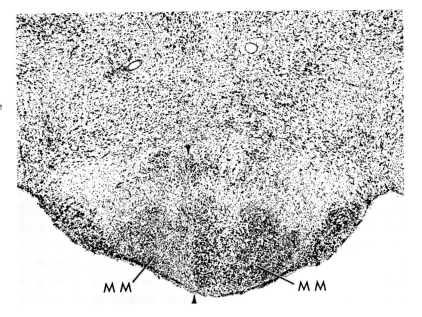

8–81 Mamillary body of same brain as in Fig. 8–80, retrograde transneuronal degeneration of cells in left mamillary nuclei **(MM)** that project their axons to degenerated area of thalamus. **Arrowheads** indicate midline. Thionin stain. × 140.

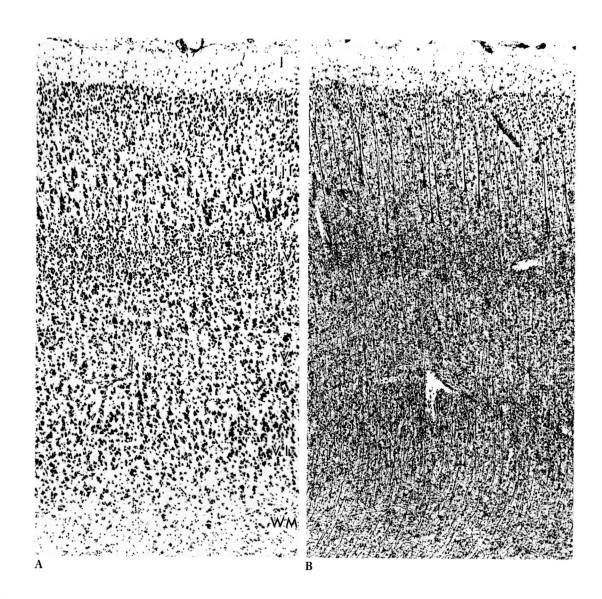

A

B

8–82 **A.** Nissl-stained preparation of paravisual cerebral cortex of a monkey showing cell layers. (I–VI) **WM,** white matter. × 70. **B.** Bodian-stained preparation of section adjacent to that shown in part A demonstrating cellular and fiber lamination. × 70.

"Cortical" and Other Laminated Structures. Where nerve cells are found on the surface of the brain, the region is called a *cortex* (Fig. 8–82A and B). Here the neurons are arranged in a series of superimposed layers with cells of similar type tending to occupy the same layer. As in the case of the nuclear masses, each cortical area is, in some respects, morphologically distinct, so that

no general account can be given that is applicable to all.

In the simplest types of cortex (like that in certain parts of the olfactory system and in the hippocampal formation), the principal cells have their somata arranged in a single, compact lamina, while their principal dendrites are regularly oriented in a second overlying layer. The various extrinsic inputs to the cortex terminate on these dendrites and are so arranged that the afferents from different sources contact different segments of the dendritic tree (Fig. 8–83). Various inter-neurons, usually of an inhibitory kind, are found in a third, deeper layer and their axons usually terminate on the cell somata or the proximal

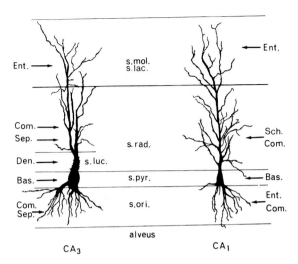

Ent.

s.mol.
s.lac.

Ent. →

Com. →
Sep. →

Den. →   s.luc.

Bas. →

Com.
Sep. →

s.rad.

s.pyr.

s.ori.

alveus

← Ent.

← Sch.
   Com.

← Bas.

Ent.
Com.

CA₃   CA₁

8–83 Drawings of two types of pyramidal cell found in the mammalian hippocampus to illustrate the principle that afferents from different sources are usually spatially segregated on the surface of complex neurons. **Ent, Com, Sep:** entorhinal, commissural, and septal afferents. (From Gottlieb, D. I., and Cowan, W. M. 1972. Z Zellforsch. Mikrosk. Anat. 129:413.)

parts of the dendrites of the principal cell type. This type of spatial segregation of afferent inputs is most clearly seen in simple cortical areas such as this, but it may well be the case in most neurons that receive synapses from two or more sources. The output from such a cortex is represented by the collected axons of the principal cells, which generally enter a zone of subcortical white matter.

Most cortical areas are considerably more complex than this. For example, in all but a few regions of the cerebral cortex (the so-called *neocortex*) there are five superimposed cellular layers and a relatively cell-free outer zone, or molecular layer, just beneath the surface (Fig. 8–82A). Within each cellular layer, there are often several different cell types, although for heuristic reasons it is convenient to regard them as belonging to only two major classes: *pyramidal cells,* so called because of the pyramidal form of the cell bodies, which lead superficially to a prominent ascending or apical dendrite; and nonpyramidal, or *stellate cells,* whose dendritic arborizations lack the rigid organization of the pyramidal cell (see Figs. 8–7, 8–8, and 8–11A and B). The pyramidal cell bodies are generally found in layers II, III, and V, and to a lesser extent in layer VI, and send their apical dendrites

into the supervening layers and their axons into the subcortical white matter. The nonpyramidal cells are found in all layers, but certain types are particularly concentrated in layer IV. Their axons are distributed within the cortex itself. Certain extrinsic inputs to the cortex (for example, those from the related thalamic nucleus) appear to terminate mainly on the nonpyramidal cells in layer IV, whereas others (such as the commissural fibers from the cortex of the opposite hemisphere) also end in layers I, II, and III. These and other inputs are then relayed to the pyramidal cells in the outer layers by nonpyramidal cells with vertical axons (Fig. 8–8). The axons of the pyramidal cells, in turn, project to other regions of the brain. Investigators have recently found that the pyramidal cells in different layers project to different parts of the nervous system: generally the cells in layers II and III were found to project to other parts of the cerebral cortex, those in layer VI to the thalamus, and those in layer V to the brainstem, basal ganglia, and spinal cord. A second important principle that has emerged from recent studies of the sensory areas of the cerebral cortex is that interrelated cells are arranged into vertical columns or slabs perpendicular to the cortical surface and passing through all layers. In each column all the cells appear to subserve one sensory submodality, or to be responsive to some special feature of a sensory stimulus. Thus, in the somatosensory cortex the cells in one column may all respond to movement of a particular joint, whereas those in another column may all respond to light tactile stimulation of the skin. Similarly, in the visual cortex, cells in one slab will respond preferentially to stimulation of the left eye, whereas those in the adjoining slab will respond to stimulation of the right eye. And within either "eye-dominance column," all the cells in a single, narrow, vertical column may respond only to visual stimuli with a particular spatial orientation. In the case of the motor cortex, the cells of a column are all connected to the same group of spinal motoneurons.

The cerebral cortex can be subdivided into a number of different areas, each having its own distinctive structure. These so-called cytoarchitectonic fields differ from each other in the number, density, and arrangement of the cells and fibers in their various layers, and the boundaries between adjoining fields are occasionally remarkably distinct (Fig. 8–84). Most of these cytoarchitectonically distinct fields also have dis-

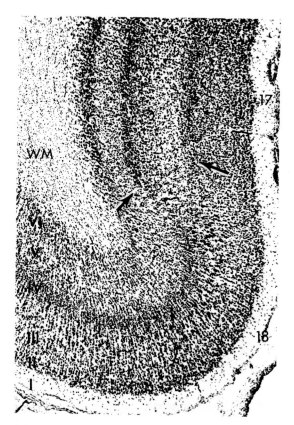

8–84 Junction of primary visual area **(17)** of monkey cerebral cortex with adjacent area **(18)**. **Arrows** show region at which trilaminar layer **IV** of area 17 gives place to unilaminar layer **IV** of area 18. Latter area also has larger cells in layer **III**, and layers **V** and **VI** are less distinct. **WM**, white matter. Thionin stain. × 23.

tinctive patterns of afferent and efferent connections, and in a number of cases it has been possible to show that functionally they are equally distinct. How these striking differences are generated during the early development of the cortex is unknown. At present the only relevant evidence we have is that the cells in the different layers are generated at different times. The first-formed cortical cells are those that finally reside in the deepest lamina (layer VI); those in the progressively more superficial layers are generated at successively later times. In addition, because many of the cells appear to display their characteristic functional properties shortly after the cortex is developed, it seems likely that the formation of their connections is genetically determined. But the "wiring pattern" seems also to be modifiable by environmental manipulation

(for example, by depriving the visual cortex of its normal functional input from one eye).

The Reaction of Neural Tissue to Injury

Because, among animal cells, neurons are distinguished by the number and variety of their processes, considerable attention has been paid to the trophic relationship between the nerve cell soma and its axonal and dendritic processes and to the long-term consequences of neuronal injury. More than a century ago the English physiologist Augustus Waller formulated what is perhaps still the only "law" in neuroanatomy when he pointed out that when an axon is interrupted, the distal segment invariably degenerates. However, it is not only in this part of the axon that degenerative changes occur. In many neurons comparably severe changes can be seen in the perikaryon; in several neuronal systems, an atrophy, or even degeneration, can be observed in the neurons that are related synaptically to the injured nerve cells.

Changes at the Site of the Lesion

After the uncomplicated interruption of an axon, there is a short period during which axoplasm leaks from the cut ends, since the axon appears to be in a state of some turgor owing to the continuous flow of axoplasm and axonal organelles. However, the leakage of axonal contents does not seem to be a serious matter, for within a short while there is a retraction of the axon and the axolemma appears to fuse over the severed ends and effectively seals them off. This is followed by a damming up of axonal material behind the fused membranes so that within 12 to 24 h there is a distinct swelling or dilatation of the axon. These swellings (which contain a variety of organelles, neurofilaments, vesicles of various kinds, mitochondria, and so forth, and stain deeply with most reduced silver methods) are termed *retraction bulbs*. The subsequent fate of the retraction bulbs depends on whether or not regeneration occurs in the cut axon. In most, if not all, parts of the central nervous systems of higher vertebrates (including reptiles, birds, and mammals) no significant regeneration occurs, and within a day or two the proximal end of the severed axon degenerates at least as far back as the axon's nearest collateral branch. In the peripheral nervous system (and to a lesser extent in the central nervous systems of fish and amphibians) numerous filopodia appear on the surface of the retraction bulb. Subsequently, large numbers of new axonal sprouts grow out from the bulb and make their way toward the distal segment of the nerve (Fig. 8–63).

At the site of the injury the supporting and certain other nonneural cells become activated and participate in the removal of the neuronal debris in the formation of a scar and possibly also in the process of regeneration. In the central nervous system the cells principally involved in this "mopping-up operation" are the local astrocytes and microglial which may be stimulated to proliferate and to become actively phagocytic. Oligodendrocytes and vascular pericytes also become reactive. And if there has been some damage to the neighboring capillaries, large numbers of blood-borne phagocytes (polymorphonuclear leukocytes and other macrophages) usually invade the tissue. After the necrotic tissue has been phagocytosed, the glial cells initiate a vigorous repair process. Astrocytic processes either expand to fill the vacated area to form a dense glial scar that bridges across the traumatized zone or, if this area is too large, they effectively seal it off as an encysted space. The oligodendrocytes, on the other hand, seem to be able to sequester large masses of cellular debris by forming myelin ensheathments around them. These glial responses, and especially the formation of a glial scar, most probably either prevent or seriously limit central neural regeneration.

In the peripheral nervous system, the Schwann cells show a similar prompt response by actively proliferating and phagocytosing the breakdown products of the neuronal degeneration. To what extent the reaction of the Schwann cells actually promotes regeneration is not known. To date, most attempts to demonstrate it experimentally have yielded equivocal results, but it is clear that they do form new sheaths for the regenerating axons.

The Reaction in the Distal Segment

In certain invertebrate nerves the surrounding sheath cells seem to be able to maintain the viability of the distal segment of a cut axon more or less indefinitely. But more often, and certainly in all vertebrates, the entire distal segment will, in time, undergo *Wallerian degeneration*. However, the earliest changes seem to appear not close to the injury, as might be expected, but at the axon terminals.

Terminal degeneration takes several forms.

The earliest changes, in the form of a swelling and possibly some loss of synaptic vesicles, can often be recognized within 12 to 24 h after axotomy. (The actual rate of appearance varies somewhat from system to system but, in general, appears to be a function of the distance of the nerve transection from the terminals: the closer to the terminals the axon is interrupted, the more rapidly the degenerative changes appear.) Subsequently, there may be a marked increase in the number of neurofilaments in the terminals, and a corresponding decrease in the number of synaptic vesicles (Fig. 8–85). The neurofilamentous hyperplasia (which is presumably a result of the polymerization of soluble filament precursor material in the axon) accounts for the increased argyrophilia of degenerating axon terminals; and because the filaments often appear as a tangled whorl around a central cluster of mitochondria and synaptic vesicles, in neurofibrillar preparations such degenerating terminals are often impregnated as ringlike structures. Later the whole terminal may become filled with filaments and, in silver preparations, appear as a swollen, degenerating end bulb.

A third reaction involves a progressive increase in the density of the axoplasmic matrix of the terminal and a concomitant loss of the remaining synaptic vesicles (Fig. 8–86). This "dark reaction" may occur as a primary response in certain nerve terminals or, in others, it may be secondary to the neurofilamentous change described above. The physicochemical nature of the axoplasmic change is unknown, but in time there is virtually a complete loss of synaptic vesicles and the mitochondria become increasingly dense and fragmented. A short while later the terminal appears to be "dissected" away from the postsynaptic membrane specialization and phagocytosed by the neighboring astrocytes; the engulfed fragments then resemble lysosomal dense bodies. Terminals undergoing this dense reaction are particularly susceptible to impregnation by certain silver methods, e.g., the Fink-Heimer modification of the Nauta technique, a feature that makes these methods extremely useful for determining the sites of termination of neural pathways.

With the exception of the neuromuscular junction, the degeneration of most peripheral nerve terminations has not been carefully studied. In the case of the neuromuscular junction, the degenerative changes are essentially comparable to those at central neuronal synapses. However, because of the more favorable circum-

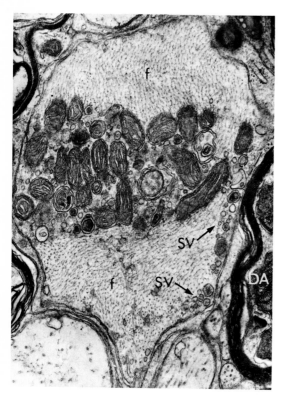

8–85 Electron micrograph showing proliferation of neurofilaments **(f)**, reduction in synaptic vesicles **(SV)**, and central clumping of mitochondria and lysosomes in an axon terminal following interruption of its parent axon. **DA**, degenerating axon. Inferior colliculus of cat. × 34,000. (From Jones, E. G., and Rockel, A. J. 1973. J. Comp. Neurol. 147:93.)

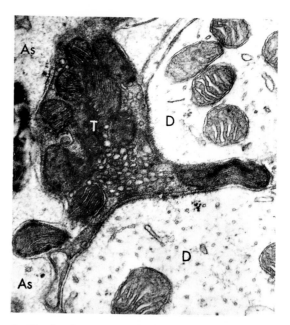

8–86 The electron-dense reaction in a degenerating axon terminal **(T)** that has been cut off from its cell soma. Note the dense clumping of the synaptic vesicles, the persistence of the postsynaptic membrane specializations on the dendrites **(D)**, and the surrounding astrocytic processes **(As)**. × 33,000. (From Jones, E. G., and Rockel, A. J. 1973. J. Comp. Neurol. 147:93.)

stances for experimental study, it has been easier to show that the cessation of transmission from nerve to muscle precedes the earliest morphological changes by several hours, and that the time required for transmission to fail varies directly with the length of the segment between the nerve section and the axon terminals.

Proximal to the terminals the axon—and in the case of myelinated fibers, the surrounding myelin sheath—seems to degenerate in a piecemeal fashion. Over most of its extent the axoplasm becomes progressively more electron-dense, the normally smooth contour of the axon becomes more and more irregular with fusiform swellings and constrictions every few microns along its length, and it finally breaks up into numerous short fragments. This accounts for the characteristic fragmented appearance of degen-

erating nerve tracts that has been used to such good effect in tracing pathways in the central nervous system (Fig. 8–93). Concurrently, the myelin lamellae (where present) are drawn away from the axolemma, and clefts appear between adjoining lamellae as the myelin sheath disintegrates. The fragmentation of the myelin sheath, and an alteration in its lipid composition, form the basis of yet another method for following neural pathways—the Marchi technique. The signal for the disintegration of the myelin sheath, when its enclosed axon degenerates, is unknown, but the fact that it occurs so consistently suggests that there is normally a close—perhaps even trophic—relationship between axons and the related myelin-forming cells.

Degenerative Changes in the Proximal Segment of the Axon

Depending on the reaction of the nerve cell soma, the axon proximal to the site of the transection may either degenerate completely or show only relatively minor changes in the region adjoining the traumatized zone. Should the parent cell die (see below), the axon will degenerate in a proximodistal sequence starting near the initial segment. Because the appearance of the degeneration is essentially the same as that seen in the distal segment, it is called *indirect Wallerian degeneration* (or, sometimes retrograde fiber degeneration, although this is misleading in that it suggests that the degenerative change proceeds backward from the lesion to the cell soma).

In cases in which the cell body survives the injury, the axon appears to degenerate only as far back as the nearest collateral branch. In the absence of regeneration of the main portion of the axon, this collateral may become hypertrophied and function as the principal conducting channel of the neuron. Regeneration, when it occurs, may begin either from near the origin of this collateral or, more often, from the retraction bulb, as described above. The actual process of axonal regeneration appears to be identical to the initial outgrowth of the axon with the interesting difference that usually several (up to 50) sprouts grow out from the cut end of the axon. The great majority of these sprouts subsequently degenerate; only one or two actually grow into the distal stump of the nerve.

The Reaction of the Nerve Cell Soma to Axotomy

Although it is commonly stated that the event termed *chromatolysis* is the characteristic response of nerve cells to interruption of their axons, a whole spectrum of reactions may in fact occur in the soma, from the death of the neuron at one end, to no discernible change at the other.

The reason for this variability is unknown: it is widely believed that the presence of axon collaterals proximal to the nerve section is responsible for preserving the integrity of the soma, and that chromatolysis is essentially a regenerative response.

Chromatolysis. This reaction is usually seen in motoneurons, in sensory ganglion cells, and in a number of large central neurons in the brainstem and spinal cord (Fig. 8–87). Characteristically it consists of a progressive breakdown of the Nissl material (from which the reaction gets its name), a tendency for the nucleus to become more and more eccentric (usually moving away from the axon hillock), and a variable amount of swelling of the perikaryon. In its fully developed state the cell appears globular, having lost its usual angular profile, with the nucleus pressing against the cell membrane and only a narrow rim of Nissl material around the perimeter of the cell or in a "cap" over the nucleus. The whole process takes about 2 weeks to develop, and if the axon regenerates the entire sequence of changes may be reversed over the next 4 to 6 weeks.

Cell Death. In many neural centers (such as the nuclei of the mammalian thalamus) and in the developing nervous sytem, axon section is followed within a few days by the death of the cell and its removal by glial action. The cytolog-

8–87 A normal motoneuron **(A)** and one showing advanced chromatolysis **(B)** after interruption of its axon. (From Bodian, D., and Mellors, R. C. 1945. J. Exp. Med. 81:469; courtesy of D. Bodian.)

A

B

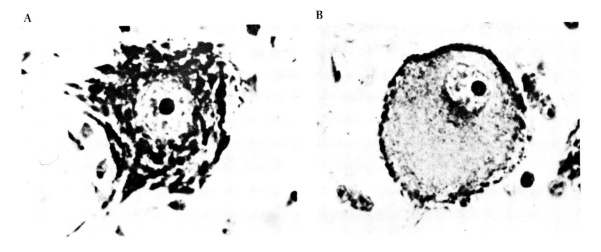

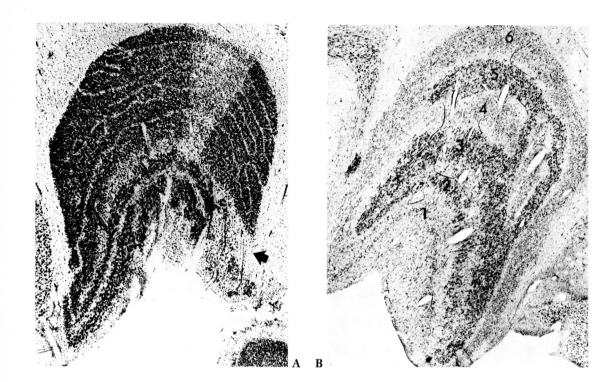

8–88 **A.** Retrograde cell degeneration involving a wedge-shaped area extending through all layers of the lateral geniculate nucleus of a monkey after destruction of a small portion of the visual cortex **(arrow).** Thionin stain. × 15. **B.** Anterograde transneuronal degeneration in monkey lateral geniculate nucleus which has resulted in severe cell shrinkage in the neurons of layers 1, 4, and 6, following removal of the contralateral eye some months earlier. Thionin stain. × 20. (Part A from Kaas, J. H., Guillery, R. W., and Allman, J. M. 1973. Brain Behav. Evol. 6:253; courtesy of J. H. Kaas.)

phied form. Whether this is because the cells have other axonal branches that escaped injury or because of some other reason remains to be determined. In still other cases, such as the large pyramidal neurons in the cerebral cortex, there may be no detectable reaction in the perikaryon even though the greater part of the axon has been amputated. In at least some instances the cell seems to be preserved by the hypertrophy of collateral branches given off close to the cell body.

ical changes vary from case to case, but characteristically the nucleus becomes increasingly pyknotic, the Nissl material is lost, and the perikaryon shrinks dramatically. In the adult nervous system these changes are accompanied by a marked glial proliferation *(gliosis),* which persists after the removal of the neuronal debris (Figs. 8–80 and 8–88A). On the other hand, in embryos the neuronal death not only occurs more rapidly but is seldom accompanied by an obvious glial reaction (Fig. 8–89).

Other Cellular Reactions. In some situations the neurons seem to persist more or less indefinitely after axon section, but in a shrunken, atro-

Transneuronal (or Transsynaptic) Degeneration

In a few neuronal systems distinct degenerative (or atrophic) changes have been observed in the neurons that are synaptically related to those whose axons were interrupted. Depending on the direction of the transneuronal effects, they may be termed *anterograde* or *retrograde.* Such effects may extend beyond the first synapse so that secondary and even tertiary transneuronal effects are recognized.

Anterograde Transneuronal Degeneration. The classic site for this type of change is the dorsal lateral geniculate nucleus of the mammalian thalamus, which receives a substantial part of its

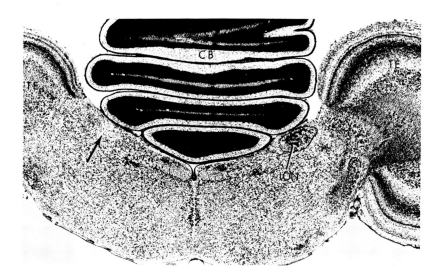

input from the ganglion cells of the retina (Fig. 8–88B). If an eye is removed, or if an optic nerve is cut, the related cells in the lateral geniculate nucleus undergo a progressive atrophy marked by the shrinkage of both the perikaryon and the nucleus, the loss of some Nissl material, and in adults, after many weeks or months, some degree of cell death. In younger animals the changes occur more rapidly, are more severe, and if sufficient time has elapsed, they may be associated with secondary changes in the neurons in the visual cortex to which the geniculate cells project. The most commonly described secondary transneuronal change in the cortex is a loss of dendritic spines, but a generalized thinning of the cortex with a loss of cells in certain layers has also been described.

Although the transneuronal changes in the visual system are the best-documented examples of this form of degeneration, it is now known to occur in many regions in both the central and peripheral nervous systems. Such degeneration is generally thought to be due either to the removal of some form of trophic substance passed from the pre- to the postsynaptic neuron or to the absence of appropriate functional activity in the postsynaptic cells.

Retrograde Transneuronal Degeneration. In some neural systems in which retrograde cell degeneration after axon section is particularly severe, such as the lateral geniculate and anterior nuclei of the mammalian thalamus, degenerative changes have also been observed in the cells that project to those nuclei (Fig. 8–81). Such retro-

8–89 Neurons whose axons are unable to form synaptic connections during development degenerate completely as shown by the absence of the nucleus of origin of the centrifugal fibers to the chick retina **(ION)** after early removal of the contralateral eye in the embryo. In the region usually occupied by the ION, there is a complete cell loss on the side opposite the eye removal **(arrow). CB,** cerebellum; **TE,** tectum. Thionin stain. × 28.

grade transneuronal changes are significantly more severe in young animals and become progressively more marked with increasing survival after the initial lesion. In the case of the anterior thalamic nuclei, it has been found in several species that if the primary lesion in the cerebral cortex occurs early enough, degenerative changes may be found not only in the mamillary nuclei (which project to the anterior thalamic nuclei) but also in one of the midbrain tegmental nuclei that sends its axons to the mamillary nuclei.

Why certain neural systems should show primary, or even secondary, retrograde transneuronal changes is not yet known; at present the only clue is that this type of degeneration is never seen unless there is appreciable cell death in the initial retrograde degeneration. This suggests that there may be a two-way interaction between neurons that are synaptically related: if a neuron is to reach full growth and survive, it must both form an adequate number of synapses on other neurons (or effector tissues such as muscle or gland cells) and receive an adequate number of synaptic inputs from other neurons. Whether these contacts are necessary simply to maintain an adequate level of activity or to provide an adequate exchange of trophic materials remains to be determined.

Methods Used in the Study of the Nervous System

Many techniques are used to study the nervous system. We shall consider only those more commonly used. Broadly, the methods fall into two classes: (1) those based on the study of *normal* neural tissue, and (2) *experimental* methods.

Methods for Normal Neural Tissue

In the study of normal neural tissue, five groups of techniques are in common use.

The Nissl Method. The staining of the Nissl material within neurons, by any one of a number of basic aniline dyes, has been used for almost a century to identify the somata of individual neurons and to analyze the distribution of populations of neurons. Several of the illustrations in this chapter (for example, Figs. 8–10, 8–84, and 8–89) are of Nissl-stained preparations; their use is essential for any cytoarchitectonic or cytological study of the nervous system.

8–90 Several weeks after interrupting a fiber bundle, all the axons degenerate and are removed by the phagocytic action of glial cells. In this section of the human spinal cord in a case of tabes dorsalis, the fibers in the gracile funiculi **(GF)** have completely disappeared. (Weigert method, to show myelinated fibers.) **AM**, arachnoid mater; **DR**, dorsal root; **VR**, ventral root. × 9.

Methods for Staining Nerve Fibers. A number of techniques more or less selectively stain the sheaths of myelinated axons. Most of them involve some prior treatment of the tissue in a mordant such as potassium dichromate, which serves to stabilize the lipids of the myelin sheaths, and subsequent staining of the pretreated myelin with a basic dye such as hematoxylin. Figure 8–90 shows a preparation stained in this way. Because of its high affinity for lipids, osmium tetroxide also provides an extremely intense stain for myelin (Fig. 8–51). Axons themselves and dendrites can be stained by various *reduced silver methods*. In a general sense these methods resemble certain photographic procedures in which silver salts are "developed" and the resulting metallic silver "fixed." In many of these methods, the tissue is pretreated in a silver nitrate solution at high pH followed by a reduction involving an acidified formalin solution. As a result, "nuclei" of metallic silver are deposited around certain cellular organelles (for example, the nuclear membrane, nucleoli, and so forth) but especially around clusters of neurofilaments. As we have pointed out, this appears to be the basis for the light-microscopic appearance of neurofibrils. These methods are sometimes called "neurofibrillar methods." Figures 8–24, 8–25, and 8–75B show preparations of this kind.

The Analytic Methods. Because of the difficulty of analyzing preparations in which all the neuronal perikarya or all the various processes are stained, two invaluable methods were developed in the latter part of the last century. They are the *supravital methylene blue method of*

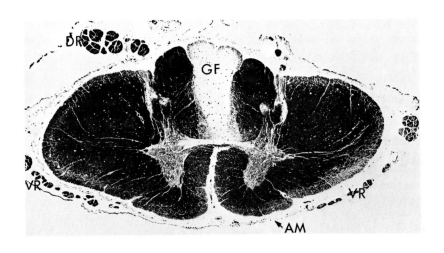

Ehrlich and the *Golgi method.* These methods have two major advantages: first, they stain only a small percentage of the neurons in any one area (commonly less than 1%); and, second, they usually stain the cells in their entirety. As Figs. 8–11 and 8–12 show, in a preparation of this kind, individual neurons stand out strikingly against a relatively clear, unstained background, and usually the full extent of the perikarya, the dendrites (including dendritic spines), and the unmyelinated segments of their axons are displayed. The reason for the selectivity of these methods is not known, nor is the mechanism of the actual staining procedures. In the case of the Golgi method (which has been the more intensively studied and is currently the more widely used of the two methods), the tissue is commonly pretreated with potassium dichromate and then impregnated in a silver nitrate solution. This results in the deposition of silver salts throughout most of the interior of the neuron, excluding the various membranous components. Despite a certain capriciousness, these methods are extremely valuable for studying dendritic organization and are among the few that are useful for analyzing local neuronal circuitry.

Intracellular Labeling of Physiologically Identified Neurons. This recent development in neurobiology represents an especially powerful addition to the older analytic methods, because it permits full visualization of neurons whose functional properties have previously been defined electrophysiologically. Briefly, the method involves using a micropipette to inject a cell with a fluorescent dye (such as Procion yellow), or an opaque substance (such as a cobalt salt), or a histochemically demonstrable enzyme (such as horseradish peroxidase). The label, usually injected into the perikaryon, diffuses or is actively transported into the dendrites and the initial portion of the axon (Fig. 8–95). In suitably prepared sections and with the appropriate optics (e.g., fluorescence microscopy is needed to visualize cells filled with Procion yellow), the entire geometry of the cell can be readily demonstrated. Alternatively, the marker molecule can be iontophoresed up the axon from its cut end and subsequently precipitated in the perikaryon and dendrites. This approach has proved especially effective for labeling motoneurons in invertebrates. A recent variant of the intracellular labeling procedure involves the use of tritium-labeled precursors of certain macromolecules (such as

[³H]amino acids or [³H]fucose), which are incorporated into proteins or glycoproteins and which are rapidly transported from the soma into the dendrites and axon of the labeled cell. After an appropriate interval to allow for the transport of the radioactive macromolecules, the distribution of the tritium label can be displayed autoradiographically.

Electron Microscopy. The introduction of the electron microscope to biology in the early 1950s added an entirely new dimension to neuroanatomical studies, not only because it offered increased resolution but, perhaps more importantly, because it displayed *all* the structures within a tissue. In this respect it differs from all the other methods commonly used. One of its earliest contributions was the demonstration that there is no extensive "ground substance" in the brain and spinal cord as was formerly believed; rather, the central nervous system resembles most other ectodermal derivatives, with only narrow (200 Å) clefts between adjoining cells and their processes. In addition, it made possible for the first time the critical study of such structures as synapses and their associated organelles, the substructure of myelin sheaths, the form of nodes of Ranvier, and the ultrastructural counterparts of such neuronal organelles as Nissl bodies, and neurofibrils. The preparation of neural tissue for electron microscopy generally involves fixation by perfusion with a buffered solution of aldehydes (formaldehyde and glutaraldehyde are commonly used), postfixation in osmium tetroxide, and embedding in an appropriate plastic. Because the sections used are generally of the order of 600 to 1,000 Å thick and the area available for study in any one section is usually only a few hundred square microns in extent, the amount of tissue that can be studied is rather limited. Within these limits, however, the method is the most critical available to the neuroanatomist. In recent years this approach has been significantly extended by the development of techniques for preparing large numbers of serial sections, by the application of the electron microscope to tissue previously stained by some other method (such as the Golgi technique or after intracellular labeling; see Fig. 8–95), and by the introduction of such special methods as freeze-etching, which permits the interior of membrane surfaces to be visualized (Fig. 8–31). The use of the high-voltage electron microscope has made it possible to study sections as thick as 1 or 2 μm; this has been particularly valuable in the analysis of Golgi-impregnated material.

Experimental Methods

Although the examination of normal material is an essential prerequisite for all neuroanatomical studies, it is seldom possible in such material to determine the connections between groups of neurons that are separated by more than just a few hundred microns. For this, one must resort to experimental material, which is basically of two kinds: the first is aimed at determining the *origin* of neuronal pathways, the second at mapping their sites of *termination*.

Retrograde Methods. For many years the method of choice for determining the origin of nervous pathways was based on the retrograde reaction seen in nerve cell somata after their axons were interrupted or their synaptic terminals destroyed (for example, see Figs. 8–80 and 8–88A). This method was particularly successful in elucidating the origin of the motor divisions of the cranial nerves, the location of spinal motoneurons supplying various muscle groups and certain of the connections of the cerebellum, and most strikingly, in establishing the pattern of projection of the various nuclei of the thalamus on the cerebral cortex and corpus striatum. Unfortunately, as we have pointed out above, not all neurons show a clear-cut reaction to axotomy, and in these cases the method not only is of little value but has often proved to be misleading. Another "retrograde" method is both more reliable and more generally applicable than the cell-degeneration approach. This method is based on the uptake of exogenous marker molecules (such as the enzyme horseradish peroxidase [Figs. 8–91 and 8–92], the reaction product of which can be readily demonstrated histochemically) by axons and especially by their terminals, and its transport back to the cell soma by the process of retrograde axonal transport. This method has proved to be invaluable for such difficult problems as the origin of the various efferent projections from the cerebral cortex, the projection of different populations of retinal ganglion cells, and the connections of various nuclear groups in the thalamus and brainstem.

Anterograde Methods. The alternative approach is aimed at determining the site and pattern of termination of the axons arising from a

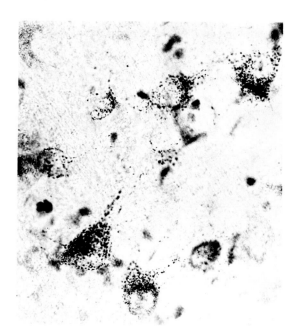

8–91 A group of neurons that have been labeled retrogradely with the enzyme marker horseradish peroxidase. Dark granules are reaction product in cell soma and dendrites. × 430. (From Jones, E. G., and Leavitt, R. Y. 1974. J. Comp. Neurol. 154:349.)

given population of neurons. Three fundamentally different strategies have been used. The first is based on the anterograde degenerative changes seen in the distal portion of axons after their interruption or the destruction of their parent nerve cell bodies by an experimental lesion. Because these changes have been described in the previous section, we need only add that the methods most widely used at present are variants of a silver technique introduced by Nauta and Gygax in 1951 and commonly called the *Nauta technique* (Figs. 8–93 and 8–94). This technique takes advantage of the increased argyrophilia of degenerating axons; and when the staining of the normal fibers is critically suppressed, the degenerating axons and axon terminals can be displayed against a relatively clear background. The most critical method for identifying degenerating axons and presynaptic processes is the use of the *electron microscope*. Indeed, this is the only method that enables one confidently to identify synaptic relationships; the presence of the various degenerative changes described on pages 359–360 (Figs. 8–85 and

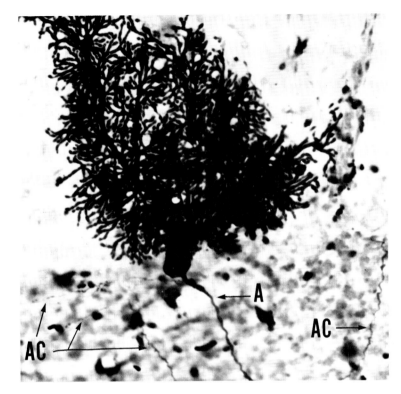

8–92 A Purkinje cell from the cerebellar cortex of a cat stained by the intracellular injection of horseradish peroxidase. **A,** axon; **AC,** axon collateral. × 25. (Courtesy of S. T. Kitai.)

8–86) in a presynaptic profile constitutes ineluctable evidence that the parent cell or its axons has been damaged.

An earlier method was introduced by Marchi in 1885 and was based on the increased affinity of disintegrating myelin sheaths for osmium tetroxide. However, because it was somewhat capricious and applicable only to myelinated pathways, the Marchi method is now only of historical interest. If enough time has elapsed between the causative lesion and the fixation of the brain, the anterograde degeneration of the pathways in question may have proceeded to the point where all the fibers have been removed by glial action. In this case their former location can

be identified, as it were negatively, by the absence of stainable fibers. Although this approach has little to commend it for experimental studies, it is still quite widely used in human neuropathology to follow the degeneration resulting from long-standing brain lesions (Fig. 8–90).

The second strategy is based on the axonal transport of materials synthesized in neuronal somata and distributed along the length of the axons to their terminals. Most commonly, various tritiated precursors, such as [3H] fucose or [3H] amino acids, are used. A concentrated solution of the labeled precursor is injected into the neuronal population whose connections are to be studied. The neurons in the immediate vicinity

8–93 Degenerating axons become intensely argyrophilic, as seen in this photomicrograph of the optic chiasm of a guinea pig 6 days after removal of the left eye. **Ve,** ventricle, Nauta-Gygax method. × 80.

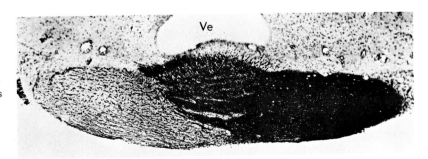

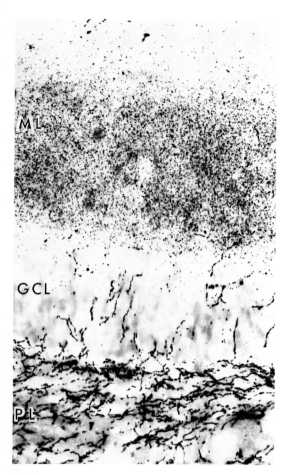

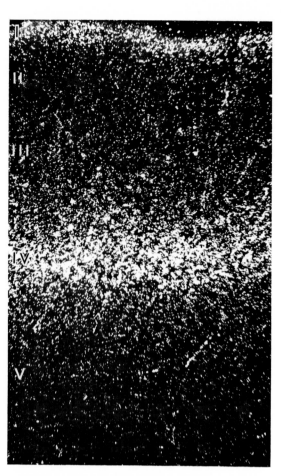

8–94 Silver-stained, degenerating axons ascending from the polymorph layer **(PL)** of the dentate gyrus through the granule cell layer **(GCL)** to end in a dense mass of terminal fragments in the deeper part of the molecular layer **(ML)**. Fink and Heimer stain, marsupial brain after destruction of hippocampal commissure. × 200. (From Heath, C. J., and Jones, E. G. 1971. J Anat. [Lond.] 109:253.)

8–95 Dark-field photomicrograph from an autoradiograph demonstrating axoplasmically transported label in axon terminals in layers I and IV of the cerebral cortex following an injection of tritiated amino acids in the thalamus. × 165.

of the injection (but not axons passing through it) take up the precursor and incorporate it into certain macromolecules (such as proteins, glycoproteins, or glycolipids), which are then transported at various velocities down their axons. The labeled axons and axon terminals can then be identified in serial light-microscopic autoradiographs (or electron-microscopic autoradiographs) of the relevant areas (Fig. 8–95). Because this method is based on an established physiological property of nerve cells and does not involve the destruction of the tissue being studied, it has a number of advantages over the degeneration methods and, in addition, appears to be somewhat more sensitive.

The third strategy is aimed at identifying specific neural pathways that act by the release of certain identified neurotransmitters. These methods are based either on the inherent fluorescence of such biogenic amines as dopamine, norepinephrine, and serotonin when exposed to formalin vapor or, for example, in the case of cholinergic and noradrenergic fibers, on the binding of fluorescent-labeled antibodies to the enzymes choline acetyltransferase and dopamine-β-hydroxylase, which are the key enzymes in the biosynthesis of acetylcholine and norepinephrine, respectively (Fig. 8–35). A somewhat different method in this category is based on the finding that neurons that release certain transmitter substances (such as γ-amino butyric acid or glycine) have a high-affinity uptake system for the transmitter. When exposed to a radioactively labeled solution of the transmitter, the neurons, and especially their axon terminals, take up the label in high concentrations; its presence in the cell or axon terminals can subsequently be demonstrated autoradiographically. Since their introduction in the late 1960s, these methods have proved extremely useful, in both the central and peripheral nervous systems, and clearly presage the development of a new phase in neuroanatomical studies that should lead in time to a complete account of the "chemical architecture" of the brain and spinal cord.

References and Selected Bibliography

General

Brodal, A., 1981. Neurological Anatomy in Relation to Clinical Medicine, 3rd ed. New York: Oxford University Press.

Cajal, S. Ramón y. 1909–1911, Histologie du Système Nerveux de l'Homme et des Vertébrés, 2 vol. Republished 1952. Consejo Superior de Investigaciones Cientificas, Madrid.

Cooper, J. R., Bloom, F. E. and Roth, R. M. 1978. The Biochemical Basis of Neuropharmacology. Third ed. New York: Oxford University Press.

Fawcett, D. W. 1981. The Cell, 2nd ed. Philadelphia: W. B. Saunders.

Jones, E. G. 1982. The Structure of Nervous Tissue, four-part tape–slide course. New York: Audio Visual Mktg., Inc.

Kandel, E. R. (ed.). 1977. Handbook of Physiology. Section I. The Nervous System, vol. I, Pts. 1 and 2, Cellular Biology of Neurons. Bethesda, Md.: American Physiological Society.

Kandel, E. R., and Schwartz, J. H. 1981. Principles of Neural Science. New York: Elsevier North-Holland.

Kuffler, S. W., and Nicholls, J. G. 1976. From Neuron to Brain. Sunderland, Mass.: Sinauer Associates Inc.

Scientific American. The brain. Vol. 241 pt. 3 (1979).

Schmitt, F. O., and Worden, F. G. (eds.). 1974. The Neurosciences Third Study Program. Cambridge, Mass.: MIT Press.

Schmitt, F. O., and Worden, F. G. (eds.). The Neurosciences Fourth Study Program. Cambridge, Mass.: MIT Press.

Shepherd, G. M. 1979. The Synaptic Organization of the Brain, 2nd ed. New York: Oxford University Press.

Siegal, G. J., Albers, R. W., Agranoff, B. W., and Katzman, R. 1981. Basic Neurochemistry, 3rd ed. Boston: Little, Brown, and Co.

Development

Angevine, J. B., 1970. Critical cellular events in the shaping of neural centers. In F. O. Schmitt (ed.), The Neurosciences Second Study Program. New York: Rockefeller University Press, pp. 62–72.

Cowan, W. M., 1978. Aspects of neural development. Int. Rev. Physiol. 17:149.

Cowan, W. M., (ed.). 1981. Studies in developmental neurobiology. Essays in Honor of Viktor Hamburger. New York: Oxford University Press.

Dennis, M. J. 1981. Development of the neuromuscular junction: Inductive interactions between cells. Ann. Rev. Neurosci. 4:43.

Hamburger, V., Brunso-Bechtold, J. K., and Yip, J. 1981. Neuronal death in the spinal ganglia of the chick embryo and its reduction by nerve growth factor. J. Neurosci. 1:60.

Hamburger, V., and Levi-Montalcini, R. 1949. Proliferation, differentiation and degeneration in the spinal ganglia of the chick embryo under normal and experimental conditions. J. Exp. Zool. 111:457.

Jacobson, M. 1978. Developmental Neurobiology, 2nd ed. New York: Plenum Press.

Rakic, P. 1974. Neurons in Rhesus monkey visual cortex: Systematic relation between time of origin and eventual disposition. Science 183:425.

Rakic, P. 1977. Prenatal development of the visual system in Rhesus monkey. Phil. Trans. Roy. Soc. Ser. B. 278:245.

Sidman, R. L. 1974. Cell-cell recognition in the developing nervous system. In F. O. Schmitt and F. G. Worden (eds.), The Neurosciences Third Study Program. Cambridge, Mass.: The MIT Press, pp. 743–758.

Sidman, R. L., and Rakic, P. 1974. Neuronal migration, with special reference to the developing human brain: A review. Brain Res. 62:1.

Tuchman-DuPlessis, H., Auroux, M., and Haegel, P. 1974. Illustrated Human Embryology, vol. III. Nervous System and Endocrine Glands. New York: Springer-Verlag New York, Inc.

Neurons

Barr, M. L., Bertram, L. F., and Lindsay, H. A. 1950. The morphology of the nerve cell nucleus, according to sex. Anat. Rec. 107:283.

Bray, D., and Gilbert, D. 1981. Cytoskeletal elements in neurons. Ann. Rev. Neurosci. 4:505.

Chan-Palay, V., and Palay, S. L. 1972. High voltage electron microscopy of rapid Golgi preparations. Neurons and their processes in the cerebellar cortex of the monkey and rat. Z. Anat. Entwicklungsgesch. 137:125.

Jones, E. G. 1975. Varieties and distribution of non-pyramidal cells in the sensory-motor cortex of the squirrel monkey. J. Comp. Neurol. 160:205.

Jones, E. G., and Powell, T. P. S., 1969. Morphological variations in the dendritic spines of the neocortex. J. Cell. Sci. 5:509.

Palay, S. L., and Palade, G. E. 1955. The fine structure of neurons. J. Biophys. Biochem. Cytol. 1:69.

Palay, S. L., Sotelo, C., Peters, A., and Orkand, P. M. 1968. The axon hillock and the initial segment. J. Cell Biol. 38:193.

Peters, A., Palay, S. L. and Webster, H. DeF. 1976: The Fine Structure of the Nervous System, 2nd ed. Philadelphia: W. B. Saunders.

Pfenninger, K. H., 1978. Organization of neuronal membranes. Ann. Rev. Neurosci. 1:445.

Schwartz, J. H. 1979. Axonal transport: Components, mechanisms, and specificity. Ann. Rev. Neurosci. 2:467.

Synapses

Bodian, D. 1937. The structure of the vertebrate synapse. A study of the axon endings on Mauthner cells and neighboring centers in the goldfish. J. Comp. Neurol. 68:117.

Cold Spring Harbor Symposia on Quantitative Biology. 1976. The Synapse, Vol. 40. Cold Spring Harbor Laboratory, New York.

Gray, E. G. 1959. Axo-somatic and axo-dendritic synapses of the cerebral cortex: An electron microscope study. J. Anat. (Lond.) 93:420.

Heuser, J. E., and Reese, T. S. 1973. Evidence for recycling of synaptic vesicle membrane during transmitter release at the frog neuromuscular junction. J. Cell Biol. 57:315.

Heuser, J. E., Reese, T. S., and Landis, D. M. D. 1974: Functional changes in frog neuromuscular junctions studied with freeze-fracture. J. Neurocytol. 3:109.

Landis, D. M. D., and Reese, T. S. 1974. Differences in membrane structure between excitatory and inhibitory synapses in the cerebellar cortex. J. Comp. Neurol. 155:93.

Uchizono, K. 1965. Characteristics of excitatory and inhibitory synapses in the central nervous system of the cat. Nature, 207:642.

Supporting Cells

Brightman, M. W., and Palay, S. L. 1963. The fine structure of the ependyma in the brain of the rat. J. Cell Biol. 19:415.

Brightman, M. W., and Reese, T. S. 1969. Junctions between intimately opposed cell membranes in the vertebrate brain. J. Cell Biol. 40:648.

Bray, G. M., Rasminsky, M., and Aguayo, A. J. 1981. Interactions between axons and their sheath cells. Ann. Rev. Neurosci. 4:127.

Bunge, R. P. 1968. Glial cells and the central myelin sheath. Physiol. Rev. 48:197.

Jones, E. G. 1970. On the mode of entry of blood vessels into cerebral cortex. J. Anat. 106:507.

Penfield, W. 1932. Neuroglia: Normal and pathological. In W. Penfield (ed.), Cytology and Cellular Pathology of the Nervous System, vol. 2. New York: Hoeber, pp. 421–479.

Peters, A. 1966. The node of Ranvier in the central nervous system. Quart. J. Exp. Physiol. 51:229.

Peters, A., Palay, S. L. and Webster, H. DeF. 1976. The fine structure of the nervous system. The Neurons and Supporting Cells. Philadelphia: W. B. Saunders.

Vaughn, J. E. 1969. An electron microscopic analysis of gliogenesis in rat optic nerves. Z. Zellforsch. Mikr. Anat. 94:293.

Vaughn, J. E., Hinds, P. L., and Skoff, R. P. 1970. Electron microscopic studies of Wallerian degeneration in rat optic nerves. I. The multipotential Glia. J. Comp. Neurol. 140:175.

Uzman, B. G. 1964. The spiral configuration of myelin lamellae. J. Ultrastruct. Res. 11:208.

Webster, H. De F. 1975. Development of peripheral myelinated and unmyelinated nerve fibers. In P. J. Dyck, P. K. Thomas, and E. H. Lambert (eds.), Peripheral Neuropathy. Philadelphia: W. B. Saunders.

Peripheral Nervous System

Barker, D.: The morphology of muscle receptors. In C. C. Hunt (ed.), Handbook of Sensory Physiology, vol. III/2, chap. 2. New York: Springer-Verlag New York, Inc., pp. 1–190.

Gershon, M. D. 1981. The enteric nervous system. Ann. Rev. Neurosci. 4:227.

Hubbard, J. I. (ed.). 1974. The Peripheral Nervous System. New York: Plenum Press.

Iggo, A. (ed.). 1974. Somatosensory system. Handbook of Sensory Physiology, vol. 2. New York: Springer-Verlag New York, Inc.

Loewenstein, W. R. 1960. Biological Tranducers. Sci. Am. 203:98.

Central Nervous System

Eccles, J. C., Ito, M., and Szentágothai, J. 1966. The Cerebellum as a Neuronal Machine. Berlin: Springer-Verlag.

Hubel, D. H., and Wiesel, T. N. 1977. Functional architecture of macaque monkey visual cortex. Proc. Roy. Soc. Lond. Ser. B. 198:1.

Jones, E. G. 1981. Functional subdivision and synaptic organization of the mammalian thalamus. In R. Porter (ed.), Int. Rev. Physiol., vol. 25, Neurophysiology IV. Baltimore, Md.: University Park Press, pp. 173–245.

Palay, S. L., and Chan-Palay, V. 1974. Cerebellar Cortex: Cytology and Organization. New York: Springer-Verlag New York, Inc.

Schmitt, F. O., Worden, F. G., Adelman, G., and Dennis, S. G. (eds.). 1981. The Organization of the Cerebral Cortex. Cambridge, Mass.: The MIT Press.

Willis, W. D., and Coggeshall, R. E. 1978. Sensory Mechanisms of the Spinal Cord. New York: Plenum Press.

Degeneration and Regeneration

Bodian, D., and Mellors, R. C. 1945. The regenerative cycle of motoneurons with special reference to phosphatase activity. J. Exp. Med. 81:469.

Cajal, S. Ramón Y. 1928. Degeneration and Regeneration of the Nervous System, W. May, (trans.). 2 vols. Oxford, England: Oxford University Press.

Gray, E. G., and Guillery, R. W. 1966. Synaptic morphology in the normal and degenerating nervous system. Int. Rev. Cytol. 19:111.

Tsukuhara, N. 1981. Synaptic plasticity in the mammalian central nervous system. Ann. Rev. Neurosci. 4:351–380.

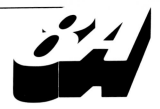

The Special Senses

Edward G. Jones

An earlier section of this book outlined some general principles of neuronal organization, dealing in particular with the ganglia of the peripheral nervous system and the nuclei and cortices of the central nervous system. Some of the more unique arrangements of neurons, often in association with special forms of ancillary cells, are found in the eye, the ear, and the nose. Although less complicated, the system of taste receptors in the mouth and pharynx is also worthy of mention.

The neural elements of the inner ear and olfactory epithelium are derivatives of placodal tissue, that is, of specialized parts of the ectoderm that develop independently of the neural tube and neural crest. From these placodes, additional supporting cells also develop. The neurons and the supporting cells of the retina are derived from an outpouching of the neural tube itself—the optic vesicle. Taste buds are derivatives of the epithelium of the tongue and pharynx. They receive their innervation from the peripheral processes of pseudounipolar neurons that develop as parts of the ganglia associated with the facial, glossopharyngeal, and vagus nerves.

Taste Buds

Taste buds first appear as small concentrations of cells in appropriate parts of the epithelium of the tongue and pharynx. They appear early in development and are innervated only after some days or weeks, but their numbers and distributions are fixed at an early age.

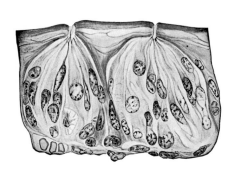

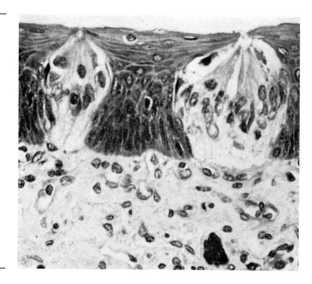

8A–1 Section on the side **(left)** and through the center **(right)** of taste buds of a camel's tongue. Methylene blue and eosin stain. (From Padykula, H. A. 1982. *In* L. Weiss (ed.), Histology, 5th edition. New York: Elsevier.)

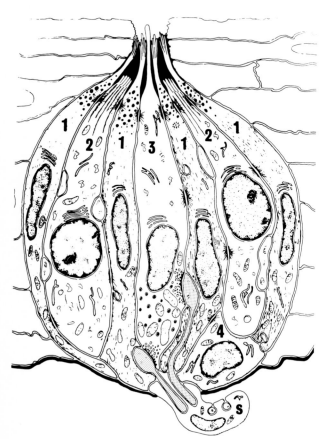

8A–2 Diagram summarizing the general features of a taste bud. The two principal cell types are the gustatory **(3)** and the supporting cell **(1)**. A basal cell **(4)** is the proliferative cell. Cell **2** is of uncertain function. Nerves enter from the underlying connective tissue and contact the gustatory cells. At the pore, many of the cells support a slender hairlike process; the bottom of the pore is filled with a dense, homogeneous substance. (Kindly provided by R. G. Murray.)

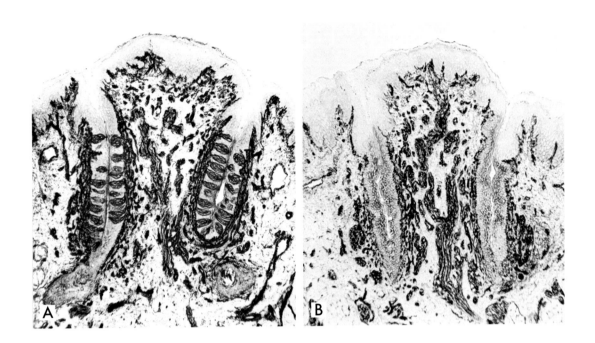

The epithelial element of each taste bud consists of two major types of nonneuronal cell: central sensory cells and peripheral supporting cells (Fig. 8A–1). The sensory cells are elongated. Their apexes, bearing small numbers of microvilli, protrude through a small open pore in the taste bud and thus come in contact with chemicals dissolved in the saliva. The bases of the cells contain small numbers of smooth and dense-cored vesicles and are contacted by the naked terminal branches of the appropriate gustatory nerve (Fig. 8A–2). There is a slight membrane density at the site of contact where the process of transduction is thought to occur. The change in membrane conductance leading to the appearance of a receptor potential is probably induced by the absorption of gustatory molecules at receptor sites on the apical part of the cell membrane.

A single branch of a gustatory nerve can innervate many taste buds. Each nerve is capable of responding to a wide range of gustatory stimuli, so it is unlikely that single taste buds are sensitive to only one taste quality, although there is some broad specificity among regional groupings of taste buds.

The supporting cells separate the sensory cells from one another and, from their complement of organelles, appear to secrete the polysaccharide-rich material that fills the pore of the taste bud. Other cells in the taste bud represent sensory and supporting cells in the process of development, for there is a continual turnover of

8A–3 **A.** ATPase activity in the taste buds of a normally innervated circumvallate papilla in a rat. × 70. **B.** Papilla 2 weeks after denervation. The taste buds have disappeared. (From Zalewski, A. A. 1970. Exp. Neurol. 30:510.)

the cell population of the taste bud throughout the life of the animal. There appears to be a resident population of germinal cells from which all the other cells of the taste bud are replaced every 10 days or so. The continued existence of the taste buds is dependent, however, on innervation; if their nerves are cut, they degenerate (Fig. 8A–3). This trophic dependence of receptor cells on sensory nerves is further emphasized by the regeneration of the taste buds following reinnervation, even by inappropriate gustatory nerves. However, regeneration in response to innervation by nongustatory nerves does not occur in mammals, indicating that the trophic influence is a highly specific one.

The Olfactory Epithelium and Olfactory Bulb

The olfactory epithelium is a thick, pseudostratified structure situated in a restricted part of the upper nasal cavity in humans but rather more extensive in other animals (Fig. 8A–4). It contains neurons, as well as supporting cells and a

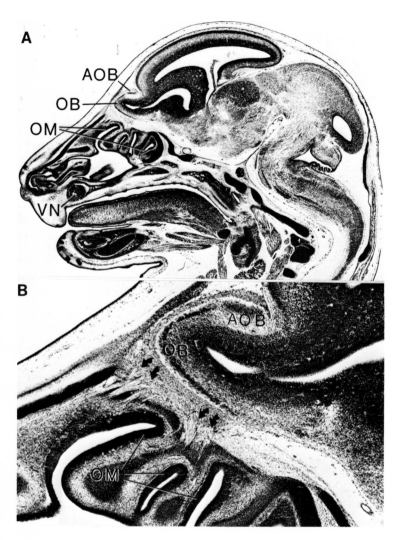

8A–4 A. The developing olfactory mucosa **(OM)** and its close association with the overlying olfactory bulb **(OB)** in a rat fetus at 17 days of gestation. Also shown is the vomeronasal **(VN)** (Jacobson's) organ, an ancillary olfactory epithelium with neurons that send axons to the accessory olfactory bulb **(AOB).** The latter is said to be absent in the postnatal human. In animals, its connections with the rest of the brain are different from those of the main bulb and suggest involvement in different aspects of olfactory behavior. **B.** Note the olfactory fila **(arrows)** penetrating the cribriform plate. Thionin stain. **A,** × 10; **B,** × 30.

population of basally placed proliferative cells (Fig. 8A–5) that replace the neurons and supporting cells throughout the life of the individual. All the cellular elements in each olfactory epithelium are derived from one of a pair of olfactory placodes. These are thickenings of the ectoderm that occur in the embryonic head process early in development and that are subsequently incorporated into the nasal cavity as it develops.

The supporting cells of the olfactory epithelium are tall, columnar cells covered with microvilli on their apical surfaces and joined by desmosomes. Their functions are uncertain. Basal cells are the deeply placed proliferative cells of the epithelium that replace the neurons and supporting cells completely about once a month.

The receptor cells of the olfactory epithelium are true neurons, unlike the receptor cells of several other sense organs, such as the ear, in which the receptor cells are not usually so classified. They are vertically oriented bipolar neurons (Fig. 8–8) with a single dendrite reaching to the free surface of the epithelium. This single dendrite ends in an expanded, ciliated knob that protrudes into the covering layer of mucus (Figs. 8A–5 and 8A–6). In this position, its membrane is presumed to contain receptor molecules that interact, probably stereochemically, with odoriferous molecules in the fluid. It has been suggested that absorption of an odoriferous molecule at such a receptor site results in the formation of a transient hole in the membrane

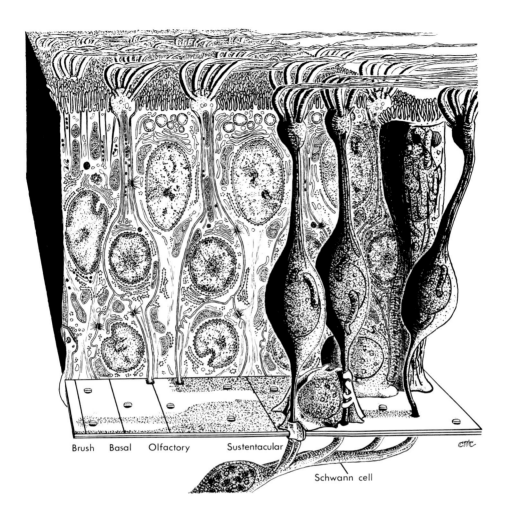

Brush   Basal   Olfactory   Sustentacular

Schwann cell

8A–5 Olfactory epithelium, showing three-dimensional and ultrastructural aspects. (From Sorokin, S. 1982. *In* L. Weiss (ed.), Histology, 5th edition. New York: Elsevier.)

through which ions such as Cl^- and K^+ may pass; thus depolarizing the cell and setting up a receptor potential. Individual receptor cells, like those in taste buds, respond to a wide range of stimuli.

The cell body of the olfactory receptor neuron is small. From its base a thin, naked axon emerges and joins with the unmyelinated axons of many other receptor neurons. Finally, after penetrating the basal lamina, the bundle becomes ensheathed in Schwann cells (Fig. 8A–5). The bundles, or fila, join with others to form the fasciculi of the olfactory nerve. These traverse the cribriform plate of the ethmoid bone to make synapses in the overlying olfactory bulb of the appropriate side of the brain (Fig. 8A–4). There is little known about the transmitter agent used at this synapse. The olfactory axons are rarely thicker than 0.2 microns, are unmyelinated, and,

in the olfactory fila and fasciculi, many are usually in direct contact with their neighbors, unlike unmyelinated axons in a peripheral nerve in which Schwann cell processes separate the individual fibers. This has led some workers to suggest the possibility of ephaptic or electrotonic interactions between the olfactory fibers. The olfactory axons presumably degenerate when olfactory receptor neurons die and are replaced by new axons growing from new receptor neurons. Hence, the synapse in the olfactory bulb must be made and broken many times during the lifetime of an individual.

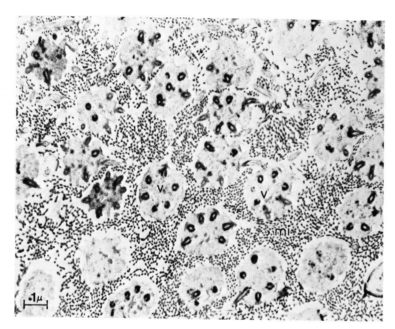

8A–6 A section tangential to the surface of the frog's olfactory mucosa showing the olfactory vesicles that give rise to the cilia of the receptor neuron **(v)** and the intervening microvilli **(mi)** of the supporting cells. (From Graziadei, P. P. C. 1971. *In* L. M. Beidler (ed.), Handbook of Sensory Physiology, IV/I. New York: Springer.)

The olfactory bulb is a relatively simple neural network with well-worked-out circuitry. It consists of several concentric layers (Figs. 8A–7 and 8A–8). A key element in the organization is the deeply placed, single row of medium-to-large mitral cell bodies. These cells have a single

8A–7 Sections of the olfactory bulbs of a rabbit stained with thionin **(A)** and with the Bodian stain **(B)** showing layers. **O,** olfactory nerve layer; **GL** glomeruli; **OP,** outer plexiform layer; **M,** mitral cell layer; **IP,** inner plexiform layer; **G,** granule cell layer; **V,** obliterated ventricle. × 25. ▽

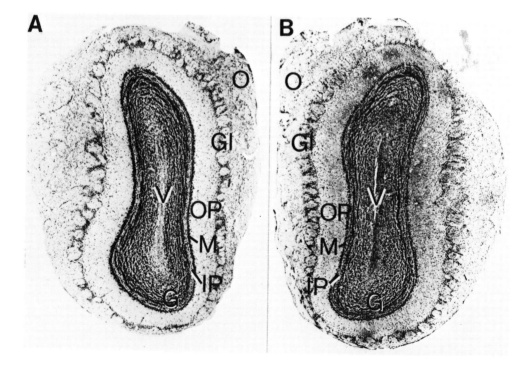

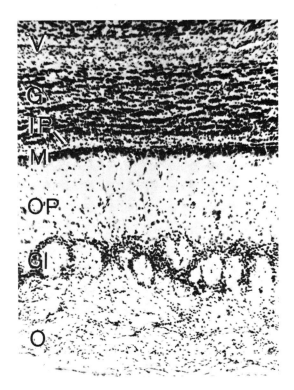

8A–8 Thionin-stained section of the olfactory bulb of a rabbit at higher magnification showing the layers seen in Fig. 8A–7. × 90.

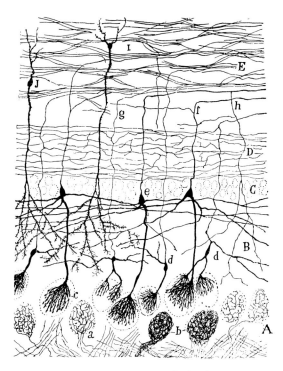

8A–9 Drawing by Ramón y Cajal of Golgi impregnated neurons in the olfactory bulb of a cat. **A.** Glomerular layer with terminations of olfactory nerve fibers **(a, b)** and of mitral cell dendrites **(c).** **B.** Outer plexiform layer with mitral cell dendrites, modified mitral (tufted) cells **(d),** and the gemmules of granule cells (unlabeled). **C.** Mitral cell layer. **D.** Inner plexiform layer. **E.** Granule cell layer with granule cells **(I, J)** and mitral cell axons **(h, l).** (From Ramón y Cajal, S. 1911. Histologie du Système Nerveux de l'Homme et des Vertébrés. Paris: Maloine.)

long dendrite that ascends toward the surface of the bulb; just deep to the layer of entering olfactory nerve fibers, the dendrite branches repeatedly to form a compact tuft (Fig. 8A–9). This tuft receives the terminations of 1,000 or more olfactory axons. Tuft and axon endings are surrounded by small cells with dendrites that also ramify among the mitral cell tuft and the axon terminations (Figs. 8A–9 and 8A–10). The whole aggregation, some 100 to 200 microns in diameter, is referred to as a *glomerulus*. The surrounding small cells are referred to as *periglomerular cells*. In Nissl preparations their stained somata outline the positions of the glomeruli (Figs. 8A–7 and 8A–8). A row of glomeruli encircles the olfactory bulb just beneath the outer covering of olfactory axons. Some evidence suggests that groups of glomeruli may receive input only from the axons of olfactory receptor neurons that are specifically activated by only one kind of odor. Because of the organization of the remainder of the olfactory bulb, to be discussed following, this would imply that different odors may be pro-

jected into the central nervous system along preferential routes, in a pattern resembling the topographic organization of the other sensory systems alluded to in Chapter 8. It would also imply that the regenerating axons of newly generated olfactory receptor neurons that respond to particular odors should find their way back to appropriate glomeruli.

The mitral cell, as well as being the principal recipient of afferent synapses in the olfactory bulb, is also the output cell, sending its axon in the lateral olfactory tract toward the cerebral hemisphere. Apart from a small version of the mitral cell, the tufted cell, all other neurons in the olfactory bulb modulate transmission at the synapse between olfactory axons and mitral cell dendrites or along the mitral cell itself. The peri-

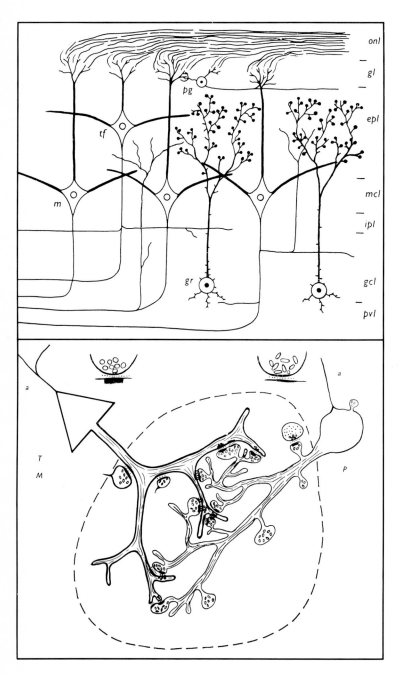

8A–10 A. Schematic figure of neural organization in the olfactory bulb. The olfactory fibers **(onl)** synapse with the terminal branches of the mitral **(m)** and tufted **(tf)** cells in the glomerular layer **(gl)** where they are associated with the small periglomerular cells **(pg)**. Granule cells **(gr)** send their peripheral processes into the external plexiform layer **(epl)** to end on the dendrites of mitral and tufted cells. The axons of the mitral and tufted cells pass into the periventricular layer **(pvl)** and give off collaterals mainly in the internal plexiform layer **(ipl)**, which ramify in the granule cell layer **(gcl)** and external plexiform layer. **(mcl,** mitral cell layer). **B.** Schematic diagram to show the dendrodendritic relationships between the mitral cell **(M)** and periglomerular cell **(P)** dendrites in an olfactory glomerulus. The mitral cell dendrites show spherical vesicles and synapse with asymmetric thickenings whereas dendrites of the periglomerular cell show flattened vesicles and symmetric thickenings. Axon terminals of periglomerular cells synapse with symmetric thickenings and flattened vesicles onto the stem dendrites. Olfactory nerve terminals (not shown) synapse on all dendrites within the glomerulus. (Part **A** from Price, J. L., and Powell, T. P. S. 1970. J. Cell Sci. 7:91. Part **B** from Pinching, A. J., and Powell, T. P. S. 1971. J. Cell Sci. 9:379.)

glomerular cell has already been mentioned. It receives olfactory axon synapses in the glomerulus into which its dendrites extend, but it sends its axon into adjacent glomeruli (Fig. 8A–10). There it ends on mitral cell dendrites in a symmetrical synapse with flattened synaptic vesicles (Fig. 8A–10). It is therefore thought to be inhibitory in function, perhaps serving to set up

surround inhibition in glomeruli around those activated by a particular odor. It has been suggested that the transmitter agent at this synapse is either glutamic acid decarboxylase (GABA) or dopamine.

In the glomerulus into which it sends its dendrites, the periglomerular cell is also involved in a peculiar form of *reciprocal synapse* already il-

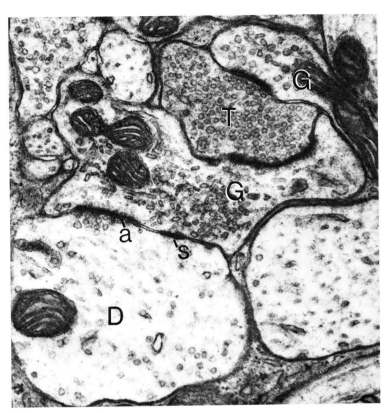

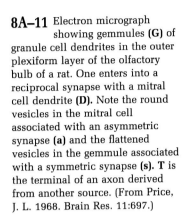

8A–11 Electron micrograph showing gemmules **(G)** of granule cell dendrites in the outer plexiform layer of the olfactory bulb of a rat. One enters into a reciprocal synapse with a mitral cell dendrite **(D)**. Note the round vesicles in the mitral cell associated with an asymmetric synapse **(a)** and the flattened vesicles in the gemmule associated with a symmetric synapse **(s)**. **T** is the terminal of an axon derived from another source. (From Price, J. L. 1968. Brain Res. 11:697.)

lustrated in Fig. 8–37. The dendrites of the periglomerular cells contain flattened synaptic vesicles and are presynaptic to mitral cell dendrites at a symmetrical synapse. Near this contact, the recipient mitral cell dendrite contains spherical synaptic vesicles and is itself presynaptic to the dendrite of the periglomerular cell at an asymmetrical synapse (Fig. 8A–10). By means of its dendritic and axonal terminations, both of which are thought to be inhibitory in nature, the periglomerular cell is well placed to serve as a modulator of transmission at the first olfactory bulb synapse.

The largest population of neurons in the olfactory bulb have their somata deep to the mitral cell layer and surround the olfactory ventricle. These are the *granule cells*. They have small somata but elongated, highly branched dendrites that extend up into the external plexiform layer that lies above the layer of mitral cell bodies. The dendrites, unlike those of the other cells in the olfactory bulb, are covered in long, bulbous spines or gemmules. The granule cells are unique in that they lack axons. By means of their gemmules, however, they enter into reciprocal synaptic relationships with the shafts of the mi-

tral cell dendrites. Each gemmule contains flattened synaptic vesicles and is the presynaptic element of a symmetric synapse onto a mitral cell dendrite (Fig. 8A–11). Within a micron or less, the mitral cell itself contains spherical synaptic vesicles and is the presynaptic element of an asymmetric synapse back onto the same gemmule. The transmitter used by the granule cells appears to be GABA; that of the mitral cell component of the reciprocal synapse is uncertain, but it may be aspartic acid. It is thought that activity at olfactory nerve synapses in the glomeruli leads to impulses that are propagated along the mitral cell dendrites and, ultimately, out of the olfactory bulb in the mitral cell axons. En route, the mitral-to-granule-cell component of the reciprocal synapse sets up an excitatory postsynaptic potential in the granule cell that leads thereafter to an inhibitory postsynaptic potential in the mitral cell via the granule-to-mitral-cell component of the reciprocal synapse. As well as providing for self-inhibition of a mitral cell, this mechanism can lead to lateral inhibition of surrounding mitral cells, because of release of transmitter from the excited granule cells at gemmules on many other mitral cells. In this way, the granule cell serves as the principal regulator of impulse traffic through the olfactory bulb.

What has just been outlined is by no means the complete synaptic circuitry of the olfactory bulb; a number of other cell types of uncertain function have been described, and there are other afferent inputs to it from other parts of the brain. As described, however, it shows how principal neurons (the mitral cells) and intrinsic neurons (the periglomerular and granule cells) interrelate with one another in the organization of a central nervous structure.

The Eye

The neural apparatus of the eye has been called an externalized part of the brain because of its structure and its origin as a brain outgrowth during development (Figs. 8A–12 and 8A–13). It commences as a vesicle that is soon inverted to form the *optic cup*. Because of the inversion, the cup comes to have two layers of neuroepithelium: an outer layer, destined to become the pigment epithelium, and an inner layer, destined to become the neural retina (Figs. 8A–12 and 8A–13). Between them, the old lumen of the optic vesicle is obliterated, as also is the lumen in the stalk of the vesicle. The stalk is the route along which axons of retinal ganglion cells grow to reach the brain and thus form the optic nerve. For an account of cellular proliferation in the neuroepithelium, see Chapter 8 and Fig. 8–28.

All other elements of the eye—lens, ciliary apparatus, iris, cornea, choroid and sclera—are derived from the mesoderm or ectoderm overlying the optic cup (Fig. 8A–13).

The neural retina of the adult is a thin sheet, no more than 300 microns thick, into which is packed a remarkable variety of neuron types. Because of the orderly arrangement of these neurons, their connectivities have been worked out in considerable detail. There is a receptor layer, three layers of cell bodies (the outer nuclear layer, the inner nuclear layer, and the ganglion cell layer), two synaptic layers (the outer plexiform layer and the inner plexiform layer), and an optic nerve fiber layer (Figs. 8A–14 and 8A–15). The basic circuit (Fig. 8A–24) is one in which

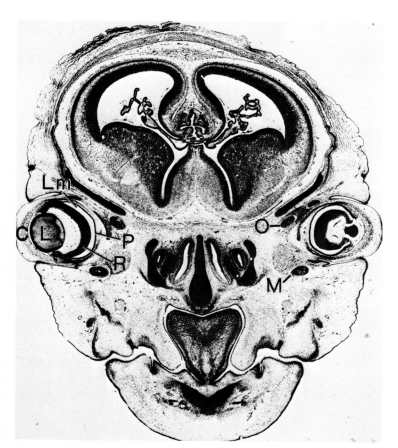

8A–12 Cross section through the head of an 18-mm pig embryo showing the developing cerebral hemispheres **(above)**, the two eyes **(laterally)**, the olfactory cavities **(middle)**, and the tongue and lower jaw **(below)**. The ophthalmic **(O)** and maxillary **(M)** divisions of the trigeminal nerve are also clearly seen. In the eyes, note the developing cornea **(C)**, lens **(L)**, and the pigment **(P)** and neural retina **(R)** layers of the optic cup. Between these layers, the lumen **(Lm)** of the old optic vesicle is still visible. Thionin stain. × 10.

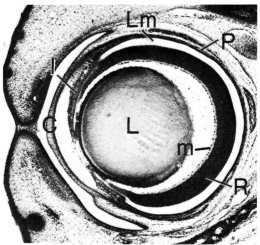

FIGURE 8A–13

FIGURE 8A–14

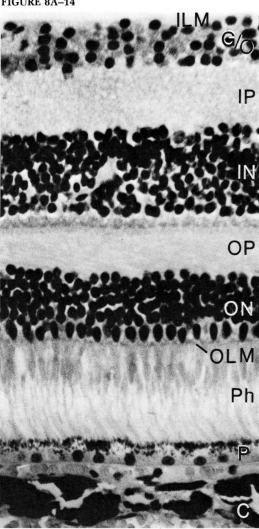

8A–13 Sagittal section through the eye of a rat fetus at 17 days of gestation. In comparison with Fig. 8A–12, the eyelids have formed, the cornea **(C)** has thinned, and an iris **(I)** is present. Note the pigment epithelium **(P)**, neural retina **(R)**, and intervening lumen **(Lm)**. The marginal layer **(m)** of the retinal neuroepithelium is seen, indicating that mitosis occurs at the old luminal surface, as in the neuroepithelium of the brain and spinal cord (cf. Fig. 8–3). Thionin stain. × 35.

8A–14 Thick section through the macular region of the retina of a monkey: **C**, choroid; **P**, pigment epithelium; **Ph**, photoreceptor layer; **OL**, outer limiting membrane; **ON**, outer nuclear layer; **OP**, outer plexiform layer; **IN**, inner nuclear layer; **IP**, inner plexiform layer; **G/O**, ganglion cell layer and optic nerve fiber layer. Hematoxylin and eosin stain × 500.

8A–15 Plastic section through the retina of a bird, showing the same layers as in Fig. 8A–14 but with greater resolution. Cone pedicles are easily seen in the outer nuclear layer **(ON)** as well as several varieties of cell somata in the inner nuclear layer **(IN)** and dendrites in the inner plexiform layer **(IP)**. Birds are unusual in having some myelin in the optic nerve fiber layer **(O)**. Toluidine blue stain. × 550.

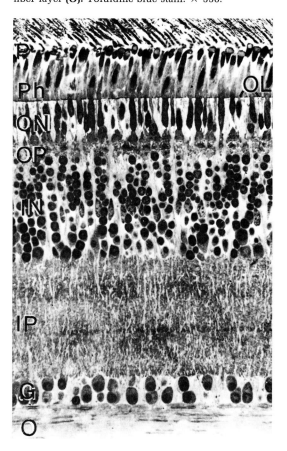

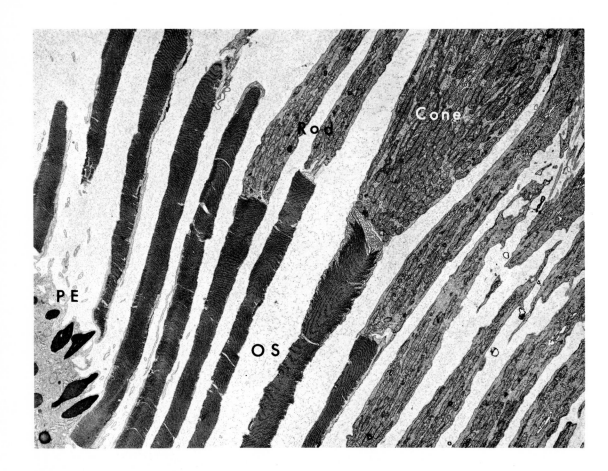

8A–16 Photoreceptor elements of the retina. Inner segments of rods and cones contain many mitochondria. Outer segments **(OS)** consist of lamellar membranes. Pigment epithelium **(PE)** envelops the tips of the outer segments. × 12,000. (From Kuwabara, T., and Cogan, D. G. 1982. *In* L. Weiss (ed.), Histology, 5th edition. New York: Elsevier.)

the photoreceptors, which have their cell bodies in the outer nuclear layer, make synapses in the outer plexiform layer with the dendrites of bipolar neurons. Bipolar neurons have somata in the inner nuclear layer; their axons enter the inner plexiform layer to make synapses with the dendrites of ganglion cells, the axons of which then run in the optic nerve fiber layer to the optic nerve and thence to the brain. The synapses in the outer plexiform layer between photoreceptors and bipolar cells and those in the inner plexiform layer between bipolar cells and ganglion cells are modulated by two types of interneurons with cell bodies that lie in the inner nu-

clear layer: *horizontal cells* act at the synapse between photoreceptors and bipolar cells; *amacrine cells* act at the synapse between bipolar cells and ganglion cells.

Photoreceptors

There has long been debate as to whether the photoreceptors should be regarded as true neurons or as receptor cells akin to hair cells of the inner ear. They show certain characteristics typical of both neurons and sensory cells. One set of features setting these cells apart from most neurons is that they have low resting membrane potentials (approximately 20 mV as compared to the 70 mV common to most neurons); they do not generate action potentials; their response to a sensory stimulus is not a depolarization but a slow hyperpolarization.

There are two kinds of photoreceptor in the retinas of most animals: rods and cones. Rods are sensitive to luminosity and respond in a graded manner proportional to the intensity of light reaching them. Cones are color receptors and are of three functional types: one sensitive to red, one to green, and one to blue light. Mainly because of their connections in the retina, cones are also responsible for visual acuity.

Rods tend to be long and thin and cones short and fat, but each has a fundamental similarity of structure (Figs. 8A–16 to 8A–21). The cell bodies of each are situated in the outer nuclear layer and extend their photoreceptive elements through the outer limiting membrane of the retina. These elements are divided into inner and outer segments. The inner segment, which is an extension of the cell body, is particularly rich in mitochondria, smooth endoplasmic reticulum, and Golgi complex. It is connected to the outer segment by a short cilium (Fig. 8A–17) that possesses the usual peripheral nine pairs of microtubules but lacks the central two pairs found in most cilia. The outer segment contains one of the visual pigments that is bleached under the influence of light (rhodopsin in the case of the rods and other pigments with different spectral sensitivities in the case of the cones). It is a membrane-bound bag filled with a large number of disc-shaped laminated plates. Each of these consists of a membranous sac compressed so that the two membranes are in contact except at the periphery of the disc. In cones, the peripheral dilatations may communicate with the extracellular space through openings in the cell membrane (Figs. 8A–20 and 8A–21). The discs are formed near the cilium of the photoreceptor and move peripherally. The outer segments are enveloped by the elongated villous processes of the adjoining pigment epithelium (Fig. 8A–22). In this region, older discs are progressively sloughed off and phagocytized by the pigment epithelium. It has been estimated that a single rod in the monkey retina may contain 1,300 discs, each surviving about 10 days.

The visual pigments form molecular monolayers in the discs of the outer segments. They are capable of trapping photons, an event that leads to isomerization of a part of the pigment molecule. This is the initial step in the bleaching of the visual pigment that leads eventually to a change (a slow hyperpolarization) in the resting membrane potential of the photoreceptors by decreasing sodium conductance of the membrane. The mechanism by which this is mediated is unclear.

Restoration of the visual pigment to an isomeric state capable of trapping photons again

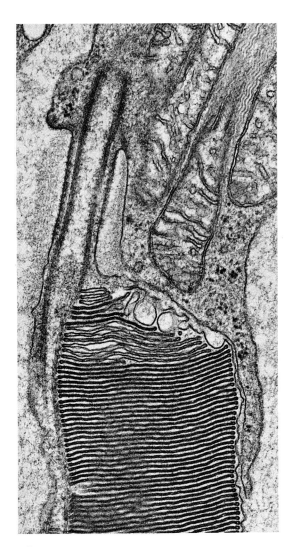

8A–17 Electron micrograph through the junctions of the outer and inner segments of a rod. The upper portion shows the inner segment containing dense concentrations of mitochondria, whereas the lower portion shows the outer segment, or photoreceptive end organ, containing laminated plates. The two portions are connected by a modified cilium. × 32,000. (From Kuwabara, T., and Cogan, D. G. 1982. *In* L. Weiss (ed.), Histology, 5th edition. New York: Elsevier.)

occurs after cessation of a stimulus. At least in the case of rhodopsin, the light-trapping component of the pigment can be synthesized from vitamin A.

The inner surfaces of the cell bodies of the photoreceptors are drawn into elongated processes that extend into the outer plexiform layer.

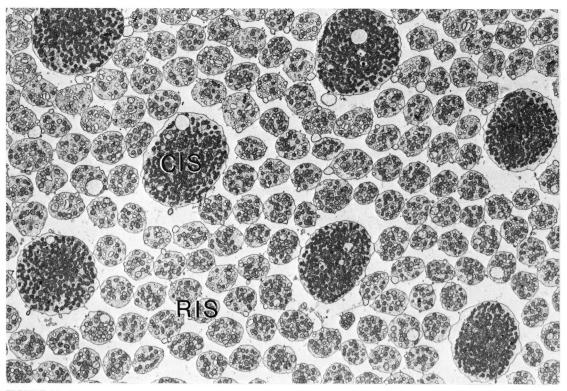

FIGURE 8A–18

FIGURE 8A–19

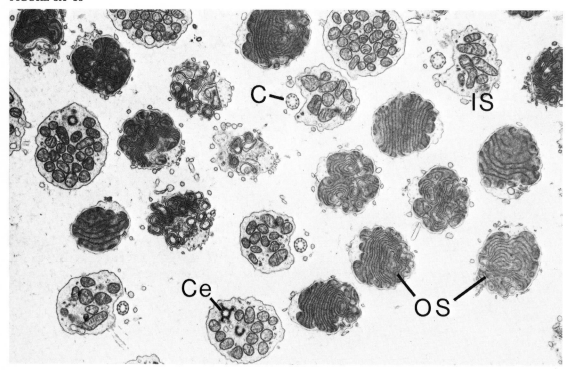

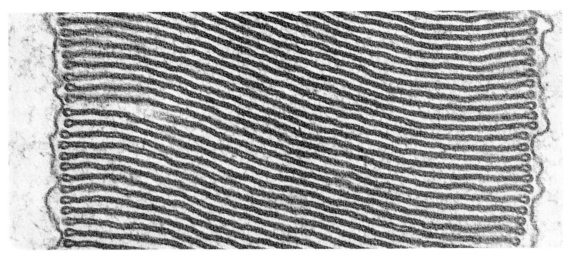

FIGURE 8A–20. See caption below.

FIGURE 8A–21

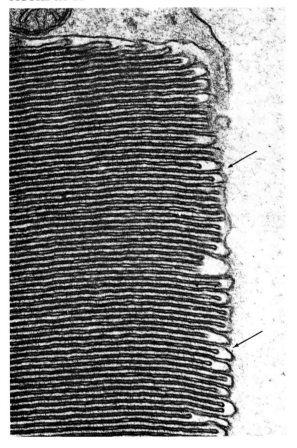

8A–18 Electron micrograph showing tangential sections of rod **(RIS)** and cone **(CIS)** inner segments from a human retina. × 4000. (Courtesy of Dr. A. I. Cohen.)

8A–19 Electron micrograph showing tangential sections of rod and cone inner segments **(IS)**, outer segments **(OS)**, occasional connecting cilia **(C)** and centrioles **(Ce)**. Human retina. × 11,000. (Courtesy of Dr. A. I. Cohen.)

8A–20 Higher magnification of a rod outer segment. Saccular discs are separated from each other and do not communicate with exterior of cell. (From Kuwabara, T., and Cogan, D. G. 1982. *In* L. Weiss (ed.), Histology, 5th edition. New York: Elsevier.)

8A–21 Cone outer segment. Many membranes of the ▷ saccular discs constitute the outer wall of the photoreceptor. The inner side of the disc can communicate with the outside of the cell **(arrow)**. × 50,000. (From Kuwabara, T., and Cogan, D. G. 1982. *In* L. Weiss (ed.), Histology, 5th edition. New York: Elsevier.)

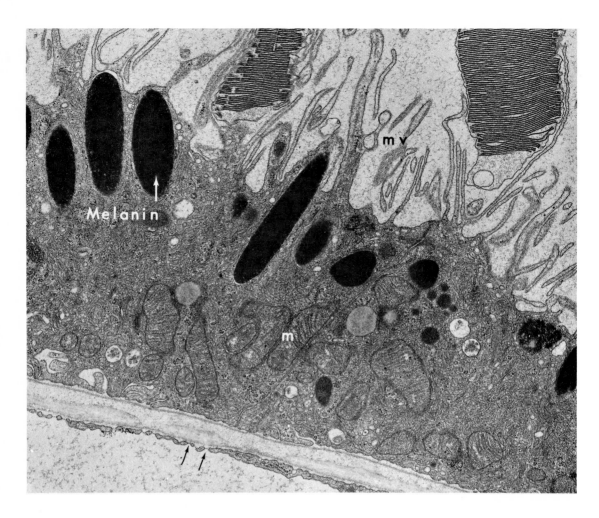

8A–22 Electron micrograph of the junction between choroid and retina. In the lower left-hand corner is a fenestrated capillary of the choroid. At center, the photoreceptor outer segments are interdigitating with microvilli of the pigment epithelium. (From Kuwabara, T., and Cogan, D. G. 1982. In L. Weiss (ed.), Histology, 5th edition. New York: Elsevier.)

Here those of rods end as small terminals called *rod spherules,* whereas those of the cones end in large flattened *cone pedicles* (Figs. 8A–23, 8A–24, and 8A–26). Rod spherules and cone pedicles enter into an unusual triadic synaptic arrangement with the dendrites of bipolar cells and with the processes of horizontal cells (Figs. 8A–23 through 8A–25 and 8A–27). The tips of the bipolar cell dendrites invaginate the spherule or pedicle; opposite the dendrite tip, in the cytoplasm of the spherule or pedicle, there is a synaptic ribbon flanked by clear synaptic vesicles

(see Fig. 8–37). On each side of the dendrite tip is the process of a horizontal cell (Fig. 8A–23). Thickenings occur in the membranes of all four opposed processes. At this synapse, the graded hyperpolarization induced in the photoreceptor by incident light is conveyed to both the bipolar and the horizontal cells. It is thought that, in the absence of stimulation, horizontal cells may be depolarized by a continual release of transmitter from the photoreceptors; the effect of light, therefore, may be to reduce the release of transmitter at the ribbon synapse, leading to a hyperpolarization of the horizontal cells. Some bipolar cells are hyperpolarized in response to light; others are depolarized. It is not clear how the change in the membrane potential of the bipolar cells is effected by the rod spherule or cone pedicle nor how the horizontal cell processes are involved.

The outer plexiform layer exhibits an important kind of neuronal specificity in which rods

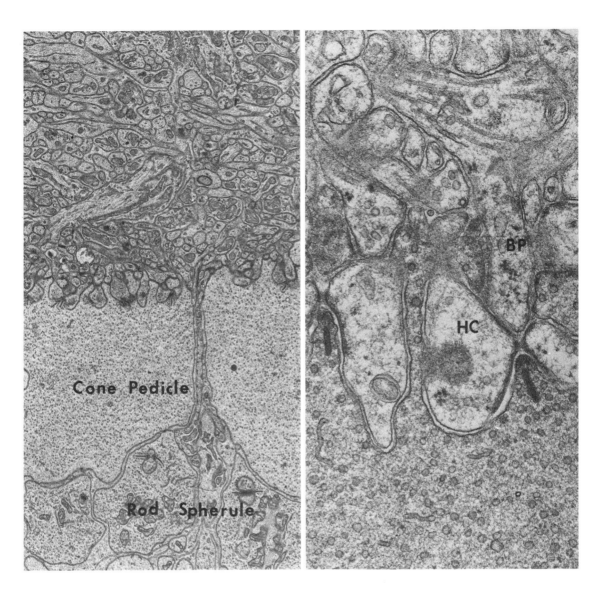

8A–23 **A.** Outer plexiform layer showing **(left)** cone pedicles and rod spherules. × 6300. At higher magnification **(right)** is a synapse between large horizontal cell processes **(HC),** the dendrite of a bipolar cell **(BP),** and the cone pedicle that contains numerous vesicles and synaptic ribbons. × 37,000. **B.** Diagram of a synaptic junction at a cone pedicle. Under each synaptic ribbon in the cone terminal are three processes. Horizontal cell processes **(H)** are more deeply inserted. The bipolar dendrite **(MB)** is separated from the membrane underlying the synaptic ribbon by a space of about 800 to 1,000 Å, which is bounded by the horizontal cell processes. **FB** is a further bipolar cell dendrite. (Part **A** from Kuwabara, T., and Cogan, D. G. 1982. *In* L. Weiss (ed.) Histology, 5th edition. New York: Elsevier. Part **B** from Dowling, J. E., and Boycott, B. B. 1966. Proc. R. Soc. Lond. B. 166:80.)

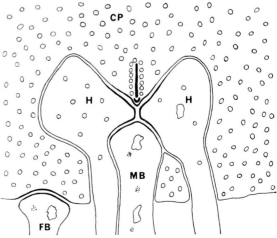

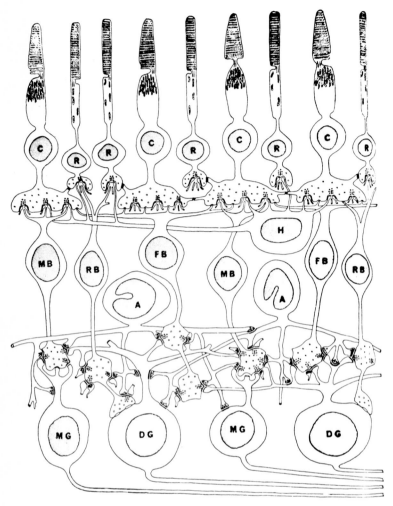

8A–24 A summary diagram of the synaptic circuitry in the retina: **R**, rod; **C**, cone; **MB** midget bipolar cell; **MG**, midget ganglion cell; **H**, horizontal cell; **A**, amacrine cell; **DG** diffuse ganglion cell. (From Dowling, J. E., and Boycott, B. B. 1966. Proc. R. Soc. Lond. B. 166:80.)

and cones contact only particular kinds of bipolar cells and horizontal cells. Some bipolar cells are contacted only by rod spherules and by the axonal processes of those horizontal cells that possess such processes. Other bipolar cells are contacted only by cone pedicles and by the dendrites of horizontal cells. There is less convergence of receptors onto cone bipolar cells than onto rod bipolar cells. In parts of the retina, cone bipolars receive 5 to 6 cone pedicles, whereas rod bipolars receive as many as 50 rod spherules. Some large bipolar cells seem to receive both rod spherules and cone pedicles, but their relationships to horizontal cells is unclear. Horizontal cells are of two types (Fig. 8A–25). Each has radiating dendrites with short processes invaginated into the bases of cone pedicles at triads.

One type, however, also possesses a relatively long, thin axon that at several hundred microns from the dendritic field expands into a branched set of processes virtually as large as the dendritic field itself. Its short processes are invaginated into the bases of rod spherules at synaptic triads.

Neither horizontal cells nor bipolar cells are capable of generating action potentials. The influence of the photoreceptors is thus transmitted to the ganglion cells (the output cells of the retina) by graded electrical potentials. These may be modified by lateral interactions with horizontal cells. In the case of the rod-to-bipolar pathway, because of the extensive lateral spread of the axonal processes of the horizontal cells, such lateral interactions can involve bipolar cells attached to rods over a considerable area. The

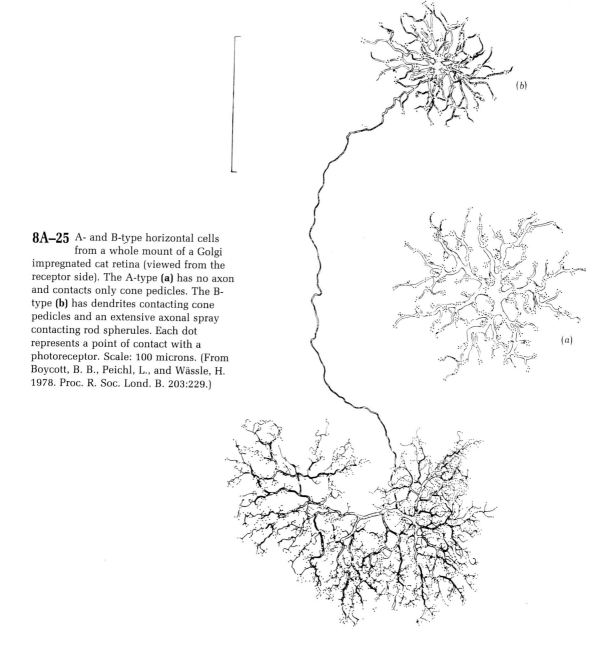

8A–25 A- and B-type horizontal cells from a whole mount of a Golgi impregnated cat retina (viewed from the receptor side). The A-type **(a)** has no axon and contacts only cone pedicles. The B-type **(b)** has dendrites contacting cone pedicles and an extensive axonal spray contacting rod spherules. Each dot represents a point of contact with a photoreceptor. Scale: 100 microns. (From Boycott, B. B., Peichl, L., and Wässle, H. 1978. Proc. R. Soc. Lond. B. 203:229.)

cone-to-bipolar pathway may be subject to lateral interactions over a far less extensive area, in keeping with its role in visual processes involving a high degree of spatial resolution.

The graded potentials mediated by the bipolar cell axons reach the dendrites of ganglion cells in the inner plexiform layer. The principal synaptic type here is also a ribbon synapse, but in mammals the arrangement is a dyad rather than a triad (Fig. 8A–28). The synaptic ribbon is in the axon terminal of a bipolar cell. Opposed to this are two processes: the dendritic tips of a ganglion cell and of an amacrine cell. The amacrine cell process also contains synaptic vesicles and makes synapses back onto the bipolar cell terminal as well as onto the ganglion cell den-

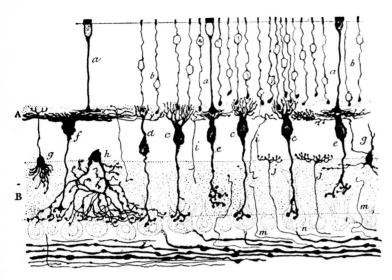

8A–26 Drawing by Ramón y Cajal of Golgi-impregnated neurons in the retina of a mammal: **a,** cones; **b,** rods; **c, d,** rod bipolar cells; **e, f,** cone bipolar cells; **h,** amacrine cell; **m, n,** ganglion cell axons. Cells, **g,** and axons, **j,** have not been recognized subsequently in mammals. (From Ramón y Cajal, S. 1911. Histologie du Système Nerveux de l'Homme et des Vertébrés. Paris: Maloine.)

drite and onto adjacent amacrine cell processes. Even more complicated synaptic arrangements occur in the inner plexiform layer of nonmammals.

Amacrine cells (Figs. 8A–27 and 8A–29) resemble the granule cells of the olfactory bulb in that they lack axons and mediate their synaptic effects by means of presynaptic dendrites. These effects are exerted directly on the ganglion cells or indirectly through effects on bipolar or other amacrine cells. They control transmission at the bipolar-to-ganglion cell synapse and significantly affect the receptive field properties of the ganglion cells. With the photoreceptors, the amacrine cells are the most important influences

over ganglion cell behavior. It is becoming clear that there may be many types of amacrine cells, each containing different neurochemical transmitters, such as GABA, dopamine, and various peptides. In the retinas of some species, each neurochemical type may have a unique dendritic arborization—either widespread and diffuse or narrow and confined to one or two substrata of the inner plexiform layer—and it may only connect with particular forms of ganglion cells or other amacrine cells. The complexity of the functional interactions with ganglion cells and with other amacrine cells that this implies is considerable.

A further cell that should be mentioned is the

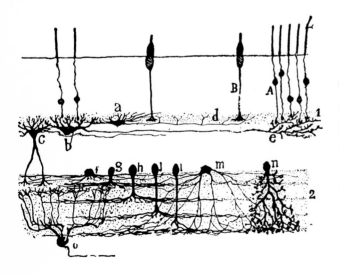

8A–27 Drawing by Ramón y Cajal of Golgi-impregnated neurons in the retina of a mammal, showing mainly horizontal **(a, b, c)** and amacrine **(f, g, h, j, l, m, n)** cells of various forms. Note the variations in amacrine cell dendrites. **A,** rods; **B,** cones; **o,** ganglion cell. (From Ramón y Cajal, S. 1911. Histologie du Système Nerveux de l'Homme et des Vertébrés. Paris, Maloine.)

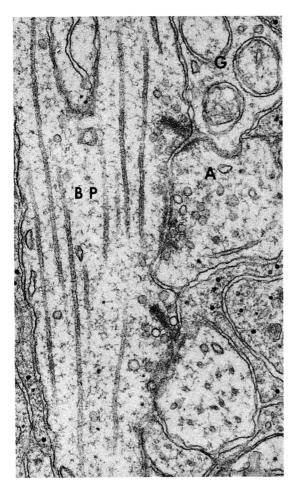

8A–28 Axon terminals formed by bipolar cells **(BP)** in the inner plexiform layer contain synaptic ribbons and clustered vesicles. Other cell components of the dyad synapse are ganglion cell dendrites **(G)** and amacrine cell presynaptic dendrites **(A)**. × 48,500. (From Kuwabara, T., and Cogan, D. G. 1982. In L. Weiss (ed.), Histology, 5th edition. New York: Elsevier.)

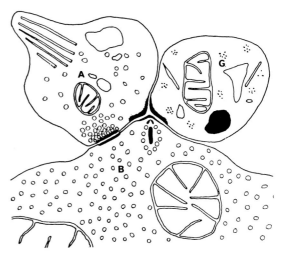

8A–29 A diagram of the dyad synaptic contacts made by bipolar terminals **(B)** with ganglion cell dendrites **(G)** and amacrine cell processes **(A)**. Frequently, the amacrine cell process makes a synaptic contact back onto the bipolar terminal, forming a reciprocal contact. (From Dowling, J. E., and Boycott, B. B. 1966. Proc. R. Soc. Lond. B. 166:80.)

interplexiform cell (not illustrated). This is a cell like an amacrine cell that has its cell body in the inner nuclear layer but with processes to both inner and outer plexiform layers. Some interplexiform cells are dopaminergic.

Ganglion cells (Figs. 8A–24 and 8A–30) are the only retinal cells with axons that conform to the usual morphological criteria and that are capable of conducting action potentials. Their cell bodies lie in a thin sheet, but they have a variety of dendritic arborizations that are either diffuse or localized with most of their branches within a particular sublamina of the inner plexiform layer in a manner similar to that of the amacrine cell (Fig. 8A–30). The sizes of the ganglion cells and especially of their dendritic trees vary greatly, from a few tens of microns to several hundred microns in extent.

The extent of the dendritic tree probably corresponds to the region of photoreceptors from which the ganglion cell receives its input. The effect of shining a light on this region may, however, be to increase ("on") or decrease ("off") the ganglion cell's discharges. Whether the effect is "on" or "off" probably depends on inputs from different populations of "on-" and "off-" type bipolar cells, that is, by inputs from bipolar cells that are either depolarized or hyperpolarized by stimulation of the photoreceptors with which they are connected.

Surrounding the "on" or "off" center of the ganglion cell's receptive field is an annular area, stimulation of which has the converse effect ("off" or "on") on the ganglion cell's discharges. The retinal circuitry leading to the formation of this antagonistic, surrounding part of the receptive field is unclear, but, undoubtedly, lateral interactions involving amacrine and horizontal

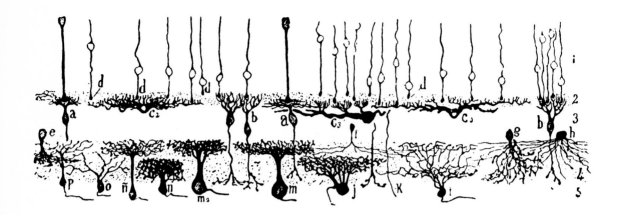

8A–30 Drawing by Ramón y Cajal of Golgi-impregnated neurons in the retina of a mammal mainly showing variations in ganglion cell sizes and dendritic arborizations (**j–p**). **a, b,** bipolar cells; **c,** horizontal cells; **d,** rod spherules; **e–h,** amacrine cells. (From Ramón y Cajal, S. 1911. Histologie du Système Nerveux de l'Homme et des Vertébrés. Paris, Maloine.)

cells are involved. The antagonistic, center-surround type of receptive field is one of the fundamental tenets of retinal physiology.

In many mammals, the sizes of ganglion cell somata can also be correlated with a particular physiological property. Large (30-micron-diameter) ganglion cells are the equivalents of the so-called Y cells recorded electrophysiologically: these are unable to summate light stimuli in a linear fashion; have large, fast-conducting axons; and respond to stimulation of their receptive fields with brisk, transient discharges. Medium (20-micron-diameter) ganglion cells are the equivalents of X cells: they summate photic stimuli in a linear fashion; have smaller, less rapidly conducting axons; and discharge briskly and tonically. The smallest cells (15 microns in diameter) are the equivalents of W cells, which have a variety of responses to light stimuli; have small, very slowly conducting axons; and discharge sluggishly. The importance of these observations rests in the fact that the first two properties at least do not converge in the regions of the brain in which the ganglion cell axons terminate; instead, they are relayed independently to the visual cortex.

The axons of retinal ganglion cells, as they proceed through the retina toward the optic nerve head (Fig. 8A–32), are unmyelinated. They lie in compartments bounded by astrocyte-like processes that are derived from the glial cells of the retina, the Müller cells. Once in the optic nerve, the axons become associated with oligodendrocytes and acquire a myelin sheath, as shown in Fig. 8–38.

The Müller cells of the retina are structurally similar to astrocytes in their watery cytoplasm; ability to store glycogen; relative lack of organelles, except filaments; and tendency to form foot processes at interfaces. The cell bodies are relatively large and situated in the inner nuclear layer. From there, vertical processes extend toward both the vitreal and the photoreceptor surfaces of the neural retina. At the vitreal surface, foot processes expand beneath the basal lamina. The stacks of such processes, rather like the glia limitans of the brain and spinal cord (see Chapter 8), are referred to as the *inner limiting membrane* (Figs. 8A–23 and 8A–24).

At approximately the level of junction between the cell bodies and inner segments of the photoreceptors, the processes of the Müller cells are joined to one another and to the adjacent photoreceptors by zonulae adhaerentes. The line of such junctions, when visualized light microscopically, is referred to as the *outer limiting membrane* (Fig. 8A–24). The junctions can probably be regarded as providing some form of structural support to this part of the retina. Beyond it, the photoreceptors protrude into the potential space formerly occupied by the lumen of the optic cup deep to the pigment epithelium (Figs. 8A–12, 8A–13, and 8A–22). Through this potential space, the photoreceptors are nourished by diffusion from the choroidal capillaries, because the retinal vessels, ramifying primarily in the optic nerve fiber layer, penetrate the neural retina only as deep as the inner nuclear

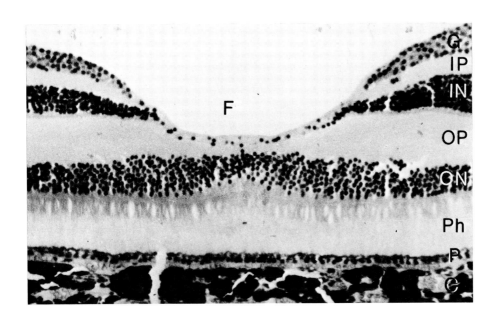

8A–31 Section through the fovea **(F)** of a monkey retina showing high cell density but lateral displacement of all cells except the photoreceptors. Layers identified as in Figs. 8A–14 and 8A–15. Hematoxylin and eosin stain. × 240.

layer. Along the potential space, the neural retina may detach from the pigment epithelium, leading to necrosis of the photoreceptors unless promptly corrected.

Regional Variations in the Retina

Up to this point, we have described the neural retina in general terms, but its structure is far from homogeneous. All its layers are absent at the point of exit of the optic nerve (Fig. 8A–32). This is called the *optic disc*, which also affords entry to the central artery of the retina and can be visualized ophthalmoscopically as a pale, round area.

At its peripheral margins, where it meets the pigment epithelium and the ciliary body (Fig. 8A–13), the neural retina is also particularly thin and the cells in its three nuclear layers are widely dispersed. At this level, rods far outnumber cones in the photoreceptor layer.

The neural retina is at its thickest in a region at the optical center of the retina, termed the *macula lutea* in primates. There are comparable regions in other mammals. The macula (in humans, 3 microns to the temporal side of the optic disc and approximately 2 mm² in area) is thick because of its particularly high concentration of photoreceptors and other retinal neurons. At the center of the macula is a deep, avascular pit, the *fovea centralis* (Fig. 8A–31). The fovea is formed by the lateral displacement of all the elements overlying the inner and outer segments of the photoreceptors. Light thus reaches the photoreceptors unimpeded. In the floor of the fovea, these are all cones, though they are so small and slender that they resemble rods. Because of the particularly high concentration and close spacing of photoreceptors in the floor of the fovea, it is the region of greatest visual acuity. The laterally displaced cone cell bodies, bipolar cells, and ganglion cells in the walls of the fovea are also particularly small and are often referred to as *midget cells*. Each midget ganglion cell maintains connections with a relatively small number of bipolar cells and, through them, with a smaller number of cones than elsewhere in the retina. This relationship, which has sometimes been estimated to approach a 1:1 ratio, is also a major factor in the high spatial resolution of visual stimuli.

Rods only become apparent toward the perimeter of the fovea, but they rapidly increase in number toward the periphery of the macula. There, cones decline in number and in humans fall from about 150,000/mm² at the fovea to about 5,000/mm² at 10° of retinal angle beyond it. At

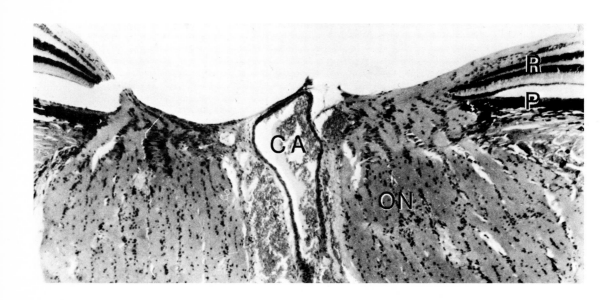

8A–32 Section through the optic nerve head of a monkey retina showing the optic nerve **(ON)**, central artery **(CA)**, pigment epithelium **(P)**, and layers of retina **(R)**. Hematoxylin and eosin stain. × 100.

10° out, rods increase in density to about 160,000/mm² and, though gradually declining in number, still outnumber cones by at least six times toward the periphery of the retina. At the periphery, many more photoreceptors ultimately converge on single ganglion cells than at the fovea, so visual acuity declines.

The Internal Ear

The neural apparatus of the internal ear is associated with both the cochlear and vestibular components of the membranous labyrinth (Fig. 8A–36). Each arises by subdivision of the otocyst, a small cavity lined by neuroepithelium derived from placodal tissue and growing in association with the eighth cranial nerve (Figs. 8A–33 through 8A–35), the cells of which are also derived from the same placode. The cochlea is concerned with hearing, the vestibular apparatus with subjective sensations of space and motion. The vestibular apparatus also plays an important role in reflexes that stabilize the posture of the body against gravity and the positions of the eyes during movements of the head, thus preventing movement of images on the retina and blurred vision.

The Vestibular Apparatus

The vestibular system takes its name from the *vestibule,* a bony cavity in the interior of the petrous temporal bone. In the vestibule lie two thin-walled, saclike dilatations of the membranous labyrinth, the *utricle* and *saccule* (Figs. 8A–36 through 8A–38). The utricle and the saccule communicate with the three *semicircular ducts,* which form the rest of the vestibular labyrinth (Figs. 8A–36 and 8A–38). The saccule lies anteriorly and inferiorly in the vestibule and is continuous with the cochlear duct by means of the narrow *ductus reuniens.* The utricle lies posteriorly and dorsally in the vestibule and is joined to the saccule by a further narrow duct. Opening into the utricle are the two ends of each of three *semicircular ducts,* the greater parts of which are contained within individual canals in the petrous temporal bone above and behind the vestibule. Dilatations of the anterior ends of the lateral and anterior ducts and of the posterior end of the posterior duct as they enter the utricle are referred to as *ampullae.* The three semicircular ducts lie at right angles to one another (Fig. 8A–36). The lateral duct lies in a plane more or less parallel to the base of the skull and is therefore tilted upward by about 30° in relation to the true horizontal when the head is held with the eyes directed straight forward. The anterior canal is in a plane directed from anterolateral to posteromedial (45° to the sagittal plane). The posterior canal, at right angles to this, is in a plane from anteromedial to posterolateral (55° to the frontal

8A–33 Horizontal section through the developing
hindbrain and pharyngeal arches of a 12-mm
pig embryo showing the otocyst **(O)** and the
developing ganglia of the trigeminal **(V)**, facial **(VII)**,
auditory **(VIII)**, and glossopharyngeal **(IX)** nerves.
Carmine stain. × 65. ▷

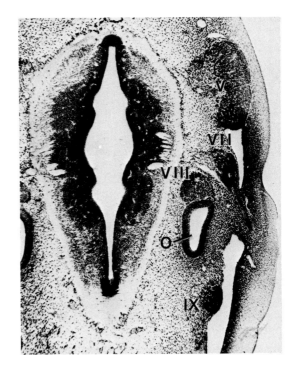

8A–34 Parasagittal section through the head of a rat
fetus at 17 days of gestation showing the
developing vestibular labyrinth **(V)** embedded in the
cartilaginous precursor of the petrous temporal bone.
Also seen are the developing eye **(E)**, brain **(B)**, upper
jaw **(UJ)** and neck **(N)** muscles, and the follicles **(F)** of
vibrissae of the upper lip. Thionin stain. × 13. ▽

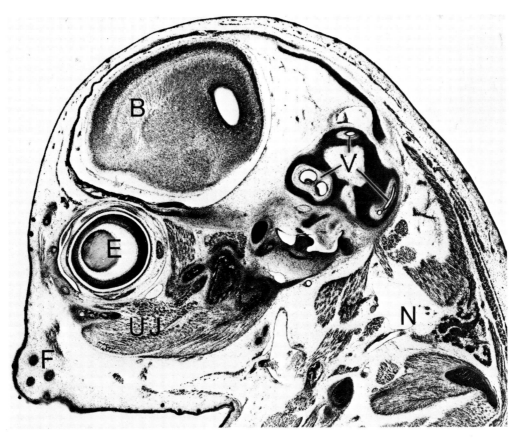

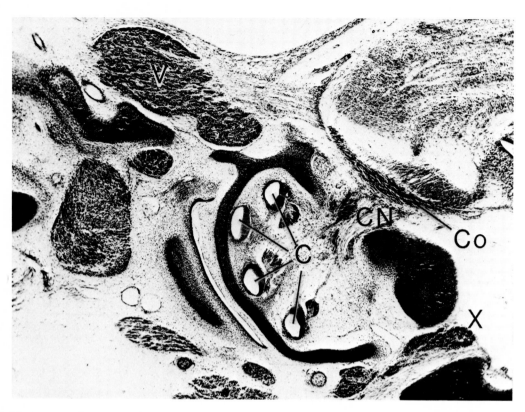

8A–35 Parasagittal section medial to that shown in Fig. 8A–34 demonstrating the developing cochlear duct **(C),** which is already coiled and associated with clusters of neurons of the spiral ganglion. The cochlear division of the auditory nerve **(CN)** and the cochlear nuclei **(Co)** in which its central branches end are also seen, together with the trigeminal **(V)** and vagal **(X)** ganglia. Brainstem is at upper right. Thionin stain. × 60.

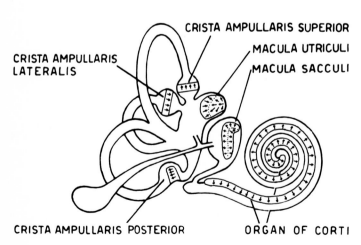

8A–36 Schematic drawing of the membranous labyrinth. Within each sensory area the orientation of the stereocilia of the sensory cells is indicated. (From Flock, A. 1982. *In* L. Weiss (ed.), Histology, 5th edition. New York: Elsevier. Modified from Ebner. Reproduced with permission of W. Engelmann.)

8A–37 Horizontal section through part of the petrous temporal bone of a dog. Brainstem **(B)** at lower right, middle ear cavity **(ME)** at upper left. The auditory nerve **(AN)** can be seen with the vestibular ganglion **(VG)** in the internal auditory meatus. At upper right are the sectioned coils of the cochlear duct, with elements of the spiral ganglion **(SG)** at the base of the spiral lamina. At bottom left is the vestibule containing portions of the utricle **(U)** and saccule **(S)**, with the stapes **(St)** in the oval window. The macula **(m)** of the saccule is visible on the medial wall of the vestibule in the sagittal plane of the head. Hematoxylin and eosin stain. × 20.

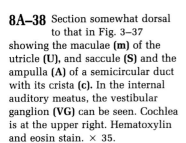
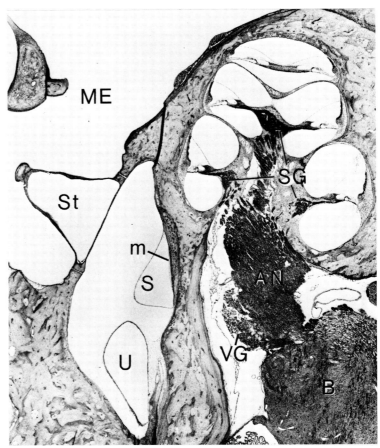

8A–38 Section somewhat dorsal to that in Fig. 3–37 showing the maculae **(m)** of the utricle **(U)**, and saccule **(S)** and the ampulla **(A)** of a semicircular duct with its crista **(c)**. In the internal auditory meatus, the vestibular ganglion **(VG)** can be seen. Cochlea is at the upper right. Hematoxylin and eosin stain. × 35.

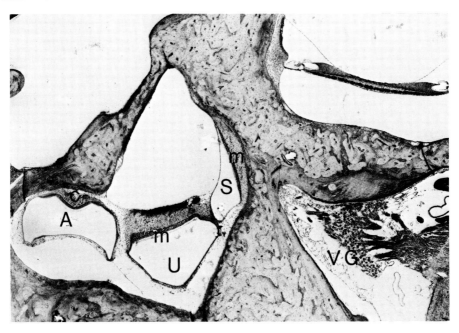

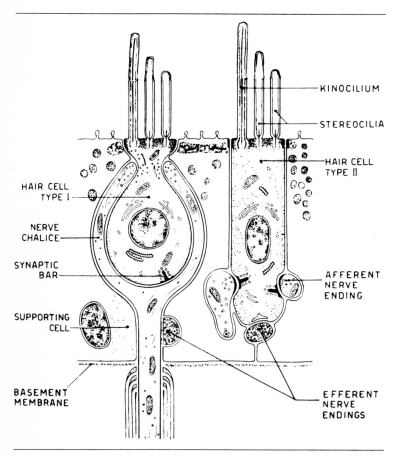

KINOCILIUM

STEREOCILIA

HAIR CELL
TYPE II

HAIR CELL
TYPE I

NERVE
CHALICE

SYNAPTIC
BAR

AFFERENT
NERVE
ENDING

SUPPORTING
CELL

BASEMENT
MEMBRANE

EFFERENT
NERVE
ENDINGS

8A–39 Schematic drawing of vestibular sensory cells. (From Flock, A. 1982. *In* L. Weiss (ed.), Histology, 5th edition. New York: Elsevier. Modified from Wersäll. Reproduced with permission of Pergamon Press.)

plane). The anterior duct of one side is approximately parallel to the posterior duct of the other; during normal vestibular function, the parallel, crossed pairs operate together.

The labyrinth is filled with *endolymph*, a fluid containing a high concentration of potassium and in the vestibular labyrinth apparently secreted by cells lining its wall. The endolymph is probably not responsible for the nourishment of the vestibular receptors but instead maintains the ionic composition of their environment in a state suitable for the sensory transduction process.

Hair Cells

The basis of vestibular, as of cochlear, sensory function is a specialized receptor cell of the membranous labyrinth, the *hair cell* (Fig. 8A–39). The hair cell is not traditionally classified as a neuron, but it is capable of maintaining a rest-

ing membrane potential, gives rise to receptor potentials in response to appropriate stimuli, and forms morphologically identifiable synapses on the nerve fibers that innervate it.

The hair cell is activated as the result of movements of the endolymph within the vestibular labyrinth. The structural and functional characteristics of the hair cells in the mammalian vestibular system differ only in details from those of hair cells in the cochlea, and they are virtually identical to the hair cells of the lateral line receptors in fish and amphibia.

All hair cells have an apical surface directed toward the interior of the membranous labyrinth and a basal surface in contact with the basal lamina lining the outer surface of the labyrinth. The apical surface of vestibular and lateral line hair cells is characterized by the possession of a single, long *kinocilium* and 60 to 100 shorter *stereocilia* (Fig. 8A–39 and 8A–40). The kinocilium resembles a typical cilium with a central pair of

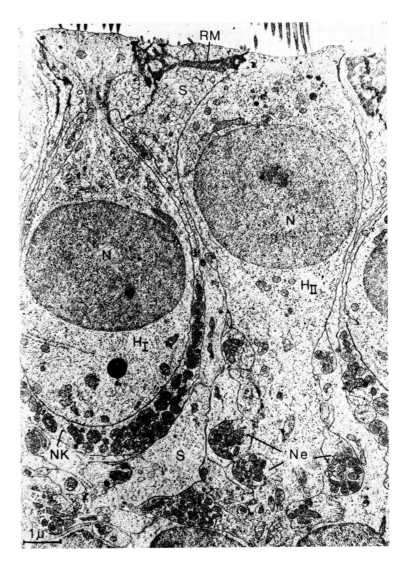

8A–40 Type I and type II hair cells from the normal macula of the utricle of a cat. **N,** nucleus; **Ne** nerve ending; **NK,** nerve calyx; **RM,** reticular lamina; **S,** supporting cell. (From Babel, J., Bischoff, A., and Spoendlin, H. 1970. Ultrastructure of the Peripheral Nervous System and Sense Organs. St. Louis: Mosby.)

microtubules surrounded by nine double microtubules, but it is immobile. It has a typical basal body with an adjacent centriole oriented at right angles to it. From the basal body protrudes a basal foot. The stereocilia are typical microvilli and, when seen in surface view, form a regular hexagonal lattice (Fig. 8A–41). Seen from the side, the stereocilia increase in length in a staircase fashion toward the kinocilium (Fig. 8A–39). Hair cells are present only in certain specialized and easily recognized parts of the vestibular labyrinth, to be described following, and, where present, their kinocilia and stereocilia are embedded in an overlying proteinaceous membrane (also to be described following) that trans-

mits movements of the endolymph to the cilia. The bases of the stereocilia are embedded in a zone of increased cytoplasmic density, the *cuticular plate*, near the apex of the hair cell. The basal body of the kinocilium protrudes deeper into the cytoplasm through a hole in the cuticular plate. Near this, there tends to be an aggregation of mitochondria.

Hair cells are directionally selective mechanoreceptors for which the exciting stimulus is shearing displacement of the cilia in the direction of the kinocilium. This leads to the generation of a receptor potential and to an increased probability of firing in the afferent nerves to which the hair cells are coupled. Displacement

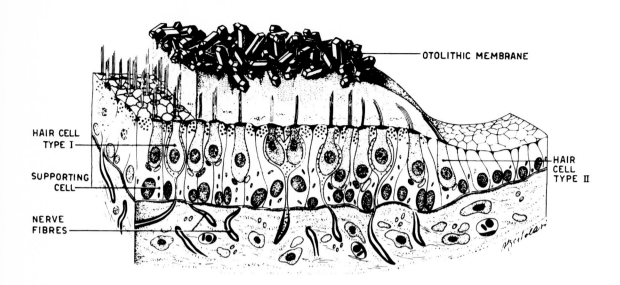

OTOLITHIC MEMBRANE

HAIR CELL
TYPE I

SUPPORTING
CELL

NERVE
FIBRES

HAIR
CELL
TYPE II

8A–41 The macula and its otolithic membrane.
(From Flock, A. 1982. *In* L. Weiss (ed.),
Histology, 5th edition. New York: Elsevier. Courtesy
of Iurato. Reproduced with permission of Pergamon
Press.)

of the cilia away from the kinocilium leads to
inhibition. The sensitivity of hair cells to small
displacements in the appropriate direction is
particularly great; the subjective experience con-
sequent on this can be quite alarming. The response of the hair cell to displacements of its
cilia in the appropriate direction is, over a wide
range, proportional to the degree of displacement. A shearing movement of the bases rather
than a bending of the sterocilia and kinocilium
appears to be the effective stimulus, but the nature of the transduction process that leads from
this to the change in membrane conductance responsible for the receptor potential is unknown.
The basal foot of the kinocilium has sometimes
been thought to play a critical role, since it is
inevitably polarized in the plane of the preferred
stimulus direction.

At its base, the hair cell is in contact with one
or more endings of afferent and efferent nerve fibers (Figs. 8A–39 and 8A–40). In the majority of
hair cells in the vestibular labyrinth and all those
in the cochlea and in the lateral line organs (type
II hair cells), the hair cell forms the presynaptic
element of a conventional synapse on small endings of peripheral processes of vestibular ganglion cells. Each peripheral process has the

structure of an axon and branches to innervate
several hair cells. At the region of contact, there
are synaptic vesicles in the hair cell, often aggregated about a synaptic ribbon, and the membrane
thickenings are asymmetric in the direction of
the afferent ending. Unlike most sensory receptors (see Chapter 8), receptor potentials and afferent impulses do not both occur in the nerve
fiber. Instead, the receptor potential generated in
the hair cells leads by a typical excitatory synaptic event to the generation of action potentials
in the afferent axon innervating them.

Found only in the vestibular labyrinth of
mammals is a second type of hair cell (type I)
that is larger and more flask-shaped than the
more common type II hair cell (Fig. 8A–39). The
type I cell is innervated by a single, large afferent
nerve ending that encloses the greater part of the
hair cell as in a chalice or cup. The membrane
contacts between type I hair cells and this large
ending are gap junctions rather than conventional synapses, and, in this case, the transmission of the receptor event to the afferent fiber
may be electrical.

Both kinds of hair cells also receive the terminals of a particular set of *efferent* axons whose
parent cell bodies reside in the brainstem. The
axon terminals form typical asymmetric synapses (Fig. 8A–40). In the case of type II hair
cells, the hair cell itself is the postsynaptic element, but in the case of type I hair cells, the large
afferent terminal is the postsynaptic element.
This unique group of efferent axons is particularly rich in the enzyme acetylcholinesterase,

suggesting (but by no means proving) that their transmitter substance may be acetylcholine. In any case, stimulation of these fibers invariably leads to inhibition of discharge in afferent fibers innervating the hair cells.

An unusually high concentration of potassium in the endolymph bathes the apexes of the hair cells. This would obviously provide less than optimal conditions for the generation of action potentials were the endolymph to communicate with the extracellular fluid at the base of the hair cell. A barrier to this appears to be provided by the *supporting cells* of the membranous labyrinth. These cells, among which the hair cells lie, extend processes around the apexes of the hair cells, embedding the hair cells in a relatively firm, electron-dense *reticular membrane* (Fig. 8A–39 and 8A–40). In this, supporting cell processes are linked to one another and to the adjoining hair cells by occluding tight junctions. Other functions of the supporting cells are uncertain. Their cytoplasm is filled with large, moderately electron-dense, membrane-bound bodies, the exact nature of which is unknown.

Receptor Regions of the Vestibular Labyrinth

Hair cells and the characteristic supporting cells with which they are associated are confined to five localized regions of the vestibular labyrinth in mammals. These are the *macula of the utricle,* the *macula of the saccule,* and the *crista* or crest within each of the ampullae of the semicircular ducts (Fig. 8A–36). In each of these regions, the elongated hair cells and the tall supporting cells cause the wall of the labyrinth to be thickened. Elsewhere, the wall is composed of a single layer of low cuboidal or squamous cells, many of which resemble the secretory cells of the choroid plexus and may produce the endolymph.

The *maculae* of the utricle and saccule have an identical structure (Figs. 8A–41 and 8A–42). Each consists of a thickened, plaquelike region some 3 mm × 2 mm in extent. That of the utricle is in a plane parallel to the base of the skull; that in the saccule, at right angles to it (close to the sagittal plane). The gelatinous membrane sur-

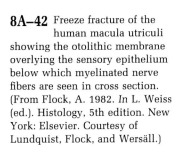

8A–42 Freeze fracture of the human macula utriculi showing the otolithic membrane overlying the sensory epithelium below which myelinated nerve fibers are seen in cross section. (From Flock, A. 1982. *In* L. Weiss (ed.). Histology, 5th edition. New York: Elsevier. Courtesy of Lundquist, Flock, and Wersäll.)

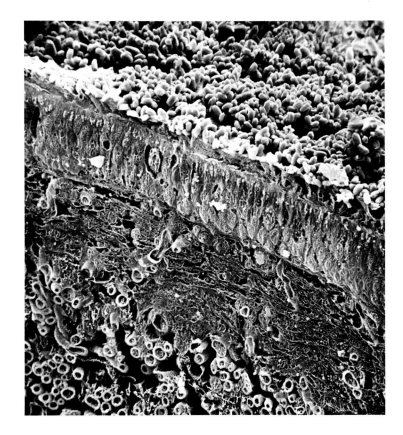

mounting the macula is referred to as the *otolithic membrane* (Figs. 8A–41 and 8A–42), since it contains large numbers of small, hexagonal crystals of calcium carbonate *(otokonia)*. The cilia of the hair cells are embedded in the protein matrix of the otolithic membrane; shearing stresses are set up in them as a result of movements of the membrane as it slides over the surface of the macula during tilting, inversion, or linear acceleration of the head.

The hair cells of the maculae are concerned primarily with static aspects of vestibular function and, when stimulated, lead to slowly adapting discharges in the nerve fibers innervating them. They are activated by movements of the otolithic membrane caused by gravitational force, as in tilting movements of the head, and by linear acceleration of the head or whole body, as in forward movement in an automobile. The orientation of the kinocilia of macular hair cells (and thus the preferred stimulus direction) is not random but highly systematic and predictable (Fig. 8A–36). It is sometimes referred to as the "hair cell map." Hence, hair cells in different maculae or in different parts of the same macula will be stimulated during movements of the head in different directions.

The *crista* of the ampulla of each semicircular duct *(crista ampullaris)* is an elevated ridge rather than a plaquelike structure (Fig. 8A–43), but its organization is very similar to that of the maculae. Hair cell density is greatest on the slopes of the crista that descend to a flattened part of the ampulla, the *planum semilunatum*. Overlying the whole crista is a gelatinous membrane, the *cupula*, that more or less seals the ampulla so that under normal circumstances there is little or no flow of endolymph from the ampulla into the utricle. The cupula lacks otokonia, and the cilia of the hair cells lie in tiny canals within it.

The hair cells of a crista are affected by sliding movements of the cupula set up by inertial movements of the endolymph caused by angular acceleration of the head in the plane of the canal in which that crista lies. Thus, the cristae of the two lateral semicircular ducts are most affected by rotation in the horizontal plane of the body when the head is tilted forward about 30°.

All the hair cells in one crista are oriented in the same direction. But the orientation of hair cells and, thus, the direction of preferred stimuli by the moving endolymph is specific for each crista (Fig. 8A–36). The kinocilia of the cristae in the horizontal canals are all oriented toward the utricle so that the preferred stimulus here is movement of the endolymph toward the utricle (utriculopetal flow). In the cristae of the anterior and posterior ducts, hair cell orientation is away from the utricle, and these hair cells are excited by movement in the opposite direction (utriculofugal flow). Since the semicircular ducts of the two sides are arranged in parallel pairs, this means that with rotation in one direction, the hair cells of one crista of the pair are stimulated while those of the other are inhibited.

The cupula of the crista behaves rather like a torsion pendulum; movements as small as a few angstroms may be sufficient to excite the underlying hair cells. After being displaced by the inertial movements of the endolymph in a direction opposite that in which the body and/or head is rotated, the cupula takes some 20 to 30 sec to recover its original position. During this time, a person experiences a sense of rotation in the opposite direction and may be subjected to certain reflex effects.

The Vestibular Nerve

The cells of origin of the vestibular nerve are true bipolar cells, derived from the otocyst and situated in the adult in the vestibular (Scarpa's) ganglion (Figs. 8A–37 and 8A–38). Unlike the cochlear (spiral) ganglion, which lies within the modiolus in the interior of the petrous temporal bone, the vestibular ganglion is situated outside the temporal bone in the internal auditory meatus. From this, two or more trunks, composed of the peripheral processes of the bipolar cells, penetrate the interior of the temporal bone and individual branches are distributed to each of the receptor areas of the vestibular labyrinth. The central processes constitute the vestibular division of the eighth cranial nerve ("auditory nerve") and pass toward the brain stem in close association with the cochlear division and the facial nerve.

It has been determined that the human vestibular nerve contains 1,400 to 2,000 nerve fibers, on average 8 to 10 microns in diameter. All are myelinated and arise from cell somata that are themselves enveloped in myelin formed by the Schwann cells of the vestibular ganglion. The peripheral processes, which tend to be somewhat thinner than the central, are also myelinated and should be regarded as axons, not dendrites. Each branches quite extensively to supply several hair

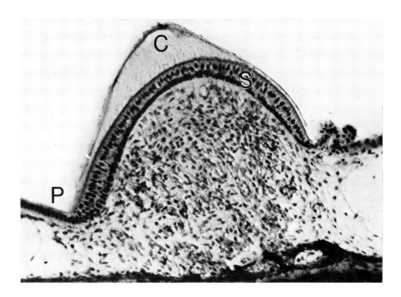

8A–43 **A.** Photomicrograph of the crista of the ampulla of a semicircular duct in the vestibular labyrinth of a dog. **C,** cupula; **P,** planum semilunatum; **S,** sensory epithelium. Hematoxylin and eosin stain. × 350. **B.** Sensory epithelium of the crista ampullaris showing hair cells with apical stereocilia embedded in the cupula. (Part **B** from Flock, A. 1982. *In* L. Weiss (ed.), Histology, 5th edition. New York: Elsevier. Courtesy of Wersäll.)

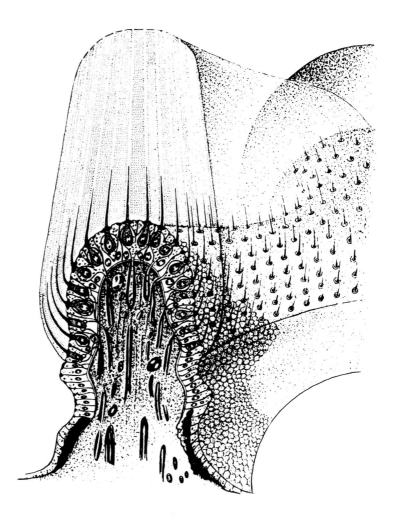

cells in one macula or crista. It is probable that action potentials are only generated in the peripheral process as the result of activity in all or most of the hair cells that its branches supply. Accompanying the large numbers of fibers that constitute the afferent component of the vestibular nerve is the much smaller efferent and presumed cholinergic component mentioned earlier.

The Cochlea

The coiled *cochlear duct* is the auditory equivalent of the vestibular labyrinth. It lies in the bony cochlea, coiled about the modiolus. Centrally, it is attached to the bony spiral lamina that projects from the modiolus (Figs. 8A–36 through 8A–38). Peripherally, it is attached by a *spiral ligament*

to the wall of the bony cochlea at a thickening of the periosteum referred to as the spiral prominence; in part of this region, the wall of the duct is thickened and multilayered and the underlying periosteum is highly vascular. The two spe-

8A–44 Cross sections of the cochlear duct of a dog.
Note nerve fibers crossing tunnel **(arrow). B,** basilar membrane; **D,** Deiters' cells; **G,** spiral ganglion; **HC,** cells of Hensen and Cladius; **IH,** inner hair cells; **N,** nerve fibers; **OH,** outer hair cells; **P,** pillar cells; **S,** stria vascularis; **SG,** spiral ganglion; **SL,** spiral lamina; **SM,** scala media; **SP,** spiral promontory; **ST,** scala tympani; **SV,** scala vestibuli; **T,** tunnel; **TM,** tectorial membrane; **V,** vestibular membrane. Hematoxylin and eosin stain. **A** × 150; **B** × 470.

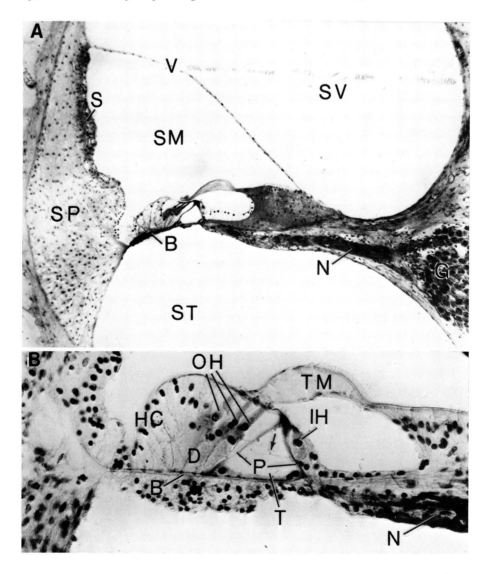

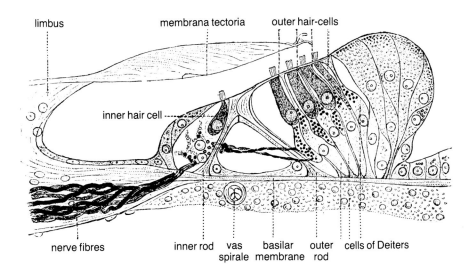

limbus   membrana tectoria   outer hair-cells

inner hair cell

nerve fibres   inner rod   vas spirale   basilar membrane   outer rod   cells of Deiters

8A–45 Schematic drawing by G. Retzius of the human organ of Corti. (As reproduced by Schäfer, E. A. 1894. *In* E. A. Schäfer and G. D. Thane (eds.). Quain's Elements of Anatomy. London: Longmans, Green.)

cializations form a structure, the *stria vascularis* (Fig. 8A–44), which resembles a choroid plexus and through which the endolymph filling the cochlear duct is probably secreted. Secretion of ions by the stria vascularis maintains a large (90-mV) positive endocochlear potential.

Unlike in the vestibular labyrinth, hair cells are situated along the full length of the cochlear duct in a specialized region of its wall called the *organ of Corti*.

In cross section, the cochlear duct is triangular (Figs. 8A–37 and 8A–44). Its base or lateral wall, containing the stria vascularis, has already been mentioned. The wall that abuts on the scala vestibuli of the bony cochlea is referred to as the *vestibular (Reissner's) membrane*. It is attenuated and made up of a single layer of flattened epithelial cells on a basal lamina that adjoins the scala vestibuli. The remaining wall, forming the organ of Corti (Figs. 8A–44 and 8A–45), is much more complicated. As well as hair cells, the epithelium shows several forms of supporting cells and additional morphological specializations. All the cells rest on the spiral lamina or on the *basilar membrane*. The basilar membrane is composed of the basal lamina of the cochlear duct, together with bundles of collagen fibers and connective tissue cells that line its external

surface, adjoining the scala tympani of the bony cochlea. In the connective tissue is a small terminal branch of the internal auditory artery. The basilar membrane is narrowest in the basal turn of the cochlea and widest at the apex, changing in humans from a width of 0.16 mm to 0.52 mm over a distance of approximately 30 mm.

As seen in cross section (Figs. 8A–44 and 8A–45), there is a triangular *tunnel of Corti* in the region where the basilar membrane meets the spiral lamina. This is formed from a pair of *pillar cells* (or rods of Corti) inclined toward another so that their apexes meet. Their bases are expanded feet; their cell bodies are rigid and contain a lattice of microtubules that end in desmosome-like junctions at the apexes of the cells. The apex of the outer pillar cell locks into that of the inner pillar cell and is then expanded laterally as a thin, flattened plate, the *phalangeal process*, over the outer hair cells. The phalangeal processes of all the outer pillar cells form part of the *reticular membrane* in which the apexes of the outer hair cells are embedded (Figs. 8A–45 and 8A–49). The rest of the reticular membrane is formed by more laterally placed supporting cells of a different type. These are the *cells of Deiters* (Figs. 8A–44 and 8A–45). Beyond them again are the supporting cells of Hensen and of Claudius.

Internal to the row of inner pillar cells is a single slanted row of (in humans) some 3,500 *inner hair cells* (Figs. 8A–44 through 8A–46). External to the outer pillar cells are three slanted rows of some 20,000 *outer hair cells*. As with vestibular hair cells, the apical cytoplasm of the

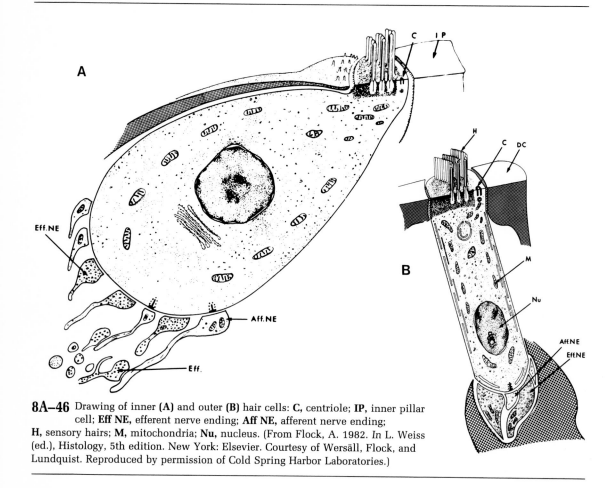

8A–46 Drawing of inner **(A)** and outer **(B)** hair cells: **C,** centriole; **IP,** inner pillar cell; **Eff NE,** efferent nerve ending; **Aff NE,** afferent nerve ending; **H,** sensory hairs; **M,** mitochondria; **Nu,** nucleus. (From Flock, A. 1982. *In* L. Weiss (ed.), Histology, 5th edition. New York: Elsevier. Courtesy of Wersäll, Flock, and Lundquist. Reproduced by permission of Cold Spring Harbor Laboratories.)

cochlear hair cells contains a densely staining cuticular plate in which are embedded the basal portions of 50 to 100 stereocilia. The stereocilia usually occur in three or more rows in which the stereocilia increase in length stepwise in the direction of the stria vascularis (Fig. 8A–46). Unlike the vestibular hair cells, the tallest stereocilia are not succeeded by a kinocilium. There is, however, a centriole in the position in which a kinocilium would be expected (Figs. 8A–46 and 9–47). The inner and outer hair cells are thus morphologically polarized like their vestibular counterparts and are excited by a displacement of the stereocilia in the direction of the centriole. The rows of stereocilia of inner hair cells are straight; those of outer hair cells are in the form of a V or W with the centriole at its apex (Figs. 8A–48 and 8A–49).

The stereocilia lie free of the reticular lamina, which, as in the case of the reticular lamina of the receptor regions of the vestibular labyrinth, probably serves to isolate the underlying hair cells and afferent nerve terminals from the endolymph in which the concentration of potassium is particularly high. The tips of the stereocilia are embedded in the *tectorial membrane* (Fig. 8A–44), a gelatinous flap secreted by cells at its attachment to the spiral lamina. The tectorial membrane resembles the cupula of a crista ampullaris so that stresses set up in it by the vibration of the basilar membrane are communicated to the stereocilia of the hair cells.

Vibrations in the air, set up by auditory stimuli, are communicated to the perilymph of the scala vestibuli and scala tympani by movements of the stapes in the oval window. These vibra-

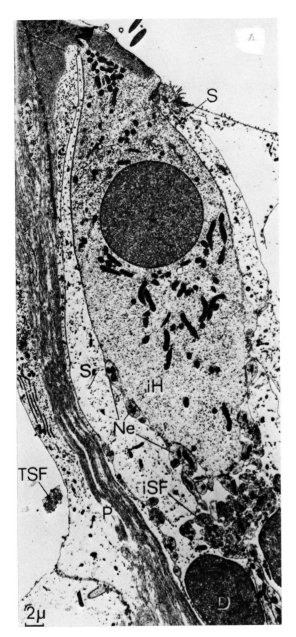

8A–47 Electron micrograph of an inner hair cell **(iH)** from the cochlea of a cat. **D, iSF, TSF,** nerve fibers; **Ne,** nerve endings; **S,** supporting cells. (From Babel, J., Bischoff, A., and Spoendlin, H. 1970. *In* Ultrastructure of the Peripheral Nerves and Sense Organs. St. Louis: Mosby.)

tions are, in turn, communicated to the basilar membrane. Sound stimuli set up a wave of vibration that travels along most of the length of the basilar membrane. However, a sound stimulus of a particular frequency, at least in the middle range of audible frequencies, tends to cause maximal deflection of the basilar membrane at a particular region. This moves from apex to base of the cochlear duct as the frequency of the sound stimulus increases. It has been suggested that, as the basilar membrane is deflected toward the relatively stiff tectorial membrane, the stereocilia of the hair cells would be displaced and that shearing stresses set up in their bases in the direction of the centriole would thus lead to depolarization of the hair cells and to the generation of receptor potentials.

The bases of the cochlear hair cells lie below the reticular membrane (Figs. 8A–45 and 8A–49) in what is assumed to be an ionic environment more suitable for the induction of action potentials in the nerve fibers that innervate them. The cochlear hair cells are surrounded by supporting cells but at intervals are in contact with the terminations of the peripheral processes of neurons of the cochlear (spiral) ganglion. Unlike those of the vestibular ganglion, the cell bodies of the bipolar neurons of the spiral ganglion are actually contained within the substance of the petrous temporal lobe, where they occupy the spiral lamina of the bony cochlea and their myelinated peripheral processes, which resemble axons, enter the organ of Corti through small orifices. There they lose their myelin sheaths.

Approximately nine-tenths of the nerve fibers appear to innervate inner hair cells. The remaining axons cross the tunnel of Corti and innervate the outer hair cells (Fig. 8A–50). Each axon ending in relation to the single row of inner hair cells appears to innervate only one hair cell (Fig. 8A–50), but each hair cell receives the terminations of up to 20 axons. By contrast, an axon ending in relation to the three rows of outer hair cells branches to innervate at least 10. It is the inner hair cells, therefore, that appear to have the neural organization suitable for a receptor system of high spatial resolution. They can be likened to the cones connected with single midget bipolar cells and single midget ganglion cells in the fovea of the retina.

The synaptic arrangements at the bases of both inner and outer cochlear hair cells resemble those of type II hair cells in the vestibular labyrinth (Figs. 8A–51 and 8A–52). The base of the

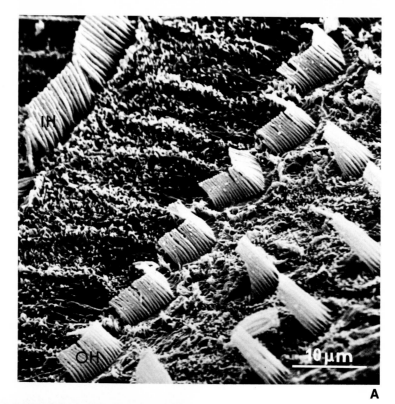

A

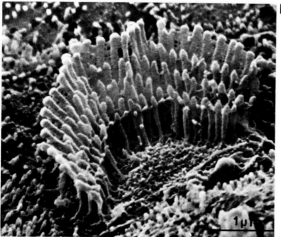

B

8A–48 **A.** Bundles of stereocilia of inner **(IH)** and outer **(OH)** hair cells project from the surface of the organ of Corti. Supporting cells of the reticular lamina have microvilli. (From A. Flock, *In*: L. Weiss (ed.), Histology, 5th edition. New York: Elsevier, 1982.) **B.** Bundle of stereocilia of an outer hair cell seen from the modiolus side. Human. (From Flock, A. 1982. *In* L. Weiss (ed.), Histology, 5th edition. New York: Elsevier. Courtesy of Lundquist, Flock, and Wesäll. Reprinted with permission from Urban and Schwarzenberg, Vienna.)

hair cell contains clear and dense-cored vesicles and makes several conventional asymmetric synaptic contacts with the terminals of the peripheral processes of the neurons of the spiral ganglion. These processes are relatively undistinguished, containing only a few mitochondria and some smooth-walled cisternae. The afferent nerve endings are vestibular cells that are also postsynaptic at an asymmetric synapse to the small terminals of *efferent* nerve fibers with parent cell bodies that are situated in the contralateral side of the brain stem. It is thought that most of these efferent nerves end in relation to the outer hair cells (Fig. 8A–50). They are pre-

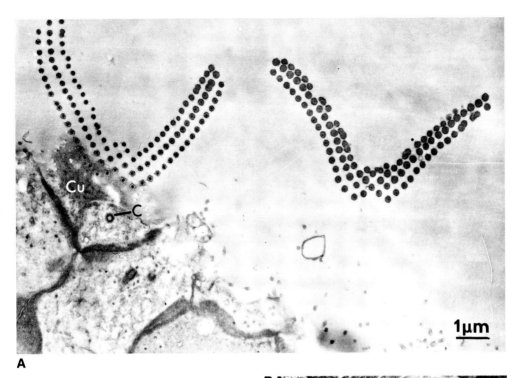

A

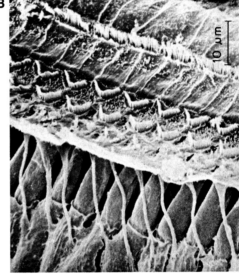

B

8A–49 **A.** Section through the stereocilia of one outer hair cell and through part of the cuticular plate **(Cu)** and the centriole **(C)** of its neighbor. (From Flock, A. *In* L. Weiss (ed.), Histology, 5th edition. New York: Elsevier. Courtesy of Flock, Kimura, Lundquist, and Wersäll. Reproduced by permission of American Institute of Physics, New York.) **B.** Phalangeal cells have slender twisted processes that reach the surface of the organ of Corti where their heads form the reticular lamina. (From Flock, A. 1982. *In* L. Weiss (ed.) Histology, 5th edition. New York: Elsevier. Courtesy of Wersäll, Flock, and Lundquist. Reproduced with permission from Killisch-Horn Verlag.)

sumably capable of depolarizing the afferent nerve terminal, thus making it less easy for a subsequent receptor potential to generate action potentials in the afferent fiber. Stimulation of the efferent (or olivocochlear) fibers is associated with the inhibition of cochlear afferent fiber discharge mainly in response to relatively low intensity sounds. It has, therefore, been proposed that under normal conditions the efferent fibers occlude responses to lower intensity background noise without affecting responses to higher intensity and presumably closer sounds, such as when concentrating on a conversation with a nearby speaker in the middle of a cocktail party.

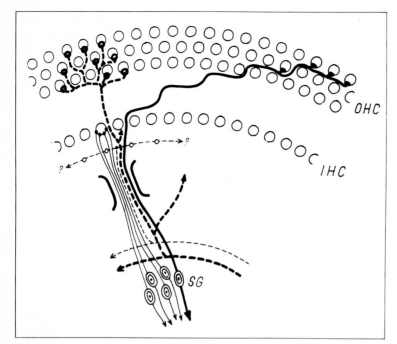

8A–50 Innervation pattern of the organ of Corti in the cat. Interrupted lines are afferent fibers; full lines are efferent fibers. **OHC,** outer hair cells; **IHC,** inner hair cells; **SG,** spiral ganglion. (From Flock, A. 1982. *In* L. Weiss (ed.) Histology, 5th edition, New York: Elsevier. Courtesy of Spoendlin. Reproduced with permission from Karger.)

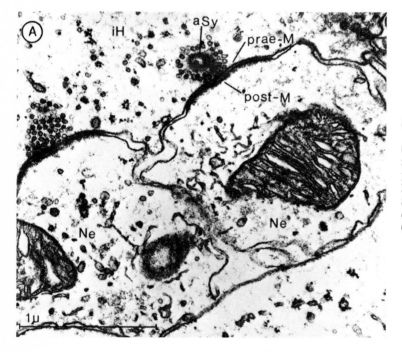

8A–51 Afferent nerve endings **(Ne)** on an inner hair cell **(iH)** of a guinea pig. **aSy,** synaptic ribbon; **PraeM, post M,** pre- and post-synaptic membranes. (From Babel, J., Bischoff, A., and Spoendlin, H. 1970. Ultrastructure of the Peripheral Nerves and Sense Organs. St. Louis: Mosby.)

The origin of the efferent fibers from the side of the brain opposite each cochlea reflects the fact that the most direct pathways from each cochlea to the centers for auditory perception are crossed in the central nervous system.

The Cochlear Nerve

The central processes of the bipolar neurons in the spiral ganglion (Fig. 8A–53) are myelinated axons resembling those of dorsal root ganglion

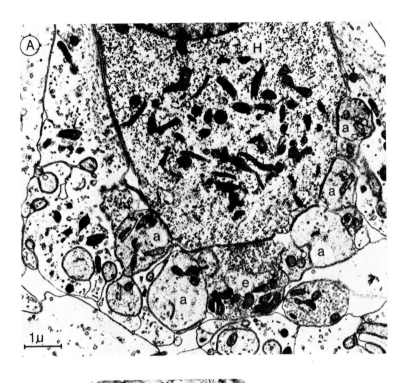

8A–52 Base of an outer hair cell **(H)** in the cochlea of a guinea pig, with afferent **(a)** and efferent **(e)** nerve endings. (From Babel, J., Bischoff, A., and Spoendlin, H. 1970. Ultrastructure of the Peripheral Nerves and Sense Organs. St. Louis: Mosby.)

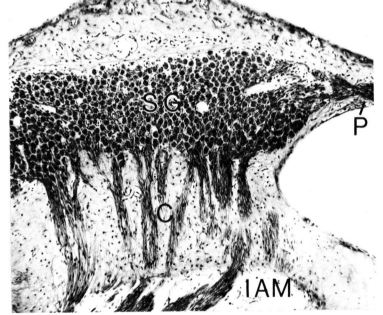

8A–53 Neurons of the spiral ganglion **(SG)** in the cochlea of a dog with peripheral processes **(P)** entering part of the spiral lamina and central processes **(C)** entering the internal auditory meatus **(IAM).** Hematoxylin and eosin stain. × 240.

cells. They enter the interior of the skull through the internal auditory meatus and there, joining the central processes of cells in the vestibular ganglion, pass in the vestibulocochlear or "auditory" nerve to the cochlear nuclei of the medulla oblongata (Figs. 8A–35 through 8A–37). There are approximately 30,000 axons in the auditory component of the human eighth cranial nerve. Other species with higher auditory acuity have many more. In cats there are some 50,000.

References and Selected Bibliography

General

Mountcastle, V. B. (ed.). 1980, Medical Physiology, 14th ed. 2 vols. St. Louis: Mosby.

Ramón y Cajal, S. 1911. Histologie du Système Nerveux de l'Homme et des Vertébrés, vol. 2. L. Azoulay (trans.) Paris: Maloine.

Shepherd, G. M. 1979. The Synaptic Organization of the Brain, 2nd ed. New York: Oxford University Press.

Taste and Olfaction

Beidler, L. M. (ed.). 1971. Handbook of Sensory Physiology IV/1 Chemical Senses—Olfaction; IV/2 Chemical Senses—Taste. New York: Springer.

Beidler, L. M., and Smallman. 1965. Renewal of cells within taste buds. J. Cell Biol. 27:263.

Clark, W. E. LeGros. 1957. Enquiries into the anatomical basis of olfactory discrimination. Proc. R. Soc. Lond. B. 146:299.

Graziadei, P. P. C., and Metcalf, J. F. 1971. Autoradiographic and ultrastructural observations of the frog's olfactory Mucosa. Z. Zellforsch. Mikroskop. Anat. 116: 305.

Pfaffman, C. (ed.). 1969. Olfaction and Taste. New York: Rockefeller University Press.

Rall, W., Shepherd, G. M., Reese, T. S., and Brightman, M. W. 1966. Dendro-dendritic synaptic pathway for inhibition in the olfactory bulb. Exp. Neurol. 14:44.

Ribak, C. E., Vaughn, J. E., Saito, K., Barber, R., and Roberts, E. 1977. Glutamate decarboxylase localization in neurons of the olfactory bulb. Brain Res. 126:1.

Sharp, F. R., Kauer, J. S., and Shepherd, G. M. 1977. Laminar analysis of 2-deoxyglucose uptake in olfactory bulb and olfactory cortex of rabbit and rat. J. Neurophysiol. 40:800.

Zalewski, A. A. 1974. Neuronal and tissue specifications involved in taste bud formation. Ann. N.Y. Acad. Sci. 228:344.

Retina

Boycott, B. B., Kolb, H. 1973. The connections between bipolar cells and photoreceptors in the retina of the cat. J. Comp. Neurol. 148:98.

Cohen, A. I. 1972. Rods and Cones. In M. G. F. Fuortes (ed). Handbook of Sensory Physiology VII/1B. Physiology of Photoreceptor Organs. New York: Springer.

Daw, N. W., Ariel, M., and Caldwell, J. H. 1982. Function of neurotransmitters in the retina. Retina 2:322.

Dowling, J. E., and Boycott, B. B. 1966. Organization of the primate retina: electron microscopy. Proc. R. Soc. Lond. B. 166:80.

Hubbell, W. L., and Bounds, M. D. 1979. Visual transduction in vertebrate photoreceptors. Annu. Rev. Neurosci. 2:17.

Kaneko, A. 1979. Physiology of the retina. Annu. Rev. Neurosci. 2:169.

Lam, D. M. K. 1976. Synaptic chemistry of identified cells in the vertebrate retina. In The Synapse. Cold Spring Harbor Symp. Quant. Biol. 40:571.

Polyak, S. 1948. The Retina. Chicago: University of Chicago Press.

Raviola, E. 1976. Intercellular junctions in the outer plexiform layer of the retina. Invest. Ophthalmol. 15:881.

Rodieck, R. W. 1973. The Vertebrate Retina. Principles of Structure and Function. San Francisco: Freeman.

Stell, W. K. 1972. The morphological organization of the vertebrate retina. In M. G. F. Fuortes (ed.). Handbook of Sensory Physiology, vol. VII/2: Physiology of Photoreceptors. New York: Springer, p. 111.

Auditory and Vestibular Systems

Babel, J., Bischoff, A., and Spoendlin, H. 1970. Ultrastructure of the Peripheral Nervous System and Sense Organs. St. Louis: Mosby.

Bekésy, G. von. 1960. Experiments in Hearing. E. G. Wever (ed.). New York: McGraw-Hill.

Davis, H. 1961. Some principles of receptor physiology. Physiol. Rev. 41:391.

Flock, A. 1971. Sensory transduction in hair cells. In. O. Lowenstein (ed.). Handbook of Sensory Physiology, vol. 1. Principles of Receptor Physiology. New York: Springer.

Smith, C. A., and Tanaka, K. 1975. Some aspects of the structure of the vestibular apparatus. In R. F. Naunton (ed.). The Vestibular System. New York: Academic Press.

Wersäll, J., Flock, A., and Lundquist, P. G. 1965. Structural basis for directional sensitivity in cochlear and vestibular sensory receptors. Cold Spring Harbor Symp. Quant. Biol. 30:115.

Wilson, V. J., and Melvill Jones, G. 1979. Mammalian Vestibular Physiology. New York: Plenum.

Index

Note: an italicized page number indicates that subject entry appears on the page in an illustration